T0260242

BENDING
THE COST CURVE
IN HEALTH CARE

The Johnson-Shoyama Series on Public Policy

Taking a comparative and international perspective, the Johnson-Shoyama Series on Public Policy focuses on the many approaches to major policy issues offered by Canada's provinces and territories and reflected in their intergovernmental relationships. Books in the series explore particular policy issues, and while research-based, are intended to engage informed readers and students alike.

BENDING THE COST CURVE IN HEALTH CARE

Edited by
Gregory P. Marchildon
and Livio Di Matteo

UNIVERSITY OF TORONTO PRESS

Copyright © University of Toronto Press 2015

Higher Education Division

www.utppublishing.com

All rights reserved. The use of any part of this publication reproduced, transmitted in any form or by any means, electronic, mechanical, photocopying, recording, or otherwise, or stored in a retrieval system, without prior written consent of the publisher—or in the case of photocopying, a licence from Access Copyright (Canadian Copyright Licensing Agency), One Yonge Street, Suite 1900, Toronto, Ontario M5E 1E5—is an infringement of the copyright law.

LIBRARY AND ARCHIVES CANADA CATALOGUING IN PUBLICATION

Bending the cost curve in health care : Canada's provinces in international perspective / edited by Gregory P. Marchildon and Livio di Matteo.

(The Johnson-Shoyama series on public policy)

Includes bibliographical references and index.

Issued in print and electronic formats.

ISBN 978-1-4426-0976-1 (bound).—ISBN 978-1-4426-0975-4 (pbk.).— ISBN 978-1-4426-0977-8 (pdf).—ISBN 978-1-4426-0978-5 (epub)

1. Medical care, Cost of—Canada—Provinces. 2. Medical care—Canada— Provinces—Cost control. 3. Medical care—Canada—Provinces—Finance. 4. Medical policy—Canada—Provinces. 5. Medical care—Cost control—Case studies. I. Di Matteo, Livio, author, editor II. Marchildon, Gregory P., 1956–, author, editor III. Series: Johnson-Shoyama series on public policy

RA410.55.C35B48 2014   362.1068'10971   C2014-902305-7
                                                    C2014-902306-5

We welcome comments and suggestions regarding any aspect of our publications— please feel free to contact us at news@utphighereducation.com or visit our Internet site at www.utppublishing.com.

North America
5201 Dufferin Street
North York, Ontario, Canada, M3H 5T8

2250 Military Road
Tonawanda, New York, USA, 14150

ORDERS PHONE: 1-800-565-9523
ORDERS FAX: 1-800-221-9985
ORDERS E-MAIL: utpbooks@utpress.utoronto.ca

UK, Ireland, and continental Europe
NBN International
Estover Road, Plymouth, PL6 7PY, UK
ORDERS PHONE: 44 (0) 1752 202301
ORDERS FAX: 44 (0) 1752 202333
ORDERS E-MAIL: enquiries@nbninternational.com

Every effort has been made to contact copyright holders; in the event of an error or omission, please notify the publisher.

The University of Toronto Press acknowledges the financial support for its publishing activities of the Government of Canada through the Canada Book Fund.

Printed in the United States of America.

Contents

Part III: Provincial Experiences in Canada

Part IV: What Can Canada Learn from the International Evidence?

Illustrations

Tables

Figures

Introduction and Overview

This is the first thematic volume in the Johnson-Shoyama Series on Public Policy, sponsored by the Johnson-Shoyama Graduate School of Public Policy, an interdisciplinary centre for advanced education, research, outreach, and training with campuses at the University of Regina and the University of Saskatchewan. Published by the University of Toronto Press, this series focuses on the provincial role in policymaking to "improve our comparative understanding of the administration, development and governance of public policy in the Canadian provinces" (Atkinson et al., xi–xii). However, this comparative understanding must be based on an understanding of similar policies in other countries and regions around the world.

Since the bulk of health-care financing, management, and delivery is within the purview of provincial governments, we brought together scholars focused on the provincial experience with an eye to determining what, if anything, was unique about the cost drivers and the policy interventions in their particular jurisdiction. We also asked some notable scholars to address health-care questions that all provinces are grappling with. For the comparative dimension, we invited prominent scholars from countries with tax-based health-financing systems to relate policy lessons of relevance to provincial decision-makers in Canada.

Based on a set of guidelines, the selected authors had prepared first drafts of their chapters by the summer of 2012. We then held an international conference titled "Bending the Cost Curve in Health Care" in Saskatoon on September 27–28, 2012, to present our initial findings to a mixed audience of scholars and decision-makers. Our authors revised their chapters in light of what they had learned, after which they were subjected to a peer review and further revision. The resulting volume represents a careful reflection by the leading scholars in the field on the challenges of ensuring the long-term fiscal sustainability of health care.

The question of sustainability

The sustainability of public-sector health-care spending has been at the forefront of a roiling policy debate for years in Canada. Unfortunately, this debate has tended to generate far more heat than light as participants argue about the most elemental facts that underpin their respective arguments. As public theatre, the sustainability debate offers the pretext for advocates outside government to present their preferred policy solutions to a problem that remains ill defined. In many cases this debate often collapses into an argument concerning the future role of the public or private sector in health-care funding and delivery.

At the same time, governments—particularly provincial governments, which raise most of the revenues for health care and spend the largest share of their budgets on health services—do face a real dilemma. Every additional dollar raised and spent on health care is a dollar that could be earmarked for other public goods and services, including education, social services, transportation infrastructure, and payment on public debt. Indeed, the notion of crowding out has become an entrenched part of the conventional wisdom inside and outside provincial governments. Despite this conventional wisdom, studies have not yet found a robust relationship between increased health spending and reduced provincial spending on other public goods and services (Landon et al. 2006).

Nonetheless, it remains true that provincial decision-makers feel enormous pressures as health care grows in size relative to other parts of their expenditure budgets. Moreover, as residents criticize their governments for the quality and timeliness of health services, provincial authorities are caught between the public's demands—to improve quality, add access and providers, and improve infrastructure—and the requirement to demonstrate value for money, minimize tax burdens, and avoid deficits. While this is a daunting challenge, it is one that provincial governments can better address if they can understand the nature of the cost drivers in health spending—their single largest expenditure item—within their own jurisdiction. In addition, provincial governments should have better information on the possible options that would be most effective in terms of bending the cost curve, as well as the limits of those alternatives.

Most provincial governments are not interested in crude cost-cutting exercises. They remember only too well what happened when that cost-cutting approach was applied to health spending in the early to mid 1990s. These cuts reduced both quality and access and, in any event, were not sustained in the long run (Tuohy 2002). As a consequence, and in the face of future declines in the growth of federal health transfers, provincial decision-makers now want to bend the health-care cost curve in a way that will not block access or damage quality. Instead, they want permanent and persistent efficiencies, which will require that they, and the regional health authorities and other health-care organizations they fund, provide more appropriate but lower-cost services, substitute providers where possible, and rein in provider remuneration, which has been growing well above the general rate of inflation.

First, however, it is essential to understand health-spending trends in Canada. The dimensions and trends of aggregate public-sector health-care spending at the national level are well documented, but unique trends at the provincial level have not yet been studied in detail, despite the fact that these are the policy-relevant trends faced by individual provincial governments.

Public-sector health spending: Canadian trends and provincial outliers

The growth of public-sector health spending in Canada from 1975 until 2008 can be divided into three phases: the first, from 1976 to 1991, was marked by rapid growth, averaging 2.6% a year in real (inflation-adjusted) terms. This was followed by a short but severe period of fiscal retrenchment from 1992 to 1996, when governments dealt with fiscal deficits in part by constraining or reducing their respective health budgets. The third was a growth phase that averaged 3.5% per year (after adjusting for inflation), from 1997 until 2008. While it is still too early to call, Canada—like most

Figure 0.1 Real per capita public-sector health expenditures in Canada, 1975–2013 (1997 dollars)

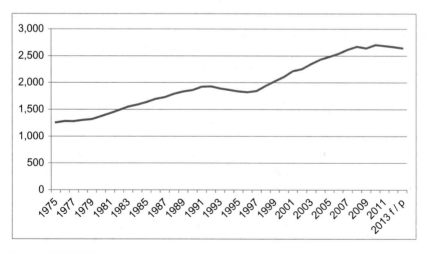

Source: CIHI 2013.

advanced industrial countries—appears to have entered a new phase of dampened growth since the fiscal crisis and recession of 2008–09.

As a share of Canada's overall economy, public-sector health-care spending reached a peak of 8.5% of gross domestic product (GDP) during the recession year of 2009. The health-to-GDP ratio declined slightly to 8.1% in 2011, based on forecast figures, as a result of post-recession economic recovery. This ratio is higher than in the late 1970s, when it was just over 5%, which reflects a trend to spend more on health care as income rises.

In recent years these trends have caused many to question the sustainability of provincial government health spending, given that it is increasing at rates above those for government revenue, GDP, and federal transfers (Di Matteo 2010; Di Matteo and Di Matteo 2009; Dodge and Dion 2011; TD Bank Financial Group 2010). The drivers of increased public-sector health-care spending and its sustainability have also been the focus of several research studies over the past few years (CIHI 2011; Constant et al. 2011). However, there has been much less comparative research on drivers and trends specifically at the provincial level, despite the fact that provincial government health spending constitutes the bulk of public-sector spending in Canada.

While there has been an upward trend in the spending common to all the provinces and some convergence in spending over time, this trend masks some of the expenditure variations across provinces—an inevitable function of Canada's federal diversity. By extension, there should also be differences in the impact of respective cost drivers across the provinces, and provincial government management practices and policy interventions when it comes to health-care spending, that can serve as sources of insight and policy guidance on bending the cost curve.

Health spending and cost drivers: A national summary

According to the most recent national health-expenditure release by the Canadian Institute for Health Information (CIHI 2013), total health expenditures in Canada were C$200.1 billion in 2011, with forecasts of $205.9 billion in 2012 and $211.2 billion in 2013, generating annual increases of 2.9% and 2.6% respectively. When adjusted for inflation, total health expenditures had risen to $136.8 billion in 2011, which represents a 0.7% increase when compared to 2010. In constant (1997) dollar terms, the rates of growth are 1.1% in 2012 and 0.9% in 2013.

When provincial/territorial government health spending is examined, C$126 billion was spent in 2010 and $130.7 billion in 2011, with forecasts of $135 billion in 2012 and $130 billion in 2013, representing about 65% of total health spending. The provincial and territorial governments account for about 92% of all direct public-sector health expenditures, a figure that excludes federal transfers through the Canada Health Transfer and equalization payments. When Canadian public-sector health spending is converted into inflation-adjusted terms and divided by population (see Figure 0.1), it shows that since 1975, real per capita provincial/territorial government health spending has more than doubled, rising from C$1,203 to a forecast of nearly $2,645 in 2013.

A CIHI (2011) analysis of cost drivers focusing on the period 1998 to 2008 found that total public-sector spending on health care increased at an average annual rate of 7.4%. Population growth contributed an average of 1% per year to the increase in health expenditures, while population aging contributed only 0.8%, making demographic factors relatively modest contributors at 1.8%. Health-sector inflation contributed 2.8% per year of the annual average rate, while other factors such as technology and increased utilization contributed the remaining 2.8%.

Health spending: A more differentiated provincial/territorial view

As we would expect, given the decentralized nature of the Canadian federation, there is considerable diversity across the provinces in terms of spending levels and expenditure growth, partly as a result of differences in ages and population density. Total nominal health expenditure per capita in Newfoundland and Labrador in 2013 is expected to reach $7,132, followed by Alberta ($6,787), while the lowest per capita spending is forecast for Québec ($5,531) and British Columbia ($5,775). Meanwhile, in 2013, total health expenditure as a percentage of provincial GDP is expected to range from a low of 8.3% in petroleum-rich Alberta to a high of 16.6% in Prince Edward Island. For the Far North, the ratio of health expenditure to territorial GDP is estimated at 20.9% for Nunavut, 12.6% for Yukon, and 9.0% for the Northwest Territories. Health expenditure per capita is highest in the territories because of an expansive geography and low population densities, and for this reason the territories are not included in the provincial comparisons that follow.

When only government spending per capita is considered and adjusted for inflation, there are also significant differences across the provinces and territories. Figure 0.2 illustrates real per capita government health spending for the provinces, demonstrating the upward trend over time as well as some of the differences among the provinces.

Figure 0.2 Real per capita government health-care expenditures, 1975–2013 (1997 dollars)

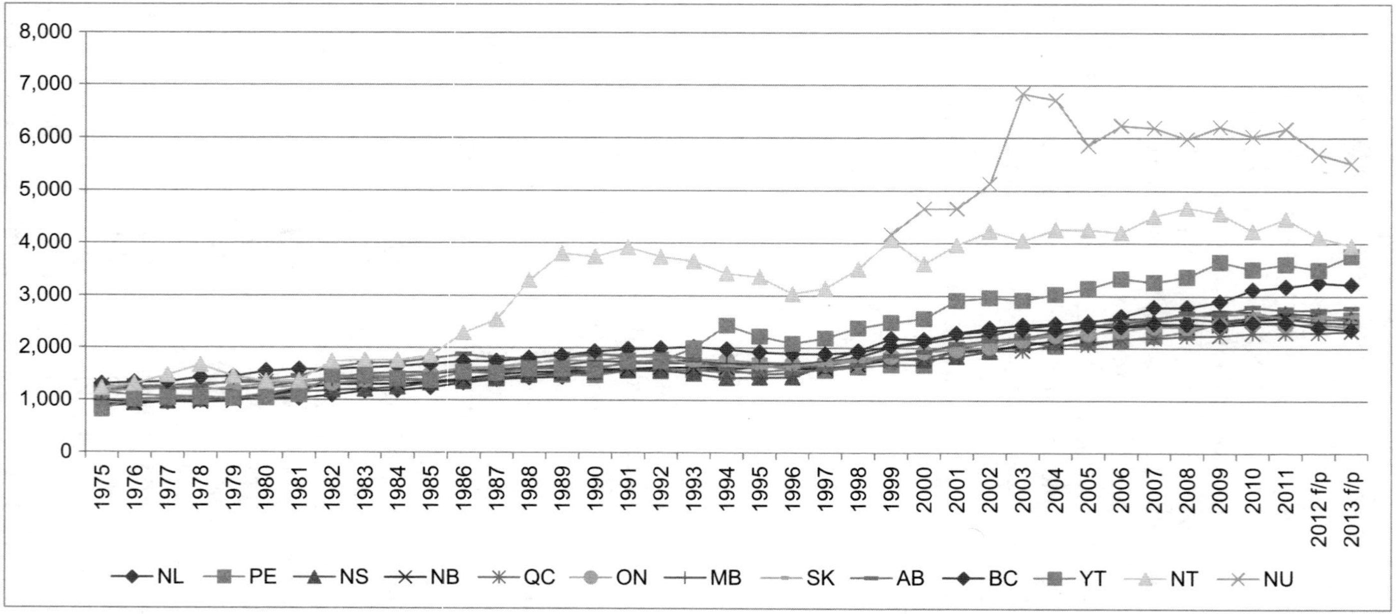

Source: CIHI 2013.

Figure 0.3 Ranked per capita provincial government health spending, 2011 (1997 dollars)

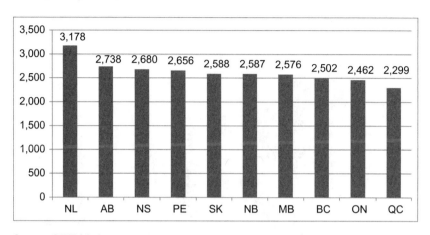

Source: CIHI 2012.

Figure 0.3 ranks real per capita provincial government health spending in 2011, showing that the spending in 1997 dollars ranges from a high of C$3,178 in Newfoundland and Labrador to a low of $2,299 in Québec.

Even when analysis is restricted to only the provinces, there are substantial differences not only in total real per capita government health spending but also in expenditure growth rates. Figure 0.4 ranks the average annual growth rates in real per capita provincial government health spending for the 1975–2011 period. Growth rates were highest in the Atlantic provinces of Newfoundland and Labrador, New Brunswick, and Nova Scotia, at over 3%, and lowest in the more urbanized provinces of Ontario, British Columbia, and Québec.

Differences also extend to expenditure envelopes within provincial health budgets. For example, hospital spending is the largest single category of public-sector health spending for Canada's provinces; it grew from an average of real per capita C$641 (1997 dollars) in 1975 to $1,137 in 2009, the start of the recession. In 2009, hospital spending ranged from a low in real per capita 1997 dollars of $917 in Québec to a high of $1,543 in Newfoundland and Labrador—a 68% difference between highest and lowest provinces. In the case of physicians, average real per capita provincial government spending rose from $210 in 1975 to reach $486 in 2009. The range here was from a low of $413 in British Columbia to a high of $602 in Ontario—a 46% difference. Finally, in the case of drugs, average real per capita provincial government spending rose from $21 in 1975 to $190 by 2009; the range in

Figure 0.4 Average annual growth rate of real per capita provincial government health spending (per cent), 1975–2011

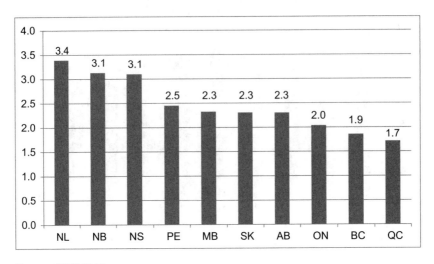

Source: CIHI 2012.

provincial drug spending was from a low of $150 in British Columbia to a high of $247 in Ontario—a difference of 65%.

Why the differences?

On a real per capita basis, why does the government of Newfoundland and Labrador spend 68% more than Québec's on hospitals? Why does the Ontario government spend 65% more on drugs in its public plan than the government of British Columbia? Are there differences in the impact of cost drivers across the provinces, or are there other institutional (including program design) or economic factors that come into play? Understanding the reasons for these marked differences has potentially important policy implications for provincial and territorial decision-makers as they try to bend the cost curve downward.

A recent CIHI (2011) analysis of underlying cost drivers isolated the following factors: population growth, aging populations, inflation in health human resource costs, growing rates of utilization, and technological extension. Despite the very different policy implications they hold for individual provincial governments, there has not been a great deal of research done to determine the impact of these individual factors on provincial health-spending growth.

Figure 0.5 Average annual growth rate of population (per cent) for Canada's provinces, 1976–2011

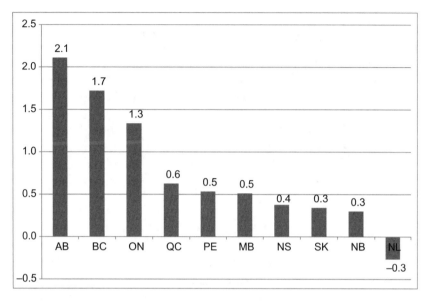

Source: CIHI 2012.

Based on the CIHI (2011) study, we know there are very important differences across the provinces when it comes to some of the basic drivers such as population growth, aging, health-specific inflation, and technology. In the case of population, the average annual growth rate of population over the period 1975 to 2011 has ranged from a high of 2.1% in Alberta to a low of minus 0.3% in Newfoundland and Labrador (see Figure 0.5). This would imply that the cost-driver pressures of an expanding population would be the greatest in Alberta and the lowest in Newfoundland and Labrador.

When it comes to aging, in 2011 the highest proportion of population aged 65 years and over was in Nova Scotia, at 16.5%, while the lowest was again in Alberta, at 10.9% (see Figure 0.6). The implication is that the cost pressures of an aging population (holding all other factors constant) should be strongest in Nova Scotia and the other Atlantic provinces and weakest in Alberta and the three northern territories, where Canada's most youthful populations are located.

In the past five years, physician expenditure has been one of the fastest-growing categories of government health spending—the most obvious example of inflationary pressures well above the general rate of inflation. The most important cost driver of this growth has been fee-for-service

Figure 0.6 Per cent of population aged 65 years and older, 2011

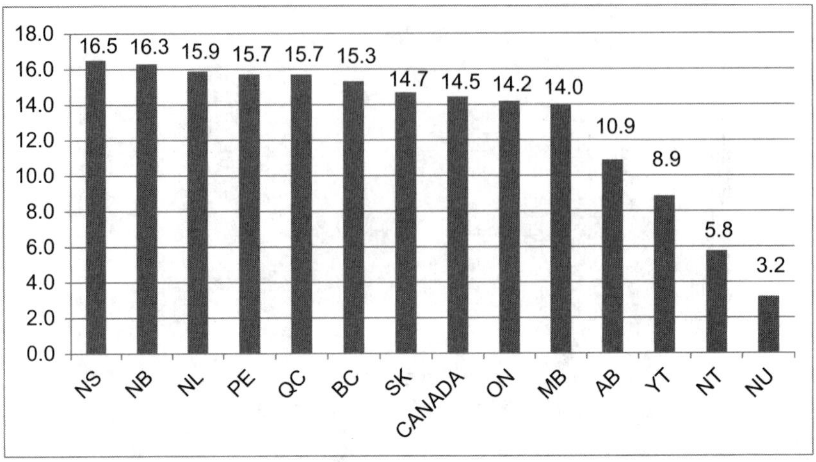

Source: CIHI 2012.

remuneration rather than utilization. However, because of the method of remuneration, this increase also correlates highly with recent increases in the number of physicians in Canada.

When the total number of physicians (both family and specialist) per 10,000 population is examined by province (Figure 0.7), it shows an increase in the per capita number of physicians over time in all of the provinces, with the biggest percentage increases in Newfoundland and New Brunswick and the smallest in Ontario and Manitoba. In 2009 the ratio of physicians to population was highest in Nova Scotia and lowest in Prince Edward Island. These differences could be expected to have implications for cost differences related to physician numbers and their associated services.

Technological change is one of the most important cost drivers but has been difficult to quantify, with most measurement approaches ascribing it as a significant component of residual growth categories. For example, the United States Congressional Budget Office (2008) has cited several studies (see Newhouse 1992 and Cutler 1995) showing that technology-related changes in medical practice contributed anywhere from 38% to 65% or more to the growth of real health-care spending per capita in the United States. Naturally one would expect expenditures to be correlated with the diffusion and use of technology, and the availability and use of technology also differ significantly by province. For example, the number of magnetic resonance imaging scans (MRIs) per 1,000 of population in 2011–12 ranged from a high of 61.3 in Ontario to a low of 31.8 in Prince Edward Island (Figure 0.8).

Figure 0.7 Total physicians per 10,000 population, by province, 1975 and 2009

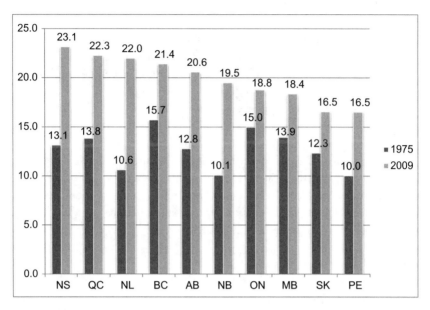

Source: CIHI 1975, 2009.

Figure 0.8 Number of MRI exams per 1,000 population, by province, 2011–2012

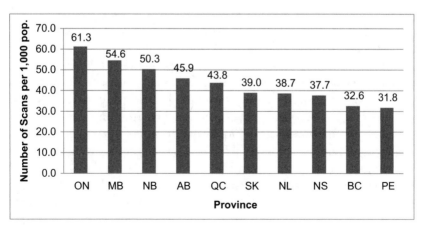

Source: CIHI 2013.

Concluding thoughts

Public-sector health-care spending in Canada, in particular provincial government health spending, has been growing rapidly since the retrenchment of the early 1990s, and its sustainability is a chronic policy issue. As a result of its constitutional past, Canada really has not one but 13 public health-care systems linked by a federal transfer and oversight mechanism whose effectiveness is open to debate. The diversity of spending across Canada's provinces and territories means that there will also be diversity in the drivers of expenditures across the provinces and territories in terms of their relative importance. It also means that when it comes to bending the cost curve, there will not be a "one size fits all" solution that can be applied across all the provinces. As a result, to bend the cost curve it becomes necessary to understand the provincial and regional experiences. As well, it is useful to look at the diversity of world experiences to see what lessons can be applied to the varied Canadian context.

Overview of the chapter contributions

This volume begins with a series of essays on understanding the nature of the sustainability problem. Part One provides the very broad political and economic context in which any efforts to bend the cost curve must be made or will be made in future years.

One of the most well-known health economists in the world, Uwe Reinhardt presents his mature reflection on this central issue, one that he has been addressing in one form or another for almost 50 years. As a young German who immigrated to North America in the early 1960s, Reinhardt attended the University of Saskatchewan during the doctors' strike of 1962 and witnessed the introduction of universal medicare in that province. He subsequently pursued graduate studies in the United States, later taking a permanent academic appointment at Princeton University. In simple but penetrating language, he explains the general rationale for cost control and the potential approaches to containment of health-care costs, including a review of payment systems and approaches to controlling the price that governments and consumers pay for health providers and services.

Payment systems are the subject of the chapter written by health economists Jeremiah Hurley and Jinhu Li. In recent years governments have experimented with incentive-based payments—colloquially known as "pay-for-performance" (P4P)—that are intended to both improve quality and restrain cost at the same time. The assumption here is that higher-quality services will, at least over time, control costs by improving health and reducing inappropriate utilization and unnecessary complications. Since the research evidence on this relationship remains sparse, Hurley and Li analyze the results from Ontario's primary-care payment changes, the largest P4P experiment in Canada. Their conclusion is bracing: P4P in this case was not an effective way to improve quality and appears to have increased rather than decreased costs. Moreover, these results are consistent with international evidence on the impact of P4P on costs, although both authors admit the limited and incomplete nature of the studies. Nonetheless, Hurley and Li conclude that if targeted financial incentives are not relied upon in isolation, but instead made part of a larger health reform, they may still have some positive impact on bending the cost curve.

John Richards and Colin Busby address the issue of aging in the context of what they feel has been the fiscal drift of governments since the mid 1990s. They review two effects, the first being the expenditure effect of having a larger population of high-needs elderly patients—or, as some pundits put it, a larger population of extremely demanding baby boomers. The second is the GDP effect: that is, the impact of having a diminishing share of the population in the active labour force. Their analysis leads to the conclusion that population aging will in fact cause significant problems for single-payer financing in Canada, contrary to other analyses. This is in part because of significant tax reductions by both provincial and federal governments from the mid 1990s until 2012. According to Richards and Busby, these governments reduced their taxation efforts by the equivalent of 7 per cent of national GDP, putting Canada in the lowest tax quartile of OECD countries. Common sense tells us that we cannot expect to have a western European–style welfare state—including its most expensive component, universal health care—at American rates of taxation. As a result, Richards and Busby recommend a modest increase in taxes in the medium term.

In Part Two, pan-Canadian analyses of cost drivers common to all provinces are presented. The section begins with an analysis of the common provincial determinants of growth in health spending. Technology, particularly as encompassed by new pharmaceuticals, and wage inflation are among the most important cost drivers faced by all governments. All governments also operate within a particular federal-provincial context that influences fiscal decision-making by all parties.

Using a regression model, Livio Di Matteo and Herb Emery examine the extent to which provincial health-expenditure differences are due to differences in non-policy-amenable variables (demography, geography, etc.) as opposed to factors that can be altered through policy interventions. One clear result is that smaller provincial populations are correlated with higher per capita health expenditures. As shown by Di Matteo and Emery, the provinces with more of their population spread out in rural and remote areas face a higher cost structure for the delivery of health services. This is particularly true for provinces in which smaller urban populations are combined with larger high-need populations, such as those living in remote aboriginal communities in the rural and northern parts of Saskatchewan and Manitoba, as well as in Labrador. This is an inescapable situation in any circumpolar region with low population density, an extreme climate, and a sizeable indigenous population with poor health status (Young and Marchildon 2012).

Di Matteo and Emery also find that the physician–population ratio is a positive and significant determinant of provincial health-care expenditures. In fact, adding just one more physician per 10,000 people is associated with a 1 per cent increase in real per capita provincial government health spending. This result is not surprising, given the central role that physicians play in provincial health systems. Indeed, it could be argued that because of the manner in which universal medicare was introduced, physician decision-making is less fettered in Canada than in most other advanced industrial countries (Tuohy 1999). Family physicians act as de facto gate-keepers, controlling referrals for diagnostic tests and further physician care through specialists. Doctors also have almost exclusive authority to write scripts for prescription drugs. In effect, provincial governments negotiate physician supply directly with medical associations through the funding of seats in medical schools and physician remuneration.

For years Steve Morgan and a team of researchers at the Centre for Health Services and Policy Research (CHSPR) at the University of British Columbia have been conducting high-quality research on pharmaceutical policy. Between 1998 and 2007, real per capita drug spending grew at an average of 6 per cent per year. The single most important cost driver was the increased number of prescription drugs purchased by Canadians, the cost of which was heavily subsidized for certain categories of residents (e.g., seniors and recipients of social assistance) by provincial governments (CIHI 2011). The extent to which cost is policy amenable can be seen in the significant variation across provinces in terms of prescription drug spending and growth trends. Historically, most cost-control reforms have been on the supply side. To the extent that demand-side policies have been relied upon, increases in patient copayments and co-insurance have tended to target those with the least information for making rational decisions. Instead, Morgan and his colleagues argue in favour of physician-based incentives. They also argue in favour of a more integrated approach to public-sector pharmacare, in which the provincial governments collaborate with the federal government to achieve a higher degree of bargaining power, potentially achieving a policy result similar to the pharmaceutical schemes in Australia and New Zealand.

Human resources constitute the single largest spending component in health care. Labour economists Phil Leonard and Arthur Sweetman address three potential approaches open to governments to address human resource costs. The first is the option of simply reducing service levels; this is the least desirable method, since this type of cost cutting undermines the basic objectives of publicly financed health care. The second option is reducing the growth in remuneration of providers so that it is roughly consistent with the general rate of inflation. The third option, improving efficiency and productivity, holds the greatest promise in terms of bending the cost curve in the long run, but it is also the most difficult to implement, monitor, and evaluate. This last approach likely requires development of what the authors call an "efficiency culture" in various health workplaces, a change that lies at the heart of the "lean" reforms initiated by various provincial governments, and particularly by the Saskatchewan government.

Katherine Fierlbeck's chapter presents three distinct approaches to containing health-care costs in Canada. The first is one in which the federal government—through conditional fiscal transfers—is the principal actor, ultimately directing cost containment, with the provinces as its agents implementing the details. This is the approach tentatively attempted through the first ministers' agreements on health reform in 2003 and 2004, with their special-purpose transfers, and is an effort whose success has been limited (Marchildon 2013; Senate of Canada 2010). The second approach is that adopted by current federal Conservative administration in which the federal government backs off or removes conditionality, thereby encouraging the provincial governments to assume full accountability and responsibility for their own cost-containment efforts. The third approach is decentralized coordination. Although this form of intergovernmental accountability may be more common in the European Community, Fierlbeck argues that the approach could be instructive when it comes time to reshape the governance of health care in Canada to facilitate bending down the cost curve.

A long-time health-policy and federalism scholar, Pierre-Gerlier Forest examines the impact of the federal stewardship role on provincial governments. As he puts it, while the provinces are the main agent on the supply side of health, the federal government remains a major determinant of the demand side of health, despite its recent insistence on a more limited role. Its role includes, for example, the surveillance and control of epidemics, immigration, taxation and income redistribution, health and safety regulation, drug use, and the price of patented pharmaceuticals. The inescapable conclusion is that, despite the primacy of provincial jurisdiction, health remains, and will continue to be, a shared responsibility between the federal government and the provinces.

Part Three drills down into the provincial experience. Authors were asked to identify any cost drivers or institutional factors that were unique or particularly influential in determining the growth of health spending. They were also expected to isolate any recent policy interventions aimed specifically at bending the cost curve.

Raisa Deber and Sara Allin recount Ontario's experience with physician payment incentives. Although it was hoped that these reforms would both improve the quality of primary care and eventually reduce the growth in fee-for-service payments—which encourage rapid visits and unnecessary referrals and prescriptions, and therefore extra costs—physician spending grew dramatically. As a consequence, the Ontario government's very recent efforts have been directed at slowing the rate of growth in physician remuneration through some tough negotiations with the Ontario Medical Association.

In their chapter on Québec, François Béland and Claude Galand describe the centrality of fiscal controls that has been at the heart of cost-containment initiatives in Québec. This fiscal discipline has been achieved through hard budget caps, health-budget reductions following recessions (though generally with a three-year lag), and tough collective bargaining with provider groups, including physicians. To bend the cost curve, the Québec government has relied on structural change and integrating across health sectors to achieve economies of both scale and scope. In 2003, for example, the Couillard reforms saw the integration of hospital care with public-sector primary-care groups (CLSCs) and nursing homes into 95 centres de services sociaux et de services de santé (CSSSs) which in turn were integrated into Québec's regional health authorities.

In their chapter on British Columbia, Kim McGrail and Bob Evans point out the extent to which the provincial government's concern about potential impact on demographic aging led to a focus on the elderly and chronically ill or incapacitated segments of the population. Through major investments in home care and community supports, and more recently in assisted-living facilities, the government has tried to reduce admissions to expensive hospital and long-term care homes requiring 24-hour-a-day nursing supervision.

The government of Alberta has relied on privatization since 2000 and organizational centralization since 2008 to achieve greater long-term efficiencies. However, as Stephen Duckett reviews in his chapter, outsourcing routine surgeries to private for-profit clinics not only failed to save money but probably cost the province more than the equivalent public options. In the case of a private orthopaedic clinic in Calgary, for example, joint procedures were 7% more expensive and foot and ankle procedures were roughly 32% more expensive. An Australian health economist, Duckett was hired by the Alberta government to become the first chief executive of Alberta Health Services (AHS), a single health region that was created to replace all the regional health authorities in the province. AHS has a mandate to achieve better economies of scale and scope in procurement, information technology, and managerial talent while reducing administrative overhead and eliminating unnecessary hospital beds. This turned out to be a difficult mandate for the government to uphold in the face of public pressures from individuals and groups whose interests were more aligned with increasing health-care spending (and therefore their own incomes) than with containing public-sector costs.

Gregory Marchildon reviews Saskatchewan and Manitoba in the same chapter because of the demographic and geographic similarities of the two provinces. Even though the federal government funds several health services for First Nations peoples on the many rural and remote reserves located in these provinces, the provincial health ministries are still required to provide medically necessary hospital and physician services to all residents. As a consequence of the large health disparities between Aboriginal and non-Aboriginal residents and growing First Nations and Métis populations, both provincial governments face higher costs than other governments. The two governments have focused on different approaches to bend their respective cost curves. In Saskatchewan the main emphasis has been on improving efficiency in hospital and other clinical care through more efficient use of inputs, including human resources, through a government-wide "Lean" initiative. Meanwhile, the Manitoba government has been a leader in substituting physician assistants and nurse practitioners for scarce (and more expensive) physician care.

Joe Ruggeri's chapter summarizes the experience of the four Atlantic provinces, which have older populations relative to all the other provinces. Until the recent resource boom in Newfoundland and Labrador, all these provinces were much more reliant on the federal government's health and equalization transfers for their health spending. Similar to the Québec case, the provincial governments in the Atlantic region have relied heavily on fiscal discipline to constrain their health spending, and as a consequence, health providers are generally paid less in this region than in the rest of Canada. Recently the New Brunswick government was able to impose a two-year freeze on its physician fee schedule, but given the shortage of doctors in many rural areas, there is a limit to this kind of control. Beyond medicare services, which must be provided free at the point of service to meet the conditions of the *Canada Health Act*, these provinces spend less on health services; for example, New Brunswick and Prince Edward Island have the least generous provincial drug plans in the country.

Part Four provides some relevant lessons for Canada from abroad. By virtue of geography and culture, it is inevitable that Canada will be compared to the United States, despite that country's outlier status as the highest spender on health care in the world. Gerard Anderson explains why so many efforts by federal and state governments to bend the cost curve in Medicare and Medicaid have so consistently failed over time. While US performance on public-sector cost containment may be an object lesson for countries on what not to do, there has been significant innovation in the private sector, particularly in non-profit and for-profit managed care. Despite its title, the *Affordable Care Act* (or "Obamacare," as it was known by its opponents) has not put cost containment front and centre. However, as Anderson points out, the *Affordable Care Act* has spurred experimentation through what are known as affordable care organizations (ACOs). With the appropriate incentives, ACOs may be able to deliver care to Medicare beneficiaries at a lower cost. However, Anderson remains skeptical that reforms that depend so heavily on private insurers can lead to meaningful cost control in the long run.

As a federation with a Westminster-style parliamentary system, Australia resembles Canada in several important institutional features. Drawing on his knowledge and experience in both countries, Stephen Duckett describes the similarities and differences in their respective health systems. Similar to most OECD countries, Australia has experienced a rapid growth in public-sector health spending since the 1990s. Although the rate of health-expenditure growth in Australia has been lower than in Canada, it does not take into consideration the sizeable investment in tax subsidies by the federal government since the late 1990s to encourage the purchase of private health insurance and the use of private hospitals to reduce pressures on the public system. One of the key differences is the national Pharmaceutical Benefits Scheme, a successful effort by the central government to use its power as a monopsony purchaser to control pharmaceutical expenditures, the fastest-growing component of health-care costs in Canada in recent decades. While this monopsony power has been weakening in recent years, there is still much for Canadian decision-makers to learn from the Australian experience with bending the cost curve on prescription drug spending.

Alan Maynard reviews the recent post-devolution experience of the National Health Service (NHS), in which the English NHS operates separately from those in Scotland, Wales, and Northern Ireland. While a plethora of reforms aimed at bending the cost curve and increasing productivity have been implemented in England in the past decade, Maynard is skeptical about their impact. Indeed, he is highly critical of the lack of evidence underpinning and accompanying these reform efforts, as well as the English penchant for continual structural reform—what he calls "continuous re-disorganization"—rather than a more incremental approach that builds on previous reforms. The implicit message here is that governments in Canada should avoid the temptation to continually reorganize their governance and administrative systems. Instead, they should pursue efficiency reforms that have some proven utility, based on the best international evidence. These reforms should then be evaluated at every stage so that governments can make the appropriate adjustments.

Although the five Nordic countries of Norway, Finland, Sweden, Denmark, and Iceland have health systems that are probably more dissimilar than many Canadians assume, Jon Magnussen uncovers the characteristics they unquestionably share. These include a common commitment to universality and an emphasis on equity. In addition, they all have tax-based financing and services that are free, or almost free (with modest copayments), at the point of use. There are also important differences. Hospital-based physicians, including most specialists, tend to be salaried. The public benefits package tends to be much broader than medicare services in Canada, and thus private financing forms a much smaller share of overall financing in the Nordic region, even with copayments in some countries. Finally, while some Nordic countries have a decentralized health system of regions (Denmark) or counties (Sweden and Finland), these units still have less fiscal authority, power, and responsibility than Canadian provinces. Moreover, very recently there has been a pronounced trend to greater centralization. As in Canada, the Nordic countries tend to emphasize supply-side measures to bend the cost curve, including increased use of activity-based funding (ABF) to hospitals using diagnosis-related groups (DRGs) and the introduction of new incentives to encourage health organizations and local governments not to spend beyond their budget allocations. At a time when ABF is just beginning to be introduced in British Columbia and Ontario, it would be worthwhile to review the evidence on the practice in the Nordic countries (Stabile et al. 2013; Sutherland 2011).

The level and rate of growth of health spending in the advanced Asian economies of South Korea, Taiwan, Singapore, Hong Kong, and Japan has been (with the exception of Japan in very recent years) considerably lower than the OECD average. The difficult question is whether this is the result of greater cost-effectiveness or reduced access to more expensive health-care interventions and less generous public coverage. Canadian comparisons should likely be limited to countries with universal health insurance coverage, first introduced in Japan in 1961, then in South Korea in 1989, and most recently in Taiwan in 1995. Drawing on her extensive experience, Tsung-Mei Cheng focuses her study on Taiwan, a country that based its single-payer design on the Canadian example because it offered lower administrative costs and less complexity than the alternatives. Taiwan has relied upon both supply- and demand-side controls to keep its cost curve bent downward. The measures have included increasing copayments and administrative fees, reducing fee-for-service payments to doctors whose volume of patients exceeds a threshold level, introducing ABF by diagnostic-related groups for hospitals, and phasing in hard caps on global budgets by health sector—dental care in 1998, traditional Chinese medicine in 2000, primary care in 2001, and hospital care in 2002. The government has also, albeit reluctantly, raised revenues through increasing premium rates. Despite these efforts, health spending has continued to grow faster than the economy and health revenues, precipitating an ongoing and fierce debate on the sustainability of Taiwan's single-payer system.

Conclusion

From the preceding chapter summary, it becomes apparent that bending the health-care cost curve in Canada is a complex endeavour, made ever more complex as a result of the "immeasurable majesty" of a federal system that creates diversity in public health care. On the one hand, this diversity means that there is at any given time a range of ongoing experiments and approaches that can be used to gain insight on techniques to bend the cost curve. On the other hand, this diversity also means that whatever lessons emerge, there is no "one size fits all" solution to bending the cost curve.

It is worth keeping in mind some of the more difficult conundrums facing decision-makers in Canada:

1. Bending the health-care cost curve is a long-term process that is much more than a quick cost-cutting exercise or yet another "structural re-disorganization." But the voting public is impatient for change. Moreover, governments have a time horizon that operates within four-year cycles and are expected to demonstrate substantive improvement in the short run.

2. When it comes to cost control, there must be an emphasis on prices as well as volume or numbers of health providers. Nevertheless,

attempts at cost control to date have focused mainly on volumes of services and numbers of health-care providers. Prices remain the undiscovered country. At the same time, however, one person's health spending is another person's income, and constraining prices will be vigorously opposed by those affected, even if a clear public benefit can be demonstrated.

3. While health system sustainability is as much about revenues as it is about spending, most provincial governments have seemingly determined that they are not prepared to increase general tax revenues. The basis for this decision seems to be rooted in a general public aversion to higher taxes and a need for competitive tax systems. At the same time, there is a general inconsistency in public attitudes that desire more and better public health services but with fewer or lower taxes.

4. While policy should be *evidence-informed* rather than *belief-based*, the complexity of health-system change makes it difficult to draw a straight line from one evidence-based improvement to health-system change as a whole. Indeed, improving the quality and quantity of evidence-based decision-making is perhaps the greatest challenge in systematically devising policies for bending the cost curve.

5. While comparative evidence is essential for a better understanding of the policy problem, you cannot bend the health-care cost curve by cherry-picking reforms from other jurisdictions and other political and social contexts. Ultimately, solutions are devised within the context of specific political, economic, and policy environments. Grafting quick fixes onto one health system based on experiences in another can quickly generate new problems to replace those they were intended to fix.

At the same time, we would do well to remember that health spending is also an investment in human capital, and that provincial government health spending has produced positive and visible benefits. This can be seen most readily by using avoidable-mortality data—the rate of deaths per 100,000 population that could have been avoided if the proper intervention to prevent or treat the condition had been available. In Canada as a whole, the avoidable-mortality rate of 373 deaths in 1979 had declined to 185 deaths by 2008. Of this, avoidable mortality attributed to medically treatable causes declined by 56%, while avoidable mortality attributed to preventable causes decreased by 47% (Pi et al. 2013).

As a country, we face two main challenges. The first challenge is deciding exactly what changes we want to make. As almost all our authors agree, while there remains room to increase efficiencies and gain greater value for money, bending the cost curve will also require more fundamental reforms to the way we manage and deliver services. However, decision-makers and policy advisors disagree on both the direction and the details of many of these changes. The second challenge is getting agreement on the basic values or principles we want to preserve and even enhance as we reshape policies, structures, and the regulatory environments of health care in Canada.

Addressing these challenges will fall mainly on the shoulders of our provincial governments and, by extension, on the electorates they serve. Yet, as argued in some of the chapters, the federal government also has both the responsibility and the potential to play an important role in addressing both challenges. We hope that what follows will assist Canadians in general and decision-makers in particular in making the best decisions they can for the generations to come.

References

Atkinson, M., D. Béland, G. P. Marchildon, K. McNutt, P. Phillips, and K. Rasmussen. 2013. *Governance and Public Policy in Canada*. Toronto: University of Toronto Press.

Constant, A., S. Petersen, C. Mallory, and J. Major. 2011. *Research Synthesis on Cost Drivers in the Health Sector and Proposed Policy Options*. Reports on Cost Drivers and Health System Efficiency no. 1. Ottawa: Canadian Health Services Research Foundation.

CIHI (Canadian Institute for Health Information). 2011. *Health Care Cost Drivers: The Facts*. Ottawa: CIHI.

———. 2012. *National Health Expenditure Trends, 1975–2011*. Ottawa: CIHI.

———. 2013. *National Health Expenditure Trends, 1975–2013*. Ottawa: CIHI.

———. 2009 and 1975. "Supply, Distribution and Migration of Canadian Physicians". Ottawa: CIHI.

Cutler, D. M. 1995. *Technology, Health Costs, and the NIH*. Cambridge, MA: Harvard University Press.

Di Matteo, L. 2010. "The Sustainability of Public Health Expenditures: Evidence from the Canadian Federation." *European Journal of Health Economics* 11, no. 6: 569–84. http://dx.doi.org/10.1007/s10198-009-0214-x.

Di Matteo, L., and R. Di Matteo. 2009. "The Fiscal Sustainability of Alberta's Public Health Care System." School of Public Policy Research Paper, University of Calgary.

Dodge, D. A., and R. Dion. 2011. "Chronic Healthcare Spending Disease: A Macro Diagnosis and Prognosis." Commentary no. 327. Toronto: C. D. Howe Institute.

Landon, R., M. L. McMillan, V. Muralidharan, and M. Parsons. 2006. "Does Health-Care Spending Crowd Out Other Provincial Government Expenditures?" *Canadian Public Policy* 32, no. 2: 121–41. http://dx.doi.org/10.2307/4128724.

Marchildon, G. P. 2013. *Health Systems in Transition: Canada.* Toronto: University of Toronto Press.

Newhouse, J. P. 1992. "Medical Care Costs: How Much Welfare Loss?" *Journal of Economic Perspectives* 6, no. 3: 3–21. http://dx.doi.org/10.1257/jep.6.3.3.

Pi, L., F. P. Gauvin, and J. N. Lavis. 2013. *Issue Brief: Building Momentum in Using the Avoidable Mortality Indicator in Canada.* Hamilton, ON: McMaster Health Forum.

Senate of Canada. 2010. *Time for Transformative Change: A Review of the 2004 Health Accord.* Ottawa: Standing Senate Committee on Social Affairs, Science and Technology.

Stabile, M., S. Thomson, S. Allin, S. Boyle, R. Busse, K. Chevreul, G. Marchildon, and E. Mossialos. 2013. "Health Care Cost Containment Strategies Used in Four Other High-Income Countries Hold Lessons for the United States." *Health Affairs* 32, no. 4: 643–52. http://dx.doi.org/10.1377/hlthaff.2012.1252.

Sutherland, J. M. 2011. *Hospital Payment Mechanisms: An Overview and Options for Canada.* Ottawa: Canadian Health Services Research Foundation.

TD Bank Financial Group. 2010. *Charting a Path to Sustainable Health Care in Ontario: 10 Proposals to Restrain Cost Growth without Compromising Quality of Care.* TD Economics Special Reports, 27 May. Toronto: TD Canada Trust.

Tuohy, C. H. 1999. *Accidental Logics: The Dynamics of Change in the Health Care Arena in the United States, Britain, and Canada.* New York: Oxford University Press.

———. 2002. "The Costs of Constraint and Prospects for Health Care Reform in Canada." *Health Affairs* 21, no. 3: 32–46. http://dx.doi.org/10.1377/hlthaff.21.3.32.

United States Congress. 2008. *Technological Change and the Growth of Health Care Spending.* Washington, DC: Congressional Budget Office. http://www.cbo.gov/doc.cfm?index=8947.

Young, T. K., and G. P. Marchildon. 2012. "A Comparative Review of Circumpolar Health Systems." *Circumpolar Health Supplements* 2012, no. 9: 1–112.

PART I

General Considerations on Bending the Cost Curve

one

Why We Should Bend the Cost Curve and How We Could Do It

UWE REINHARDT

Introduction

Conferences, symposia, and meetings on the "health-care cost explosion" and the need to "bend the cost curve in health care" have been held in advanced industrial countries for close to half a century now. The tone at these gatherings has invariably been ominous, regardless of the level of health spending, either absolutely or as a percentage of gross domestic product (GDP).

My first encounter with the topic of health-care cost control occurred in the late 1970s, when I was asked to offer an economist's perspective on the topic at a large, nationwide conference held in Washington, DC. At the time, the United States was allocating about 8 per cent of its GDP to health care, triggering the fear that before long that ratio might rise to an inconceivable 10 per cent (it is now close to 18 per cent). Taking it as an axiom that "something" had to be done about this impending threat lest the 10 per cent threshold be pierced, I had prepared a sober opus with numerous suggestions on how to avoid the impending disaster.

Upon reading my prepared speech at my request, Tsung-Mei Cheng, a fellow author in this volume, took issue with the thrust of my talk and asked me to explain why rising expenditures on health care are a major social and economic problem, when no one runs cost-containment conferences about spending on automobiles, on fast food, on entertainment, on tobacco, or on alcohol. In those years the United States was still spending more on entertainment, including sports, alcohol, and tobacco, than on hospital care. Remarkably, spending growth in these other sectors in the economy was and still is routinely celebrated as a manifestation of economic growth and job creation.

Although the criticism was blunt and trashed my prepared speech, it was entirely warranted. Health-policy makers, health-services researchers, and the pundits who regularly call for cost control in health care actually can make a good case for their position, but they do owe to the public—and especially to the providers of health care who book health spending as revenue—a thorough explanation of why the trajectory of health spending must be bent down through policy if it does not bend down by itself, as it actually seems to be doing at the time of this writing (Hartman et al. 2013; OECD 2012a). One objective of this essay is to provide the rationale.

After all, one must have some sympathy for the usually hard-working providers of health care, who see their oft-maligned enterprise in an entirely different light. They see in it a vibrant sector of the economy that adds immense value by ameliorating the suffering of fellow human beings and often prolonging life. They see all around them unmet needs for health care. They see on the horizon the enormous potential of technological improvements that can further enhance human well-being. They even see economists who, while they talk a good game about benefit-cost analysis and the need to ration health care when they are standing vertical and healthy, routinely check those prescriptions at the door when they enter a clinic or hospital room, there to seek succor from the health-care system.

Furthermore, physicians and other health professionals see their former college classmates now working in finance richly rewarded in return for merely outwitting other people with money (other speculators or the managers of pension funds), whether or not in the process they have made a positive contribution to society. Beyond finance, they see dubious spending and waste all around them in the economy—in defence, in the administration of law, in education at all levels, and even in the commercial sector, where executives must be paid enormous sums just to perform the duties one would expect managers to perform.

To acknowledge these divergent views on health spending, this essay begins by offering a broader perspective on the theme "Bending the Cost Curve in Health Care," which properly means "bending down the future time path of national and per capita health spending." Next the discussion turns to the several economic and demographic factors that have brought nations to a pass at which more vigilant control over health spending, including the rationing of some health care, seems unavoidable. Thereafter some thought is given to the various approaches one might take to bending down the future health-spending trajectory. The essay concludes with some speculation on future trends in health spending.

Health care in the economy

Like any other economic sector, the health-care sector plays a dual role in the economy. With its output it bestows value on the rest of society. At the same time, it offers individuals and owners of capital an opportunity to deploy their resources gainfully. A question often raised is whether the latter role adds social value in addition to the value of the output produced by the health-care sector, as politicians and labour leaders commonly assume. This question is explored further on.

The value of the health sector's output

In the introduction to an edited volume of essays by distinguished economists titled *Measuring the Gains from Medical Research*, the editors note that the "growth in longevity since 1950 has been as valuable as growth in all other forms of consumption combined." Although the researchers could not be sure how much of that decline in mortality was attributable to health care and how much to other factors such as sanitation, nutrition, control of pollution, and so on, the editors observe that "medical advances producing 10% reductions in mortality from cancer and heart disease alone would add roughly $10 trillion—a year's GDP—to the national wealth" and that "the average new drug approved by the U.S. Food and Drug Administration yields benefits worth many times its cost of development" (Murphy and Topel 2003, 2).

Much the same message was conveyed in a paper by David Cutler and Mark McClellan (2001, 24) and in Cutler's subsequent book *Your Money or Your Life* (2005), where he raises the following question:

> In 1950 medical spending was about $500 per person (adjusted for inflation). Today [2005] it is nearly $5,000. Suppose you were offered that $4,500 increase back, but in exchange you could only have medical care at the 1950s level—doctors trained at that level, hospitals with 1950s equipment, medicines from around that time, and so on? Would you accept the money? My suspicion is that most would not; we value the things medicine can do for us more than $4,500. But does that means that increases in medical costs are worth it? (Cutler 2005, xi–xii)

Seemingly inconsistently, while economists extol the average benefit-cost ratio in health care, they also routinely lament that there is enormous waste in health care. For example, in his "The Simple Economics of Health Reform," none other than Cutler estimates that "anywhere from 30 to 50 percent of medical spending is not needed to realize the outcomes we achieve—a waste of about $1 trillion annually" (2010, 3).

There is really no logical inconsistency here. The production of a person's or a population's "health" is a complicated, nonlinear function of the use of health care and of many other economic, environmental, and behavioural factors. Holding all these other factors constant, the

Figure 1.1 Hypothetical benefit-cost curve in health care

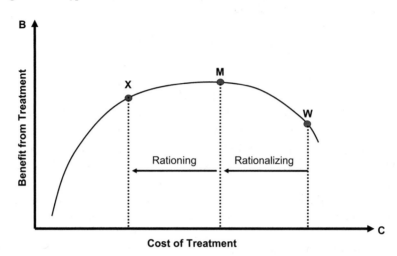

Source: Laugesen and Glied 2011, Exhibit 3.

incremental contribution that added use of health care makes to health tends to diminish fairly rapidly with greater use. In that circumstance, the *average* health benefit achieved from health care at a given level of health-care use can easily exceed in value the *average* opportunity cost of that care, even though the last few *increments* in the use of health care cost much more than the incremental value in terms of better health achieved.

Figure 1.1 illustrates this point. The graph depicts a hypothetical relationship between the cost of alternative treatments of a given medical condition and an imputed monetary value of the health benefits yielded by the alternative treatments. The graph incorporates the hypothesis that successively more resource-intensive treatments yield successively diminishing incremental health benefits and conceivably may actually harm the patient (e.g., through unnecessary surgery or radiation from excessive imaging). It is easy to see that at point M on this input-output curve the average benefit-cost ratio far exceeds the corresponding marginal benefit-cost ratio, which is 0 at that point.

Not performing procedures that add negative marginal benefits (on segment M–W)—for example, unnecessary surgery or imaging or prescription of antibiotics without compelling clinical rationale—may be called "rationalizing" health care. In general there is no disagreement on the desirability of rationalizing health care (although those who book health-care spending as revenue might be tempted to disagree). There is controversy, however,

Figure 1.2 Cost-effective supply curve for quality-adjusted life years

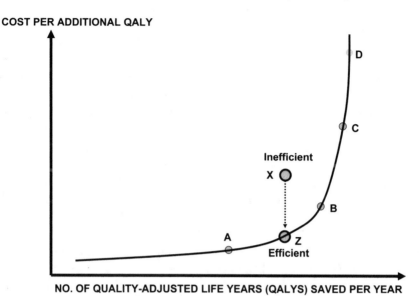

Source: Reinhardt 2012.

over segment M–X of the line in the graph: the withholding of medical interventions that do have a modest positive expected marginal health benefit *ex ante* (although not necessarily *ex post*) but whose opportunity costs exceed the value of that expected marginal health benefit. It involves what is widely decried—certainly in the United States—as "rationing" health care.

One way to reach decisions concerning the rationing of health care is to estimate the cost–effectiveness ratio associated with a proposed medical intervention, defined as the ratio of the incremental cost to the achieved incremental units of some one-dimensional index of clinical health outcome from the medical intervention in question—for example, the quality-adjusted life year (QALY) (Phillips 2009). If clinical outcome is measured by QALYs, this cost–effectiveness ratio can be viewed as the price per QALY that society has to pay when it asks the health-care sector to wrest one additional QALY from nature, given the lifestyle that members of society have chosen to adopt. One can then ask whether that price is worth paying for the value of the associated incremental benefits. Figure 1.2 can be used to illustrate this process.

The horizontal axis in Figure 1.2 presents additional QALYs "purchased" by society through the health-care sector in a given period, in increasing incremental cost per QALY from left to right. The vertical axis represents the incremental cost per incremental QALY, or the price per additional QALY.

A point such as X is inefficient in the sense that it incorporates pure waste. In an efficiently managed health system, the incremental QALY associated with point X should be attainable at a price of only Z. The distance X–Z on the vertical axis thus measures pure waste. The first task of any campaign to bend down the cost curve in health care is to drive the entire health-care system down towards the efficient QALY supply curve represented by the solid line in Figure 1.2, before the rationing of beneficial interventions is even contemplated.

But even in an efficiently run health system, with every QALY bought sitting on the efficient QALY supply curve, policymakers cannot avoid the following two troublesome questions:

1. Is there a maximum "price" above which additional QALYs will not be "bought" through health care—at least, not when the purchase would be financed from a collective pool of funds (either taxes or the premium pools of private health insurers)?
2. If there is such a maximum price, should it be the same for everyone in society, or can that price vary, perhaps by the individual patient's ability to pay?

In the United States these questions cannot even be openly broached. They are politically incorrect. Merely raising them can have one branded as a "Nazi" (Neumann 2004; *Washington Times* 2009), even though the frequently voiced demand that individuals should take greater responsibility for financing their own health care tacitly leans towards letting the maximum price to be paid for QALYs vary with the patient's ability to pay—that is, to ration even efficiently produced QALYs by price and ability to pay.

Other countries also face these two questions, explicitly but inconsistently. For example, the probability that the National Institute for Clinical Excellence (NICE) recommends against coverage of a product or procedure by the British National Health Service (NHS) decreases as the estimated cost per QALY increases. But other factors, even political considerations, also influence the decision (Parkin 2004; Rafferty 2009; Towse 2009). In other words, the judgments on which NICE bases its recommendations to the NHS depend in part on context.

While previous generations have "kicked the can down the road" on these troublesome two questions, future generations probably cannot avoid them, as economic growth in the developed nations has slowed and may continue to do so (Gordon 2012) as the distribution of income in the developed economies becomes ever more unequal, as the prevalence of obesity and its consequent illnesses continue to increase worldwide, as the number of elderly as a fraction of the population increases, and as new medical technologies, such as biological specialty drugs aimed at end-of-life care, become ever more expensive, especially for procedures aimed at saving QALYs at the end of life.

In concluding this discussion on the value of the output produced by the health-care sector, it must be conceded forthrightly that when economists talk or write about *value* in health care, they work abstractly. At the level of applied policy, there simply does not exist a consensus, even among economists and even at a conceptual level, on what the dollar value of a life-year or a quality-adjusted life year (QALY) or any clinical outcome should be. In their applied practical work, economists therefore merely assume a monetary value vaguely related to prior research—for example, $100,000 per life-year saved or per QALY (Cutler, Rosen, and Vijan 2006). The implicit assumptions here are that society is perfectly egalitarian and that taxpayers would not shrink from paying added taxes to purchase, through health care (even for the poorest person), an additional life-year, at least as long as the treatment costs fell below $100,000 per life-year (or QALY) so purchased. Economists, just like everybody else, muddle through more or less elegantly on this issue.

Health care as a creator of jobs

In many modern economies—certainly in the United States—the health-care sector has by now become a major economic locomotive and source of jobs in the economy, as is shown in Figure 1.3. These data come from a study of the employment structure of the US economy by Michael Spence and Sandile Hlatshwayo, who explored in detail the sources of the roughly 27 million net jobs added to the US economy between 1990 and 2008 (Spence and Hlatshwayo 2011).

The question is whether the jobs created by health care should be viewed as an additional value added to the economy, on top of the value of the output the health sector delivers. Politicians and unions of hospital workers seem to think so. They routinely protest the closing of hospitals or clinics in their communities, as health care has become the economic mainstay of many communities (Vladeck 1999). In this regard, these defenders of health spending are in good company, because the same argument is made whenever it is proposed to cut defence spending

Figure 1.3 Net jobs added by sector, United States, 1990–2008

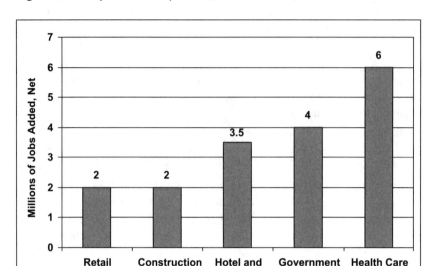

Source: Adapted from Spence and Hlatshwayo 2011, Fig. 6.

(Armbruster 2012; Schmitt and Donnelly 2011) or to close a military base—ironically, sometimes by the same commentators who favour cuts in public spending on health care or on other "entitlements" (Saletan 2012).

Sociologists also would probably impute additional social value to jobs in the health sector, because gainful employment provides the economic foundation for families and they have significant positive social spillover effects. These include reduced crime, reduced depression and alcoholism, reduced violence within families, and reduced suicides, along with superior opportunities for developing the human capital of offspring through better health care and education.

Using a narrower focus, economists are troubled by the idea of treating job creation per se as a social value on top of the value of the output produced by an economic sector. In the end, that line of reasoning might lead one to justify digging the proverbial ditches and filling them in again. Economists do recognize the positive social spillover effects of gainful employment, but they implicitly assume in their analyses that over the longer run, if someone could not find gainful employment in health care, they would find a job in some economic activity that would have roughly the same spillover effects.

Rationale for cost containment in health care

Given the high value bestowed by health care on society, along with the economic opportunities it presents to labour and capital, the question is why that sector is routinely picked on as a target for constraining spending on its output, when that imperative is never raised in connection with most other sectors in the economy. It is a fair question, although there are good reasons for singling out health care in this way, among them that much of it in the industrialized world is tax-financed. Even in the United States, over half of all health spending is now tax-financed (Woolhandler and Himmelstein 2002). Whenever public financing is involved, concern over the use of those funds and the secular growth of the financing arises naturally.

Many experts on health care also doubt, however, that the benefit-cost calculus that constrains spending in other sectors of the economy can ever work properly in health care, even if it were purely privately financed. For many goods and services produced in the economy, society is willing to let individual potential buyers do the requisite benefit-cost analysis for the decision whether or not to acquire a particular good or service, no matter how foolish the outcome of that calculus may appear to others. Furthermore, society is willing to let that decision be constrained by the individual potential buyer's ability to pay, that is, to ration goods and services among individuals by price and the individual's ability to pay.

Modern societies are manifestly unwilling to apply this thinking to health care, and not only for reasons of equity and social solidarity. There is the question of how well patients could even undertake this benefit-cost calculus. Some health economists—notably in the United States—believe that with reliable information on the prices of health-care goods and services and on their quality, individuals could function like ordinary consumers, which is why they refer to patients as "consumers." With appeal to the so-called Second Optimality Theorem, it can then be assumed that any degree of equity that society seeks in the distribution of health care can be achieved simply by redistributing purchasing power among households, as the Nobel Prize–winning economist Kenneth Arrow observed in passing but did not advocate in his seminal paper (Arrow 1963, 943).

The dominant view among health policymakers, and probably among most economists as well, is that even with modern electronic information systems, the asymmetry of technical competence and of access to information between patient and provider of health care, along with the often fragile condition of patients, severely limits the patient's ability to perform requisite benefit-cost calculus in health care for all but very simple medical interventions. This is a point that Arrow (1963) also emphasized.

Consequently there is room for supplier-induced demand (SID), by which economists mean persuading patients to accept services that a properly informed patient would not based on his or her own demand.

Furthermore, because redistribution of purchasing power to achieve equity in the use of health care typically is not politically feasible in the amounts modern health care would require, societies everywhere have made this redistribution through either a public or a private health insurance system. Insurance coverage, however, relieves patients of the need to perform the requisite benefit-cost analyses, even if they were technically capable of it. It provides the supply side of health care with even more opportunities to profitably induce demand for their services.

The growth of health spending has outpaced the growth of GDP for decades now in most developed countries, in part because the market for health care lacks adequate countervailing power on the part of the demand side. The social opportunity cost of those spending increases has become glaringly apparent. The United States, which spends almost twice as much per capita in purchase power parity (PPP) US dollars than do most other national health systems in the developed world, can serve as an illustration of these opportunity costs.

The roughly two-thirds of the American population with private insurance coverage typically obtain that coverage at their place of work. Although employers ostensibly pay the bulk of the premiums for that coverage out of company resources, economists are convinced that those outlays are recovered by employers over the longer run through lower take-home pay for employees (Summers 1989). In this connection, David Auerbach and Arthur Kellerman have reported in the health policy journal *Health Affairs* (Auerbach and Kellerman 2011, 1630) that

> [a]lthough a median-income US family of four with employer-based health insurance saw its gross annual income increase from $76,000 in 1999 to $99,000 in 2009 (in current dollars), this gain was largely offset by increased spending to pay for health care. Monthly spending increases occurred in the family's health insurance premiums (from $490 to $1,115), out-of-pocket health spending (from $135 to $235), and taxes devoted to health care (from $345 to $440). After accounting for price increases in other goods and services, the family had $95 more in monthly income to devote to non-health spending in 2009 than in 1999.

A recent research study projected the full cost of the premiums for employment-based private health insurance in the United States as a

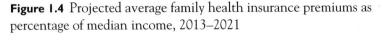

Figure 1.4 Projected average family health insurance premiums as percentage of median income, 2013–2021

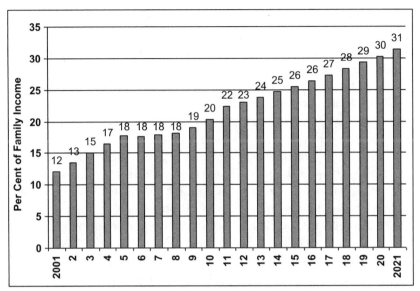

Source: Commonwealth Fund 2013.

percentage of projected median family income, implicitly assuming a full backward shift of ostensibly employer-paid premiums (Commonwealth Fund 2013). Figure 1.4 is based on Exhibit 3 of that report.

Clearly, if health insurance alone absorbed 30 per cent of the median income of an American family, the households would have to make painful trade-offs in their budgets. The opportunity cost of health spending in terms of the family's well-being and ability to educate their offspring would be high.

Although private health insurers cover about two-thirds of the American population, outlays by insurers along with out-of-pocket payments by patients account for close to only half of all personal health spending in the United States. The other half is financed by government budgets, which are increasingly constrained in size in the face of voters' unwillingness to countenance further tax increases. It is within these constrained public budgets at all levels of government that health care is now forcing troublesome trade-offs on society. It is probably so in many other developed countries as well, even with less dramatic health-spending projections.

The proper way to think of the value proposition of health care, therefore, is not the *gross value* the sector adds, which, as was noted earlier, can be considerable. Instead, one should think of the health sector's *net social value* after deducting the opportunity costs incurred to produce the gross value. These opportunity costs rise in magnitude the more constrained the budgets are from which health care and everything else is financed. They include neglect of human-capital development (education at all levels), of investments in research and development and productivity-enhancing public infrastructure, of security and national defence, and of a general standard of living.

While economists and health policymakers should have sympathy for the misgivings that health-care providers have over the push for tighter cost control in health care, providers should also understand that, from the larger macroeconomic perspective, the case for tighter cost control is compelling. It is all the more so if economist Robert Gordon (2012) is right in his previously cited conclusion that for the foreseeable future—and perhaps in the long run—the United States and, by implication, the rest of the developed economies face a permanent slowdown in economic growth, even though that hypothesis naturally is challenged by optimists (Bailey 2012; *The Economist* 2012) who see in 3-D printing, for example, a major industrial innovation that will usher in a whole new way of life for humankind, along with economic growth (Hart 2013).

Approaches to health-care cost containment

The terms *cost* and *spending* have triggered no small amount of confusion in the debate on health care. Usually one thinks of *cost* in economics as an amount per unit of something, be it a finished good or service, an entire medical treatment, or an hour of labour. By *expenditure* economists usually mean an amount per unit of time—say, a month or a year. Furthermore, economists make a distinction between the "real resource" costs and "dollar spending," which are not at all the same thing. Figure 1.5 illustrates this point.

The *real resource costs* in the lower part of the loop in Figure 1.5 include the time of health professionals, the capital equipment, and the supplies and other real resources (e.g., land) used in the production and delivery of health care. Many policies to bend the cost curve—notably in the United States—have been aimed at reducing the utilization of health care, that is, the flow of real resource costs going into health care, through greater cost sharing by patients or direct controls on utilization.

The upper part of the loop in the sketch represents generalized claims (money) on any kind of good or service produced somewhere in the world and available in the provider's locale. It does not measure what patients

Figure 1.5 Resource flows in health care: "real" vs. "financial"

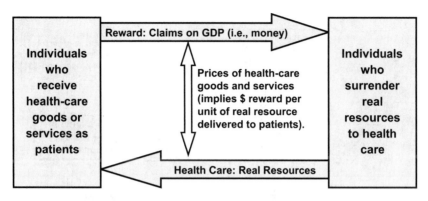

Source: Reinhardt 2012.

receive. Rather, it is the reward that the providers of real resources are paid for surrendering those resources to health care. The expenditure figures are usually expressed on a per capita basis or as a percentage of GDP. It is this *financial resource flow* whose annual growth is to be reduced by "bending the cost curve" downwards. Obviously, the real resource flow and the monetary expenditure flow are linked by the monetary rewards paid per unit of real resource surrendered (e.g., hourly reward per physician-hour worked), which express themselves to patients as *prices* for health care.

These are not pedantic distinctions. Conceptually, two health systems could bestow the same real health-care resources per capita on their population but grant their providers of health care quite different allocations of GDP as a reward. It is therefore advisable to break down the task of "bending the cost curve" into these two components: the use of real resources and the prices paid per unit of real resource.

Controlling the real resource flow into health care

Figure 1.6 summarizes, in a rough-and-ready fashion, the various tools that can be used to control the diversion of real resources from other potential uses into health care. The sketch is not exhaustive, but it presents the major tools and approaches—with some examples drawn from the United States—that can be or have been used to that end.

Policies aimed at the supply side: One time-honoured method of constraining the utilization of health care is simply to limit the physical capacity of the health-care system through regulatory means. It is the aim of classic

Figure 1.6 Alternative methods of controlling the use of real health-care resources

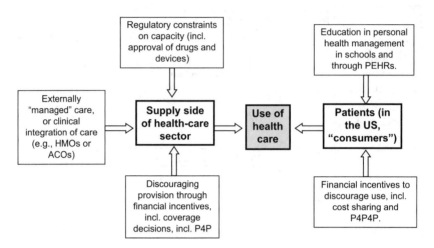

Source: Reinhardt 2012.

health-sector planning used in several countries, including Canada. In the United States, this effort finds expression through the "certificate of need" legislation that many state governments have imposed on their hospital sector (National Conference of State Legislators 2012), although rarely on other sectors of the health system. They did so in response to the federal *Health Planning Resources Development Act* (Public Law 93-641) signed into law by Republican president Gerald R. Ford in 1974.

Regulatory constraints on health-sector capacity are politically controversial—certainly in the United States—because they tend to trigger queues to resources that patients and their physicians desire access to, and thus lead to highly noticeable and sometimes irksome non-price rationing according to the queue or other administrative rules. Precisely because these constraints create an artificially limited supply, it is imperative to accompany them with regulatory constraints on the prices charged for limited-capacity services (e.g., magnetic resonance imaging machines or hospital beds). Regulatory restriction of the physical capacity of the health system in the absence of price controls combines the worst of government regulation and a free-market approach to health care.

Although some US states abandoned their "certificate of need" (CON) laws after the deregulation of health care under President Reagan, many states retain the laws to this day, with the apparent acquiescence of the politically powerful hospital lobby. The latter is understandable because, with the exception of the state of Maryland, these constraints are not accompanied by regulatory constraints on the prices for health care. The CON laws, therefore, in effect bestow on existing hospitals local monopolies that are much cherished by those hospitals. Typically, existing hospitals fight the threat of the potential entry of new hospitals with appeals to the CON laws.

Furthermore, while in most states the CON laws impose constraints on hospital capacity—for example, the number of MRIs or open-heart surgery units in hospitals—the constraints do not extend to the ambulatory sector. The result in many states has been the mushrooming of free-standing imaging centres or ambulatory surgery centres owned by physicians. If the intent of the CON laws was to constrain health-care spending, it must be doubted that this goal has been met. In any event, state hospital associations remain staunch defenders of the policy, which suggests that the revenues of existing hospitals have not suffered from this government intervention (Robeznieks 2009).

The main thrust of policies to discourage excessive use of real health-care resources that are aimed directly at the decisions of the providers of health care are financial incentives, with the triple objective of (1) improving clinical integration of the provision of health care, (2) achieving greater economy in the use of real resources in treating patients, and (3) improving in each of its many dimensions the quality of health care rendered. From a global perspective, the major alternatives to compensating the providers of health care can be summarized as in Figure 1.7, in which a distinction is

Figure 1.7 Alternative payment systems for health care

METHOD OF DETERMINING LEVEL OF PAYMENT	- BASE FOR PAYMENT -				
	Fee-for-Service (FFS)	BUNDLED PAYMENTS:		Annual Capitation per Patient at Risk	Budgets (Institutions) or Salary (Personnel, including Physicians)
		Hospital Care Only (DRGs)	Fully Bundled for Entire Episodes of Care		
Free-Market Price Setting between Individual Providers and Payers	A	B	E	H	K
Negotiations between Associations of Payers and Providers	E	C	F	I	L
Unilateral Administrative Price Setting (usually by Government)	I	D	G	J	M

Source: Reinhardt 2012.

made between the base that defines the units of health care that are priced (the columns) and the method of setting the levels of prices per unit of the base (the rows).

The method of determining the levels of compensation (the rows) depends, of course, on the political and institutional setting in which health care is embedded. The first row in the table, for example, describes the approach used in the American private commercial sector, while the third row describes the US approach for its main public insurance programs, the federal Medicare program for the elderly and federal–state Medicaid programs for the poor—an approach that has been described as Soviet pricing (Antos 2010). Ironically, that allegedly Soviet approach was imposed in 1983 on hospitals paid under the federal Medicare program by none other than that self-professed free-market devotee President Ronald Reagan, followed by President George H. W. Bush (the elder) in 1992 for physicians (Reinhardt 2010).

Regarding the base of compensating the providers of health care, current efforts among policymakers worldwide are aimed at shifting away from the time-honoured fee-for-service basis to bundled payments for entire, time-limited episodes of care across both inpatient and ambulatory procedures (Health Care Improvements Institute 2012). If episodes are not time-limited (e.g., care of chronically ill patients with multiple medical conditions or special needs patients), the preference now is for risk-adjusted annual capitation payments. More and more physicians formerly in independent practice in the United States have moved to salaried employment with larger entities such as large group practices or hospitals. Thus, for physicians salary has increasingly become the base of payment.

To safeguard the quality of care under any of these payment methods, it is proposed to make the size of the bundled payments or capitation payments a function of measurable quality indicators, the so-called pay-for-performance idea widely known as P4P. Getting these performance metrics right from a scientific basis, and getting them to be accepted as fair by providers, also remains a challenge. At the moment, it is a work in progress.

Traditional health maintenance organizations (HMOs), such as the fully integrated Kaiser Permanente health plan in California, are the ideal setting for applying any of these ideas. Because that model has had only modest success outside California, the *Affordable Care Act* signed into law by President Obama on 23 March 2010 also envisages more loosely structured organizations called "accountable care organizations" (ACOs). Any health-care delivery system that can integrate inpatient and ambulatory treatments clinically and economically through contractual arrangements can function as an ACO. The hope is that eventually they can deliver health care in return for bundled payments, although parcelling out money from the bundled payments to the various contractual partners may prove difficult and cumbersome.

How well the innovations urged by the *Affordable Care Act* will succeed remains an open question. First, determining bundled prices for entire episodes of medical care is easier said than done. There has to be some agreement among clinicians on the best evidence-based bundle of services that ought to go into the treatment of particular conditions. Even if that agreement can be reached—something not to be taken for granted—the individual components of the treatment need to be priced out to arrive at an overall bundled payment (Hussey, Ridgely, and Rosenthal 2011). Furthermore, although accountable care organizations may be able to economize on the use of real resources in treating patients, at the local level they could easily amass monopolistic power and use that power to drive up the price for whatever bundle of services is packaged for a specific clinical condition (Richman and Schulman 2011).

Even if some of the experimentation with these novel ideas in the United States ultimately fails, they bear watching from the outside. Indeed, one major contribution of US health care to the rest of the world is that it is a veritable laboratory for trying out new ideas in health care. The now widely copied bundled payment called "diagnosis-related group" (DRG) is a case in point; these groups emerged from government-funded research and demonstrations during the 1970s (Mayes 2007).

Based on my limited knowledge base, I do not think that the provincial single-payer health insurance systems in Canada have been notably innovative in reforming payment methods or health-care delivery systems. Perhaps the thought is to let other nations do the research and development and experimentation with alternative approaches and then to adopt what is suitable in Canada. If I am correct, this is disappointing, as it represents a great opportunity missed—the opportunity to show the world how to run a more efficient yet equitable health-care system.

Policies aimed at patients: Policies that may yield more economic use of real health care resources *aimed at patients* can work through several channels, including: (1) better education on personal health management in schools and universities, (2) the use of personal electronic health records (PEHRs) to provide patients with continuing education on health management and on making proper use of available health-care resources, and (3) financial incentives to discourage use of health care.

Research during the past half-century has shown convincingly that health care proper is only one of many factors driving the health status of populations and individuals, and not even the dominant one. Aside from genetic endowment, the individual's physical and socioeconomic environment and personal lifestyle weigh far more heavily (Deaton 2003; Evans, Barer, and Marmor 1994; Lalonde 1974).

During the past several decades the lifestyles typical in most advanced industrial countries have visited on future generations a mortgage, so to speak, whose full implications have yet to be understood, namely an epidemic of obesity and consequent diabetes, along with other cost-driving illnesses (Cawley and Meyerhoefer 2010; Quesenberry, Caan, and Jacobson 1998). Interactive mapping of obesity prevalence rates by US state maintained by the Centers for Disease Control presents a vivid and alarming picture of the growth in obesity in the United States (Centers for Disease Control 2010). This veritable epidemic is likely to contribute significantly to future increases in health spending (Trust for America's Health 2012).

Other nations in the OECD are not immune to these ominous trends, but so far the prevalence rates in other countries have been lower—and in some countries, much lower. In 2009, for example, the prevalence of obesity was 33.8 per cent of the population in the United States, 24.4 per cent in Canada, 14.7 per cent in Germany, 10.3 per cent in Italy, and 8.1 per cent in Switzerland, but only 3.8 and 3.9 per cent in Korea and Japan, respectively (OECD 2012b, Appendix). The relatively high prevalence in the United States can undoubtedly partially explain the paradoxical phenomenon recently reported by the US National Research Council and the Institute of Medicine in an authoritative study. It shows that life expectancy for all classes in the country is lower than it is in most other OECD countries, in spite of the much higher spending on health care in the United States (Institute of Medicine of the National Academies 2013).

Given the evident effect of lifestyle on the health of populations, it is remarkable (but, I would argue, not at all surprising) how much emphasis and money the developed nations have showered on health care proper, and how little on management consulting–style education—on personal health maintenance—given that schools and universities are ideal settings for providing that information efficiently. One reason may be that no "complex" has yet discovered a huge income flow for that endeavour, in comparison with the money flow that the health care–industrial complex has discovered in health care, just as the military-industrial complex discovered in national defence and in wars.

In connection with electronic health records, a distinction must be made between *personal* electronic health records (PEHRs), maintained and written as a link between patients and the health-care system, and those aimed at medical colleagues, which are typically referred to as "electronic health records" (EHRs) or "electronic medical records" (EMRs). It has long been dogma that EHRs can both enhance the quality of health care and lower the costs at which it is delivered. So far, however, the performance of EHRs for clinicians has been mixed and disappointing, as was found in a recent study by the RAND Corporation (Kellerman and Jones 2013). According to the RAND researchers, providers have not yet exploited the potential of that tool, and too few of such systems are interoperable within the components of larger health systems, let alone across systems.

Personal electronic health records (PEHRs) linking providers to patients would seem to be the ideal tool for engaging patients more actively and continuously in the prudent management of their own health. While they too are still a work in progress, it is clear that numerous countries in Europe and Asia are well ahead of the United States and Canada in this area. Canada in particular appears to be lagging (Schoen et al. 2012, Exhibit 1, 2808).

The final policy aimed at patients shown in Figure 1.6 is financial incentives that either discourage the use of health care of any kind or are targeted specifically at particular health-care goods and services deemed of low net value. In the United States, the latter set of incentives has come to be known as "value-based health insurance" or "value-based purchasing" (Chernew, Rosen, and Fendrick 2007). The idea here is to lower the patients' out-of-pocket cost-sharing if they seek health care from cost-effective providers or care.

A less targeted approach to financial incentives aimed at patients is what is known in the United States as "consumer-directed health care" (CDHC), a distant cousin of the medical savings accounts (MSAs) long used in Singapore (Hangvoravongchai 2002). The approach is based on private health insurance policies that impose very high annual deductibles, co-insurance, and maximum annual risk exposures for patients—often up to $10,000 a year per family. These policies are intended to provide incentives for patients to "shop around" for cost-effective health care, although so far it has been more like forcing them to act as if they were blindfolded customers pushed into a department store and asked to shop prudently for merchandise. User-friendly databases on the prices and quality of health care delivered by competing providers are the exception rather than the rule. In the United States, the significant out-of-pocket spending occasioned by these high-deductible policies can be defrayed by "health savings accounts" (HSAs), into which households can make tax-deductible deposits or employers can make deposits on behalf of employees without having it count as taxable compensation.

The structure of CDHC plans, coupled with tax-preferred HSAs in the United States, naturally favours high-income families. First, standard economic theory suggests that the self-rationing by price and ability to pay it is apt to restrict the use of health care by low-income families more than by high-income families. In effect, the CDHC model delegates the task of self-rationing health care mainly to families in the bottom half of the nation's income distribution. Second, the tax-preferred HSAs have the embedded effect of lowering the after-tax prices of health care paid for out of pocket more for high-income families than it lowers them for low-income families. As a distributive ethic, this mechanism is not easily defended. Policymakers in a political arena must be mindful of these ethical implications of the approach.

A recent study by the RAND Corporation found that, on average, high-deductible health plans cut spending for individuals, but they also reduce the use of preventive care (Beeuwkes-Buntin et al. 2011). What effect they have on the overall quality of health care received by patients is an open question, as is the question of how effectively patients can actually shop around for cost-effective health care (Ginsburg 2007). A survey of such insurance designs in several nations around the world also yielded mixed results (Hsu 2010).

In Figure 1.6, the acronym P4P4P stands for "pay for performance for patients," but it actually means "by patients." In part, the so-called value-based health insurance designs are pay-for-performance—in this case, the choice of cost-effective health-care providers (assuming that the requisite information is available to prospective patients). Charging smokers higher insurance premiums is another application of the idea. There are experiments now to extend the idea to other forms of health behaviour. For example, the insured may be offered access to lotteries with sizeable prizes for reaching certain targets for blood pressure, biomass, or exercising regularly. They may also be offered discounts on healthy foods at grocery stores that insurers have negotiated with in return for channelling customers there (Vitality Group 2013).

Whether or not improved health management through changes in lifestyle and the use of preventive health care can actually lower the growth path of annual health spending remains as yet an open question. Because so much is spent to ward off death near the end of life, it may well turn out that over the long run these measures will merely enhance the yield of health spending in terms of longer life expectancy and better quality of life (Cohen, Neumann, and Weinstein 2008; Russell 2009) but not cut overall annual health spending. But these measures could potentially be part of any strategy to bend the cost curve in health care.

Controlling the prices paid for health care

In a fascinating paper by Mark Pauly (1993), he makes the point that if costs are defined as economists would define them—that is, the value of the real resources used to produce health care—then in cross-national comparisons the United States does not actually stand out as a high spender on health care; rather, it ranks at the low end. Other countries keep their health spending per capita low mainly through monopsonistic power on the payment side of the health sector, Pauly points out, allowing them to depress prices below what they would be in a freely competitive market. The same point has been made by conservative economist John C. Goodman in his book *Priceless: Curing the Healthcare Crisis* (2012, 86). Finally, the point had been made in a much cited paper titled "It's the Prices, Stupid: Why the United States Is So Different from Other Countries" (Anderson et al. 2003).

Most developed nations have long ceased to turn over determination of prices for health care to the invisible hand of the private market (the first row in Figure 1.7 above). This approach is used mainly in the United States, and only for roughly the half of total health spending transacted in the private part of the US health system. Instead, as Pauly notes, most nations have chosen to shift more of the weight of market power in health-care price determination to the payment side, by endowing it with monopsonistic market power. This is clearly so in single-payer insurance systems. They can set prices at a level just sufficient to elicit from providers the supply of health care the policymakers deem desirable and affordable. For example, exploiting hitherto untapped monopsony power, the Canadian provinces and territories recently reached an agreement to commence, on 1 April 2013, the purchase in bulk of six popular generic drugs (Lunn 2013). In Canada, prices of generic drugs have been higher than in most other countries, including the United States (Law 2012, 4).

But considerable market power rests on the payment side also, in so-called all-payer systems under the Bismarck model of social health insurance, for example, in Germany and Switzerland. In both countries, prices are negotiated between regional associations of health insurers and the corresponding regional associations of health-care providers in what are called "quasi-markets." These negotiations are subject to overall budget constraints set by government with appeal to macroeconomic growth (the second row of Figure 1.7). These health systems control the level and growth of health spending as well as does Canada.

As already noted in connection with Figure 1.7, the United States has a bifurcated approach to price determination: unilateral price setting by government for public insurance programs, and negotiations between individual private insurers (or individual self-paying patients) and individual providers of health care in the private sector. The latter approach has had two consequences. First, the system is highly price-discriminatory. Prices for a given procedure or health-care good can vary by a factor of 10 within a state, even for a single health insurer (Reinhardt 2012, 49). In 2008, for example, the largest commercial insurer in New Jersey paid one hospital $716 for a colonoscopy and another $3,717, with others in a range between these extremes. For free-standing ambulatory surgery centres performing

Table 1.1 Fees for primary-care office visits and hip replacement

	Primary-Care Physician for Office Visit ($)		Orthopedist's Fee for Hip Replacement ($)	
	Public Payer	Private Payer	Public Payer	Private Payer
Australia	34	45	1,046	1,943
Canada	59	—	652	—
France	32	34	674	1,340
Germany	46	10	1,251	—
United Kingdom	66	129	1,181	2,160
United States	60	133	1,634	3,996

Note: Fees are calculated in purchase power parity (PPP) 2008 dollars.
Source: Laugesen and Glied 2011, Exhibit 3.

the procedure, the fee range was $443 to $1,396. For the physician component of the colonoscopy, the insurer paid a range from $178 to $431. In 2007 the largest insurer in California paid hospitals fees ranging from $1,800 to $13,700 for an appendectomy. The fees paid to hospitals for a coronary bypass graft with cardiac catheterization (DRG 107) ranged from $33,000 to $99,800. These enormous price variations appear to have no relationship to either quality or costs. The prices depend mainly on the relative market power in local markets where payers meet providers.

Second, the average prices for identical goods and services in US health care—be it a drug, a diagnostic test, an imaging service, or a particular surgery—is much higher than are comparable fees in other nations, often twice as high (International Federation of Health Plans 2011). Table 1.1, adapted from Laugesen and Glied (2011, Exhibit 3), illustrates this point.

The higher US physician fees may reflect in part the higher malpractice premiums that American physicians pay. They might also reflect higher incomes in other professions, which inevitably serve as benchmarks for physician incomes. Furthermore, they determine differential levels of national health spending per capita at a single point in time more than differential growth rates over time. But they may also include what economists call "rents," that is, price levels higher than would be needed to elicit the proper supply of health care. To the extent that this holds true for providers other than physicians, tighter control on the secular growth of health-care prices could help bend the cost curve downward, other things being equal. One approach I have already suggested would be to shift from the current price-discriminatory system towards an all-payer system such as Germany's or Switzerland's (Reinhardt 2012).

Some economists (Pauly 1993) object to a monopsonistic approach to price determination in health care on two grounds, and even to negotiated all-payer systems. First, they question its fairness vis-à-vis the providers of health care. That question is based on the implicit notion that market prices are inherently fairer to both sides of the market than are monopsonistic prices. That notion, however, is debatable in a market as problematic as the health-care market, in which market power is so heavily allocated to the supply side.

Second, these critics of monopsony on the payment side (and, for that matter, most economists) see in monopsony power the potential for serious mischief, because prices might be set too low by the payment side to elicit the desired supply of health care, leading to undesired rationing of care. In Canada, for example, located next to the more generous US market, this is a constant possibility. Here too the implicit assumption is that free-market prices will always elicit the proper supply and utilization of health care. However, I find it difficult to see that felicitous effect in the highly price-discriminatory system of US health care.

Health spending in the future

In the wake of the financial crisis and the deep recession it triggered in most developed countries, the annual growth in health spending declined drastically and even turned negative in parts of Europe (OECD 2012a). It slowed down somewhat in Canada but did not decline (CIHI 2011, Table A.3.3.1). It did not decline in the United States either, although there it slowed down noticeably, as well as attaining over 2011–12 its lowest growth rate in several decades (Hartman et al. 2013)—3.9 per cent, keeping the fraction of GDP absorbed by health care a stable 17.9 per cent of GDP. That fraction, of course, is substantially higher than comparable ratios in other developed countries. Among the three highest-spending nations in the OECD, in 2011 Canada spent an estimated 11.2 per cent of its GDP on health care, Germany 11.5 per cent, and Switzerland 11.6 per cent (OECD 2011, Table 1).

At the time of writing, there is uncertainty throughout the OECD whether the recent slowdown in the growth of health spending everywhere is a temporary response to the sharp slowdown in the growth of GDP and employment, or whether it portends a permanent downward shift in the trajectory of future health spending. Figures 1.8 and 1.9 suggest that, in the United States at least, the trajectory was bent down years ago.

As Figures 1.8 and 1.9 show, the annual growth rate of US health spending had plummeted towards the annual growth of GDP many times before, albeit never for long. What is also apparent from past US health-spending

Figure 1.8 Difference in growth of US GDP and US national health spending (per cent), 1970–2010

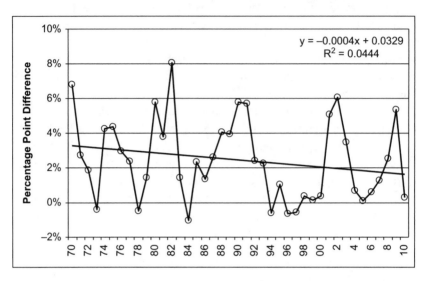

Source: Based on Centers for Medicare and Medicaid Services 2012, Table 1.

Figure 1.9 Annual growth in US real (constant dollar) health spending per capita, 1970–2011

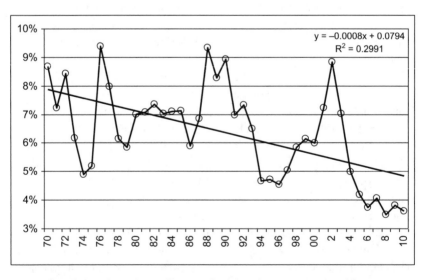

Source: Based on Centers for Medicare and Medicaid Services 2012, Table 1.

trends, however, is that the swings in short-run health-spending growth have dampened in amplitude over time and have been centred on a long-run downward-sloping trend line.

The question now is for how long that long-term trend line will extend downward in the future, and whether nations can patiently wait as the health-care sector lumbers along this gradual downward glide path towards lower spending growth or whether the mounting opportunity costs of health care in the shorter run will compel more forceful policy interventions to bend down the cost curve. As Hartman and his colleagues observe ominously about the lower growth of US health spending in 2010–11, "Overall, there was relatively slow growth in incomes, jobs, and GDP in 2011, which raises questions about whether US health care spending will rebound over the next few years as it typically has after past economic downturns" (Hartman et al. 2013, 87).

Conclusion

At the risk of oversimplifying, one can define the claim a nation's health-care sector makes on its gross domestic product (GDP) in any given year—what we usually refer to as "annual national health spending" (NHE)—as

$$\text{NHE} = (\text{price/unit of health care}) \times (\text{units of health care used/} \atop \text{capita}) \times (\text{size of population})$$

If one wants to track NHE per capita or as a percentage of GDP over time, or to compare the figure across nations at a similar stage of economic development, the population figure must be adjusted for morbidity patterns, which in turn are driven by demographic structure.

A public health policy seeking to constrain the growth of NHE over time should focus first on a careful consideration of the "units" of health care for which *price* is defined. Traditionally, in most developed economies, the unit has been the individual service. In the United States, for example, the fee-for-service schedule for physicians under the traditional government-run federal Medicare program for the elderly contains more than 9,000 service items. For hospitals, the "charge master" list of prices still used in parts of the private health insurance sector contains 20,000 items or more.

Current efforts around the world aim at redefining the "units of care" to higher levels of aggregation—the entire ambulatory and inpatient treatment of a finite episode of care, for example, such as a coronary bypass graft—or, for non-episodic chronic care, annual risk-adjusted capitation. For these measures to work, the bundles for episodic care must be carefully defined and based on empirical evidence of best practices. Furthermore, there has to be an organization capable of accepting these aggregate payments and distributing the money to the various participants in the treatment. The "new, new" concept of affordable care organizations (ACOs) encouraged in President Obama's *Affordable Care Act* of 2010 is thought of as such an organization. The ACOs are to integrate health care clinically across providers and settings in a cost-effective way. The Kaiser Permanente model, which originated in California during the Second World War, is the ultimate in ACOs.

The ACO movement in the United States may or may not be an overwhelming success, but it is worth trying. To my amazement, I do not detect even a tentative movement in this innovative direction in Canada. As hard as Canadians may try to belie it, sometimes things can be learned from the giant health-care laboratory south of the border.

There is little that policymakers can do about the size and demographic structure of the population, because it is driven by decisions made by people in the privacy of their bedrooms, as the late Senator Moynihan of New York once put it. The only marginal tweaking of population size and demography is brought about by immigration, but it has its limits.

The price for whatever unit of health care is chosen as the basis for pricing can be set unilaterally by government, as it is in the US federal Medicare system and Taiwan's single-payer system. In social insurance systems with multiple insurance carriers—for example, Germany and Switzerland—associations of insurers and counterpart providers negotiate fees that are thereafter uniformly applied to all insurers and all providers. In general, I do favour negotiated fee schedules, to give providers whose income is being determined a seat at the table and a stake in the price schedules. In my view, the worst conceivable system involves negotiations over prices between each of multiple insurers and each provider, the system that rules in the private health insurance sector in the United States—I have routinely made sport of that dubious approach (Reinhardt 2006, 2012).

Finally, it is often argued that national health spending could be reduced by focusing more on the non-medical-care determinants of ill health, an idea first put out for discussion as early as 1974, by Canada's then minister of national health and welfare Marc Lalonde, and subsequently by Robert G. Evans and colleagues (Evans et al. 1994; Lalonde 1974). By now a huge literature has emerged on that topic, whose content is beyond the scope of this paper. Suffice it to state my own view on the matter: focusing on the non-medical-care determinants of health is bound to increase both life-years and the quality of life lived, but it is unlikely to reduce NHE, other things being equal. People would live longer and healthier lives, but eventually their bodies would depreciate anyhow, triggering expensive fights with health care proper to reduce the pace of depreciation.

Furthermore, in health care, society faces a huge income-seeking medical-industrial complex that is just as powerful and persuasive as the military-industrial complex lamented by none other than former general and president of the United States Dwight Eisenhower (Eisenhower 1961). The politically powerful medical-industrial complex will fight hard, just like the defence industry, to protect its claim on the nation's GDP, and even to grow it.

References

Anderson, G. F., U. E. Reinhardt, P. S. Hussey, and V. Petrosyan. 2003. "It's the Prices, Stupid: Why the United States Is So Different from Other Countries." *Health Affairs* 22, no. 3: 89–105. http://dx.doi.org/10.1377/hlthaff.22.3.89.

Antos, J. 2010. "Confessions of a Price Controller." *The American*, 30 October. Accessed 10 January 2013. http://www.american.com/archive/2010/october/confessions-of-a-price-controller.

Armbruster, B. 2012. "Romney's Stimulus: Government Spending on the Military Will Create More Jobs." ThinkProgress Security. Accessed 20 December 2012. http://thinkprogress.org/security/2012/07/25/581571/romney-government-spending-military-jobs/?mobile=nc.

Arrow, K. J. 1963. "Uncertainty and the Welfare Economics of Medical Care." *American Economic Review* 53, no. 5: 941–73.

Auerbach, D. I., and A. L. Kellerman. 2011. "A Decade of Health Care Cost Growth Has Wiped Out Real Income Gains for an Average US Family." *Health Affairs* 30, no. 9: 1630–36. http://dx.doi.org/10.1377/hlthaff.2011.0585.

Bailey, R. 2012. "Is U.D. Economic Growth Over?" Reason.com, 16 October. Accessed 5 January 2013. http://reason.com/archives/2012/10/16/is-us-economic-growth-over.

Beeuwkes-Buntin, M., A. M. Haviland, R. McDevitt, and N. Sood. 2011. "Health-care Spending and Preventive Care in High-Deductible and Consumer-Directed Health Plans." *American Journal of Managed Care* 17, no. 3: 222–30. Accessed 9 January 2013. http://www.ajmc.com/publications/issue/2011/20113-vol17-n3/AJMC_11mar_Buntin_222to230/2.

Blendon, R. J., K. Schoen, K. Donelan, R. Osborn, C. M. DesRoches, K. Scoles, K. Davis, K. Binns, and K. Zapert. 2001. "Physicians' Views on Quality of Care: A Five Country Comparison." *Health Affairs* 20, no. 3: 233–43. http://dx.doi.org/10.1377/hlthaff.20.3.233.

Business Roundtable. 2006. *The Business Roundtable Health Care Value Index*. Executive Summary. Accessed 10 May 2014. http://businessroundtable.org/sites/default/files/The_Business_Roundtable_Health_Care_Value_Index_Executive_Summary.pdf.

Cawley, J., and C. Meyerhoefer. 2010. "The Medical Care Cost of Obesity: An Instrumental Variable Approach." National Bureau of Economic Research working paper no. 16467. Accessed 10 January 2013. http://www.nber.org/papers/w16467.pdf?new_window=1.

Centers for Disease Control (CDC). 2010. "Obesity Trends among U.S. Adults between 1985 and 2010." Accessed 7 January 2013. http://www.cdc.gov/obesity/downloads/obesity_trends_2010.ppt#533,1,Slide1.

Centers for Medicare and Medicaid Services (CMS). 2012. "NHE Summary Including Share of GDP, 1960–2010." Accessed December 2012. https://www.cms.gov/Research-Statistics-Data-and-Systems/Statistics-Trends-and-Reports/NationalHealthExpendData/Downloads/tables.pdf.

Chernew, M. E., A. B. Rosen, and A. M. Fendrick. 2007. "Value-Based Insurance Design." Health Affairs 26, no. 2: w195–203. Accessed 9 January 2013. http://content.healthaffairs.org/content/26/2/w195.full.pdf+html.

CIHI (Canadian Institute for Health Information). 2011. National Health Expenditure Trends, 1975–2011. Accessed December 2012. https://secure.cihi.ca/estore/productFamily.htm?locale=en&pf=PFC1671.

Cohen, J. T., P. J. Neumann, and M. C. Weinstein. 2008. "Does Preventive Care Save Money? Health Economics and the Presidential Candidates." New England Journal of Medicine 358, no. 7: 661–63. http://dx.doi.org/10.1056/NEJMp0708558.

Commonwealth Fund. 2013. "Confronting Costs: Stabilizing U.S. Health Care Spending While Moving Toward a High Performance Health Care System." Accessed 9 January 2013. http://www.commonwealthfund.org/~/media/Files/Publications/Fund%20Report/2013/Jan/1653_Commission_confronting_costs_web_FINAL.pdf.

Cutler, D. M. 2005. Your Money or Your Life: Strong Medicine for America's Health Care System. New York: Oxford University Press.

———. 2010. "The Simple Economics of Health Reform." Economists' Voice 7, no. 5: 1–5. http://dx.doi.org/10.2202/1553-3832.1816.

Cutler, D. M., and M. McClellan. 2001. "Is Technological Change in Medicine Worth It?" Health Affairs 20, no. 5: 11–29. http://dx.doi.org/10.1377/hlthaff.20.5.11.

Cutler, D., A. B. Rosen, and S. Vijan. 2006. "The Value of Medical Spending in the United States, 1960–2000." New England Journal of Medicine 355, no. 9: 920–27. Accessed 20 December 2012. http://dx.doi.org/10.1056/NEJMsa054744.

Deaton, A. 2003. "Health, Inequality and Economic Development." Journal of Economic Literature 41, no. 1: 113–58. Accessed 10 January 2013. http://dx.doi.org/10.1257/jel.41.1.113.

The Economist. 2012. "Productivity and Growth: What Is That?" 8 September. Accessed 5 January 2013. http://www.economist.com/blogs/freeexchange/2012/09/productivity-and-growth.

Eisenhower, D. D. 1961. "Military-Industrial Complex Speech." Accessed January 2013. http://coursesa.matrix.msu.edu/~hst306/documents/indust.html.

Evans, R. G., M. B. Barer, and T. R. Marmor, eds. 1994. Why Are Some People Healthy and Others Not? Piscataway, NJ: Aldine Transaction.

Ginsburg, P. B. 2007. "Shopping for Price in Medical Care." Health Affairs 26, no. 2: w208–16. Accessed 9 January 2013. http://dx.doi.org/10.1377/hlthaff.26.2.w208.

Goodman, J. C. 2012. Priceless: Curing the Healthcare Crisis. Oakland, CA: The Independent Institute.

Gordon, R. J. 2012. "Is U.S. Economic Growth Over? Faltering Innovation Confronts the Six Headwinds." National Bureau of Economic Research working paper no. 18135. Accessed 2 January 2013. http://www.nber.org/papers/w18315.

Hangvoravongchai, P. 2002. Medical Savings Accounts: Lessons Learned from Limited International Experience. Geneva: World Health Organization. Accessed 9 January 2013. http://www.who.int/health_financing/documents/dp_e_02_3-med_savings_accounts.pdf.

Hart, B. 2013. "Will 3D Printing Change the World?" *Forbes*, March 6. Accessed 5 January 2013. http://www.forbes.com/sites/gcaptain/2012/03/06/will-3d-printing -change-the-world/.

Hartman, M., A. B. Martin, J. Benson, and A. Catlin. 2013. "National Health Spending in 2011: Overall Growth Remains Low, but Some Payers and Services Show Signs of Acceleration." *Health Affairs* 32, no. 1: 87–99. Accessed 7 January 2013. http://dx.doi.org/10.1377/hlthaff.2012.1206.

Health Care Improvements Institute. 2012. "Bundled Payment." Accessed 1 December 2012. http://www.hci3.org/content/bundled-payment.

Hsu, J. 2010. *Medical Savings Accounts: What Is at Risk?* Geneva: World Health Organization. Accessed January 2013. http://www.who.int/healthsystems/topics/financing/ healthreport/MSAsNo17FINAL.pdf.

Hussey, P. S., M. S. Ridgely, and M. B. Rosenthal. 2011. "The PROMETHEUS Bundled Payment Experiment: Slow Start Shows Problems in Implementing New Payment Models." *Health Affairs* 30, no. 11: 2116–24. http://dx.doi.org/10.1377/ hlthaff.2011.0784.

Institute of Medicine of the National Academies. 2013. *U.S. Health in International Perspective: Shorter Lives, Poorer Health*. Accessed 10 January 2013. http://www.iom .edu/~/media/Files/Report%20Files/2013/US-Health-International-Perspective/ USHealth_Intl_PerspectiveRB.pdf.

International Federation of Health Plans. 2011. "Comparative Price Report: Medical and Hospital Fees by Country." Slide deck. Accessed 10 January 2013. http:// voices.washingtonpost.com/ezra-klein/IFHP%20Comparative%20Price%20 Report%20with%20AHA%20data%20addition.pdf.

Kellerman, A. L., and S. S. Jones. 2013. "What It Will Take to Achieve the As-Yet -Unfulfilled Promises of Health Information Technology." *Health Affairs* 32, no. 1: 63–68. http://dx.doi.org/10.1377/hlthaff.2012.0693.

Lalonde, M. 1974. *A New Perspective on the Health of Canadians*. Ottawa: Government of Canada. Accessed 10 January 2013. http://www.phac-aspc.gc.ca/ph-sp/ pdf/perspect-eng.pdf.

Laugesen, M. J., and S. A. Glied. 2011. "Higher Fees Paid to US Physicians Drive Higher Spending for Physician Services Compared to Other Countries." *Health Affairs* 30, no. 9: 1647–56. http://dx.doi.org/10.1377/hlthaff.2010.0204.

Law, M. R. 2012. "Money Left on the Table: Generic Drug Prices in Canada." Working paper, University of British Columbia Health Services and Policy Research, September. Accessed 20 January 2013. http://www.chspr.ubc.ca/pubs/journal-article/ money-left-table-generic-drug-prices-canada.

Lunn, S. 2013. "Provinces Reach Deal to Save on 6 Generic Drugs." *CBC News*, 18 January. Accessed 20 January 2013. http://www.cbc.ca/news/politics/provinces -reach-deal-to-save-on-6-generic-drugs-1.1331370.

Mayes, R. 2007. "The Origins, Development, and Passage of Medicare's Revolutionary Prospective Payment System." *Journal of the History of Medicine and Allied Sciences* 62, no. 1: 21–55. http://dx.doi.org/10.1093/jhmas/jrj038.

Murphy, K. B., and R. H. Topel. 2003. *Measuring the Gains from Medical Research: An Economic Approach*. Chicago: University of Chicago Press. http://dx.doi .org/10.7208/chicago/9780226551791.001.0001.

National Conference of State Legislators. 2012. "Certificate of Need: State Health Laws and Programs." Accessed 7 January 2013. http://www.ncsl.org/research/health/ con-certificate-of-need-state-laws.aspx.

Neumann, P. J. 2004. "Why Don't Americans Use Cost Effectiveness Analysis?" *American Journal of Managed Care* 10, no. 5: 308–12.

OECD (Organisation for Economic Co-operation and Development). 2011. Database 2011. Accessed 7 January 2013. http://www.oecd-ilibrary.org/social-issues -migration-health/total-expenditure-on-health_20758480-table1.

———. 2012a. "Health Spending in Europe Falls for the First Time in Decades." Accessed 7 January 2013. http://www.oecd.org/newsroom/healthspendingineurope fallsforthefirsttimeindecades.htm.

———. 2012b. "Obesity Update 2012." Accessed 7 January 2013. http://www.oecd.org/ health/49716427.pdf.

Parkin, D., and N. Devlin. 2004. "Does NICE Have a Cost-Effectiveness Threshold and What Other Factors Influence Its Decisions? A Binary Choice Analysis." Health Economics 13, no. 5: 437–52. http://dx.doi.org/10.1002/hec.864.

Pauly, M. V. 1993. "U.S. Health care costs: the Untold True Story." Health Affairs 12, no. 3: 152–59. http://dx.doi.org/10.1377/hlthaff.12.3.152.

Phillips, C. 2009. "What Is a QALY?" Hayward Medical Communications "What Is ..." Series, NPR09 1265. Accessed December 2012. http://www.medicine.ox.ac.uk/ bandolier/painres/download/whatis/QALY.pdf.

Quesenberry, C. P., B. Caan, and A. Jacobson. 1998. "Obesity, Health Services Use, and Health Care Costs among Members of Health Maintenance Organizations." JAMA Internal Medicine 158, no. 5: 466–72.

Rafferty, J. 2009. "Should NICE's Threshold Range for Cost per QALY Be Raised? No." British Medical Journal 338: 185.

Reinhardt, U. E. 2001. "Can Efficiency in Health Care Be Left to the Market?" Journal of Health Politics, Policy and Law 26, no. 5: 957–92.

———. 2006. "The Pricing of Hospital Services: Chaos Behind a Veil of Secrecy." Health Affairs 25, no. 1: 57–69.

———. 2010. "Medicare's Soviet Label." New York Times Economix, 12 November. Accessed 7 January 2013. http://economix.blogs.nytimes.com/2010/11/12/medi cares-soviet-label/?_php=true&_type=blogs&_r=0.

———. 2012. "Divide et Impera: Protecting the Growth of Health Care Incomes (Costs)." Health Economics 21, no. 1: 41–54. Accessed 9 January 2013. http://dx .doi.org/10.1002/hec.1813.

Richman, B. D., and K. A. Schulman. 2011. "A Cautious Path Forward on Accountable Care Organizations." Journal of the American Medical Association 305, no. 6: 602–3. http://dx.doi.org/10.1001/jama.2011.111.

Robeznieks, A. 2009. "Pros and Cons: Certificate of Need Reform Bills See Mixed Results." Modern Health Care.com, April 27. Accessed 7 January 2013. http:// www.modernhealthcare.com/article/20090427/MAGAZINE/904249983.

Russell, L. 2009. Prevention Will Reduce Medical Costs: A Persistent Myth. Garrison, NY: Hastings Center. Accessed 9 January 2013. http://healthcarecostmonitor.thehasting scenter.org/louiserussell/rss-to-pdf/makepdf.php?feed=http://healthcarecostmonitor .thehastingscenter.org/louiserussell/a-persistent-myth/%3Ffeed%3Drss2%26with outcomments%3D1&order=desc&submit=Create+PDF.

Saletan, W. 2012. "It's Not Just a Job. It's a Jobs Program." Slate. Accessed 20 December 2013. http://www.slate.com/articles/news_and_politics/politics/2012/09/romney _s_ads_against_defense_cuts_treat_military_spending_as_a_jobs_program_.html

Schmitt, G., and T. Donnelly. 2011. "Cutting Defense Won't Create More Jobs." FoxNews.com, 14 September. Accessed 2 January 2013. http://www.foxnews.com/ opinion/2011/09/14/cutting-defense-budget-wont-help-create-more-jobs/.

Schoen, C., R. Osborn, D. Squires, M. Doty, P. Rasmussen, R. Pierson, and S. Applebaum. 2012. "A Survey of Primary Care Doctors in Ten Countries Shows Progress in Use of Health Information Technology, Less in Other Areas." *Health Affairs* 31, no. 12: 2805–16. http://dx.doi.org/10.1377/hlthaff.2012.0884.

Spence, M., and S. Hlatshwayo. 2011. *The Evolving Structure of the American Economy and the Employment Challenge.* New York: Council on Foreign Relations. Accessed December, 2012. http://www.cfr.org/industrial-policy/evolving-structure-american -economy-employment-challenge/p24366.

Summers, L. H. 1989. "The Simple Economics of Mandated Benefits." *American Economic Review* 79, no. 2: 177–83.

Towse, Adrian. 2009. "Should NICE's Threshold Range for Cost per QALY Be Raised? Yes." *British Medical Journal* 338: b181. http://dx.doi.org/10.1136/bmj.b181.

Trust for America's Health. 2012. *F as in Fat: How Obesity Threatens America's Future.* Princeton, NJ: Robert Wood Johnson Foundation. Accessed 10 January 2013. http://www.healthyamericans.org/assets/files/TFAH2012FasInFatFnlRv.pdf

Vitality Group. 2013. The Power of Health. Accessed 9 January 2013. http://www .thevitalitygroup.com/.

Vladeck, B. 1999. "The Political Economy of Medicare." *Health Affairs* 18, no. 1: 22–36. http://dx.doi.org/10.1377/hlthaff.18.1.22.

Washington Times. 2009. "Health 'Efficiency' Can Be Deadly." Editorial, February 11. Accessed 10 January 2013. http://www.washingtontimes.com/news/2009/feb/11/ health-efficiency-can-be-deadly/.

Woolhandler, S., and D. U. Himmelstein. 2002. "Paying for National Health Insurance— and Not Getting It." *Health Affairs* 21, no. 4: 88–98. http://dx.doi.org/10.1377/ hlthaff.21.4.88.

two

Financial Incentives and Pay-for-Performance

JEREMIAH HURLEY AND JINHU LI[1]

Introduction

Even a cursory reading of current health policy analysis and commentary leaves the unmistakable impression that funding reform is critical to improving quality and controlling costs. In the past decade, pay-for-performance in particular has entered the pantheon of policy ideas (integrated health systems, report cards, managed care, etc.) that sweep through health policy circles, promising to cure the various ills of modern health care. The logic behind pay-for-performance runs something like the following: *Quality in our health-care systems falls below expected standards. Traditional funding methods do not selectively reward quality. Ergo, the way to improve quality is to pay for it.* The idea is compelling, drawing on deeply intuitive (if simplistic) economic and psychological views of motivation—if we want something, pay for it. And for policymakers, pay-for-performance's promises of better performance without requiring them to get involved in the difficult, messy work of changing the delivery system is attractive: give the providers the right incentives and let them figure out how best to achieve the stated objectives.

In this chapter we review the evidence regarding the effectiveness of pay-for-performance and, more generally, consider how funding reform can contribute to achieving the twin aims of improving the quality of care and restraining the growth in health-care costs. This is, of course, part of the larger question regarding the use of financial incentives to guide behaviour.

To start, funding per se should be distinguished from the active use of financial incentives as a policy instrument, or tool, for achieving specific policy objectives. Funding embodies the allocation of monies from a third-party payer (public or private) to health system organizations, providers, and programs that deliver health-care services to individuals (Hurley 2010). As such, it is an essential health system activity that unavoidably creates financial incentives. These incentives influence the behaviour of

---

1 We thank Bolanle Alake-apata for helpful research assistance.

health system actors—health-care providers, individuals, developers of medical innovations, and even the funders themselves. While any system of funding creates financial incentives, and any sensible design reflects a careful consideration of those incentives, the deliberate, active use of targeted financial incentives to communicate and induce specific desired behaviours is a distinct policy act (Giacomini et al. 1996). This distinction is not merely academic: in the one case, a policymaker merely faces reality, and design choices need not be motivated by the desire to communicate policy objectives through financial incentives; in the second case, the policymaker actively chooses to use financial incentives as the instrument for communicating policy objectives and changing behaviour.

Governments around the world, including Canada's provincial governments, emphasize funding reform as a pivotal part of efforts to improve quality, performance, and cost control.[2] In Canada, reform of physician funding emphasizes a shift from traditional fee-for-service payment to alternative methods of payment for primary care, while reform of hospital funding emphasizes a shift from global budgeting to case-based funding (often now called "activity-based" funding). Beyond these changes to base systems of funding, a number of provinces, including British Columbia, Alberta, Manitoba, Ontario, and Nova Scotia, have introduced targeted financial incentives aimed at improving quality of care, especially with respect to preventive services and the management of chronic diseases (Canadian Medical Association 2010). It is timely, therefore, to review Canadian and international evidence regarding the effectiveness of funding reform, and targeted financial incentives in particular, on system performance.

The motivating question for this paper presumes that improved quality of care and reduced rates of cost growth are mutually compatible policy goals, asking only how funding reform might further both of these objectives. But it is important to consider briefly whether they are, in fact, mutually compatible goals. The concept of quality has many dimensions and interpretations in health care. In using *quality*, we follow the Institute of Medicine, which defines it as "the degree to which health services for individuals and populations increase the likelihood of desired health outcomes and are consistent with current professional knowledge (Institute of Medicine 2001, 232). Importantly, this conception of quality

---

2 As do health-care analysts and commentators. See, for example, Drummond and Burleton (2010) and Falk et al. (2011) for recent Canadian commentaries that emphasize funding reform as part of an overall set of policies to improve quality and fiscal sustainability.

is not limited to the skill with which a given medical act is performed but includes the mix of services provided (or, in some cases, not provided) to an individual or population, and the coordination and appropriateness of those services, therefore capturing essential elements of *health system quality* and performance.

Incontrovertible evidence documents that higher expenditures (and even higher levels of service provision) do not necessarily lead to higher quality. Indeed, they often result in lower quality. Hence, reducing the rate of increase in costs need not negatively affect quality. Some of the most compelling evidence for this derives from studies of inappropriate health-care utilization and geographic variations in health-care utilization. Much of this comes from the United States, but studies from Canada and other countries concur with US findings. Reviews of appropriateness research estimate that up to one-third of all surgical procedures in the United States are clinically inappropriate or are of questionable value (Institute of Medicine 2012; McGlynn 1998; McKethan et al. 2009), and that between 21% and 47% of US health-care expenditure is of little or no value because of failures of care delivery, failures of care coordination, overtreatment, administrative complexity, pricing failures, fraud, and abuse (Berwick and Hackbarth 2012). In Canada, Wright and colleagues' widely cited study of elective surgery in British Columbia found that the vision scores of approximately 25% of patients undergoing cataract surgery indicated that the surgery was unwarranted (Wright et al. 2002). As documented by the Dartmouth Atlas of Health Care, areas with large differences in medical expenditures show small differences in quality of care or outcomes. According to the Atlas, US Medicare spending per beneficiary for people with severe chronic illness in the last two years of life varies dramatically by state and hospital referral region, even when controlling for underlying differences in patient populations. These spending differences were independent of the type or severity of the illness and were instead related to geographical variation in practice patterns (Fisher, Bynum, and Skinner 2009). Analogous studies document similar variations in countries outside the United States (Appleby et al. 2011).

But is the converse true? Will improved quality help restrain the growth in health-care costs? Maybe. Following from the evidence cited above, higher quality in some cases calls for providing fewer services, and good-quality primary care can reduce the specialist and hospital costs associated with treating ambulatory-care-sensitive conditions. But in many areas of effective care, current rates of use fall well below those that would occur in a well-performing, high-quality health-care system. Improved quality in these areas will require increased service provision at increased cost in the short term. Evidence from the United States indicates, for instance, that Americans receive just 55% of recommended treatments for preventive care, acute care, and chronic care management (McGlynn et al. 2003). The situation in Canada is no better in many of these areas—this is one of the major motivations for provincial pay-for-performance schemes targeted at preventive services and chronic care.[3] Many expect that higher quality will, over time, help control costs by eliminating inappropriate utilization; reducing complications, readmissions, and related phenomena; and improving health. But in the end this is an empirical question. A recent review concluded that sometimes quality-improvement initiatives that claim to generate savings do so, sometimes they do not, but mostly we do not know, because good research is limited (Øvretveit 2009). Regardless, we should pursue improved quality because it is the right thing to do, knowing that sometimes it will lead to higher costs but also increased benefits sufficient to justify those costs.

In reviewing the evidence on how funding reform can contribute to the twin aims of higher quality and controlling costs, we begin with evidence regarding the effectiveness of pay-for-performance, examining first the limited Canadian evidence, and then place that evidence in the context of international experience with pay-for-performance. We then consider the potential for broader funding reform to contribute to improving system performance.

Targeted financial incentives

As its use and salience in policy have increased, the precise meaning of the term *pay-for-performance* has become less clear; it is now used to refer to a wide variety of funding arrangements, some of which only tangentially link pay and performance. We adopt a relatively narrow interpretation in which *pay-for-performance* refers to the explicit use of targeted financial incentives, usually in addition to a base-payment scheme, to encourage specific behaviours intended to improve quality of care. Although the design of pay-for-performance schemes varies across jurisdictions (e.g., Canada, the United States, the United Kingdom, and Australia), a common element is explicit financial incentives designed to change specific quality-related behaviours. In the physician sector in particular, pay-for-performance is

---

3 As noted below, for example, baseline rates of coverage for the preventive services targeted by Ontario's preventive care bonus scheme varied from 15% for colorectal cancer screening to 65% for mammography. Further, only 27% of diabetic Ontarians received the optimal number of monitoring tests for cholesterol, hemoglobin, and retinopathy.

normally grafted on top of a base-payment scheme (e.g., fee-for-service, capitation, or blended payment) and pays performance bonuses to providers whose service provision meets or exceeds pre-specified thresholds (hospital-based schemes are more likely to employ a combination of bonuses and penalties). By targeting the performance bonuses on areas for which good evidence links provision to high-quality care, the incentive is intended to increase compliance with evidence-based standards for high quality of care. Pay-for-performance can target individual providers, provider groups, or health-care institutions such as hospitals and long-term care facilities, but it has been particularly prominent in primary care, targeting preventive services (e.g., flu shots, cervical cancer screening, colon cancer screening, breast cancer screening) or chronic conditions (e.g., diabetes) for which evidence indicates that rates of uptake of effective services fall well below optimal levels.

Ontario was the first province in Canada to introduce physician pay-for-performance incentives, initially in the limited context of its capitation-funded "Health Service Organizations" in 1990. In 2004 Ontario expanded both the set of services included and the number of physicians eligible to receive the performance-based bonus payments. The Ontario scheme pays primary-care physicians bonuses when their rates of provision of targeted services meet or exceed pre-specified thresholds. British Columbia, Alberta, Manitoba, and Nova Scotia have introduced targeted physician payments aimed at improving the quality of chronic disease management. These initiatives introduced new fee codes to support the delivery of services associated with high quality that have not traditionally been reimbursed. British Columbia's Full Service Family Practice Incentive Program, for example, includes a "chronic disease management" fee code that provides an annual payment of $125 to a physician for each patient with a confirmed diagnosis of diabetes or congestive heart failure whose care accords with BC clinical guideline recommendations.

Impact of pay-for-performance on quality: Evidence from Canada

The only current evaluations of Canadian incentive schemes examine the effectiveness of targeted financial incentives included within Ontario's primary-care reform initiatives.[4] Hurley and colleagues (2011)

---

4 We are not aware of any evaluations of performance-related incentives in Alberta, Manitoba, or Nova Scotia. A series of reports provides descriptive information regarding the uptake of British Columbia's performance-related codes but does not provide a rigorous evaluation of their effectiveness (the reports can be found at "General Practice Services Committee" at http://www.gpscbc.ca).

evaluated the Cumulative Preventive Care Bonus Scheme, which targets preventive services (Pap smears, mammograms, flu shots for seniors, toddler immunizations, and colorectal cancer screening), and the Special Payments Scheme, which targets designated services in each of six areas of care of interest to the Ontario Ministry of Health and Long-Term Care (obstetrical deliveries, hospital services, palliative care, office procedures, prenatal care, and home visits). Kiran and colleagues (2012) evaluated the introduction of a fee code for diabetes management assessment, intended to encourage regular comprehensive management of diabetic patients.

Ontario's cumulative preventive-care bonus payment scheme at the time included two components: (1) a contact payment fee code of $6.86 for each eligible patient that a practice contacted to schedule an appointment for one of the included preventive-care services; and (2) a cumulative preventive-care bonus paid when a physician's provision of a targeted service exceeded defined thresholds in the target population during a defined period (see Table 2.1). The Special Payments Scheme uses a similar design but provides a fixed payment if service provision for a targeted service reaches a minimum absolute level during the preceding fiscal year.

The evaluation by Hurley and colleagues (2011) exploited variations in eligibility for the incentive payments to identify their impact on service

Table 2.1 Ontario's performance-based incentive payments*

Service	Payment Criterion	Bonus Payment (as of 2006)
Preventive Care Service Enhancement Payments		
Payment for Contacting Eligible Patients to Obtain the Preventive Service		
		• $6.86 for each documented contact for eligible patients
Cumulative Care Preventive Service Bonus		
Seniors' influenza immunization	Proportion of FP's rostered patients aged 65 or over who received a flu shot during the previous flu season (generally August to December)	• 60% of target population: $220 • 65% of target population: $440 • 70% of target population: $770 • 75% of target population: $1,100 • 80% of target population: $2,200
Toddler immunization	Proportion of FP's rostered children aged 30–42 months who received a set of 5 child immunizations by the age of 30 months	• 85% of target population: $440 • 90% of target population: $1,100 • 95% of target population: $2,200

(*Continued*)

Table 2.1 (Continued)

Service	Payment Criterion	Bonus Payment (as of 2006)
Pap smear	Proportion of FP's rostered female patients aged 35–69 who received a Pap smear for cervical cancer screening during the previous 30 months	• 60% of target population: $220 • 65% of target population: $440 • 70% of target population: $660 • 75% of target population: $1,320 • 80% of target population: $2,200
Mammogram	Proportion of FP's rostered female patients aged 50–69 who received a mammogram for breast cancer screening during the previous 30 months	• 55% of target population: $220 • 60% of target population: $440 • 65% of target population: $770 • 70% of target population: $1,320 • 75% of target population: $2,200
Colorectal cancer screening	Proportion of FP's rostered patients aged 50–74 who received a colorectal screening test by fecal occult blood testing during the previous 30 months	• 15% of target population: $220 • 20% of target population: $440 • 40% of target population: $1,100 • 50% of target population: $2,200
Annual Special Payments		
Obstetrical deliveries	5 or more specified obstetrical services to 5 or more patients in a fiscal year	$3,200 (increased to $5,000 in October 2007)
Hospital services	Specified hospital services totalling $2,000 in any fiscal year provided to all patients	$5,000 (increased to $7,500 in April 2005 for those with a Rurality Index of Ontario score greater than 45)
Palliative care	Specified palliative care services provided to four or more palliative care patients in a fiscal year	$2,000
Office procedures	Specified office procedures provided to rostered patients totalling $1,200 in a fiscal year	$2,000
Prenatal care	Specified prenatal care services provided to 5 or more rostered patients in the previous fiscal year	$2,000
Home visits	100 or more home visits provided to rostered patients in the previous fiscal year	$2,000

* See Hurley et al. (2011) for additional details.

provision. Only physicians enrolled in a "primary care reform" (PCR) practice were eligible to receive the incentive payments, while physicians who remained in traditional fee-for-service practices were not eligible. Furthermore, the timing of eligibility varied across Ontario's different PCR models. The analysis focused on full-time, community-based family practitioners engaged in comprehensive practice; it employed a number of strategies to control for possible sources of bias (e.g., physicians were not randomly assigned to the PCR models, leading to possible selection bias) and confounding (e.g., PCR practices differ from the traditional fee-for-service practice with respect to more than just eligibility for P4P incentives).

The study found no response to the contact payment or to the special payment scheme, no response for one of the preventive-care services (toddler immunization), and only a modest response to the other four preventive-care services (the absolute increases in coverage rates were 2.8, 4.1, 1.8, and 8.5 percentage points respectively for seniors' flu shots, Pap smears, mammograms, and colorectal cancer screening). The study also investigated how responses varied across physicians. Although the relationships were not strong and consistent across all preventive services, younger physicians tended to respond more than older physicians; physicians in larger practices tended to respond more than physicians in smaller practices; and physicians with middle levels of baseline compliance tended to respond more than those with either low or high levels of baseline compliance.

Kiran and colleagues (2012) examined physician responses to Ontario's diabetes incentive scheme, introduced in 2002 for all family physicians (FPs). In 2002 the province created a new code—the "diabetes management assessment" fee code—to encourage regular, comprehensive management of diabetic patients. A physician could bill the code (value $37) up to three times per year per diabetic patient; this fee is approximately $6 more than a standard intermediate assessment code a physician might alternatively bill for a visit. The code required that the billing physician maintain a diabetes flow sheet that tracked cholesterol, hemoglobin, retinal eye examinations, blood pressure, weight, and other parameters relevant to diabetes management. The analysis found that uptake of the code was low (only 25% of patients with diabetes had a billing for the code during the two-year period 2006–08); that its introduction was not associated with increased compliance with three evidence-based services (retinal eye exam, HbA.sub.1c, and cholesterol measurement); and that physicians who had already been providing the best quality of care before the incentive's introduction were more likely to bill the code. The introduction of the code appears to have rewarded those who were already providing good care while having little or no effect on other physicians.[5]

Overall, Ontario's experience with targeted pay-for-performance incentives indicates that they are not an effective way to improve quality of care through increased provision of services known to be consistent with good care. How do these findings compare with international experience with pay-for-performance?

Impact of pay-for-performance on quality: International evidence

The expanded use of pay-for-performance within health-care systems internationally has witnessed a corresponding growth in the study of its effectiveness. The research itself is of mixed quality. Studies with the best research designs (i.e., randomized trials with strong internal validity) tend to be conducted on small samples and assess initiatives targeted at a small set of services, limiting their generalizability. The observational studies do not always control well for sources of bias and confounding. In general, however, most sources of bias (e.g., non-random selection into the pay-for-performance scheme) and confounding (e.g., the financial incentives were only one part of a larger initiative) would lead to overestimates of the effectiveness of pay-for-performance. Hence, to the extent that bias is present, many studies will suggest that pay-for-performance is more effective than it really is. We first discuss previous reviews of the literature on pay-for-performance and then focus on some key studies from the United States and the United Kingdom, where pay-for-performance has been embraced most enthusiastically.

The effectiveness of pay-for-performance has been assessed in a number of systematic reviews (Armour et al. 2001; Giuffrida et al. 2000; Scott et al. 2011; Town et al. 2005). Scott and colleagues (2011) included seven studies that encompassed a variety of performance schemes (e.g., single-threshold target payments, fixed fee per patient achieving a given

---

5 In an evaluation of how physician responses to a second diabetes incentive code that Ontario introduced in 2006—the "diabetes management incentive" ($60 per patient), which physicians could claim if their care for a diabetic patient met defined standards—differed between PCR physicians paid by enhanced fee-for-service and PCR physicians paid by a capitation-based blended method, Kantarevic and Kralj (2013) found that those paid by the capitation-based blend were more responsive. Although the study does not document the effect of the incentive on quality of diabetes care, since it did not examine how compliance with underlying care standards changed either among those physicians or in comparison with physicians not exposed to the incentive, it does highlight that responses to P4P can differ depending on the base payment method.

outcome, payments based on relative performance among medical groups) and service types (e.g., smoking cessation, cervical screening, mammography screening, HbA.sub.1c, childhood immunization, chlamydia screening, asthma medication). One study found no effect on quality and the remaining six showed positive but modest effects on quality of care for some, but not all, primary outcome measures. The review concluded that "there is insufficient evidence to support or not support the use of financial incentives to improve the quality of primary health care" (Scott et al. 2011, 2).

Christianson and colleagues (2007) reviewed a large number of studies of the impact of financial incentives on health-care performance. The review of published articles examining the impact of financial incentives on improving the quality of care delivered by institutional providers and health-care practitioners (particularly physicians) concluded that the evidence is mixed. Relatively few significant impacts were reported, and because payer programs often include quality-improvement initiatives in addition to incentive payments, it was difficult to assess the independent effect of the financial incentives. Overall, the authors concluded that evidence was insufficient to inform the effective design and implementation of pay-for-performance initiatives.

The two countries with perhaps the most extensive experience with pay-for-performance are the United States and the United Kingdom. Pay-for-performance in the United States is used by private health plans—Rosenthal and colleagues (2006) estimated that by 2005 over half of commercial health maintenance organizations (HMOs) were using pay-for-performance, affecting care delivered to more than 80% of HMO enrollees—by state governments in Medicaid and children's health programs, and by the federal government in the Medicare program. The 2010 *Patient Protection and Affordable Care Act* includes a number of provisions for pay-for-performance, and the Center for Medicaid and Medicare has several ongoing demonstration projects. A recent review of experience with pay-for-performance in the United States observed that programs evaluated to date have produced mixed results and that experimentation with their design continues in an effort to make them more effective (James 2012).

Two prominent hospital-based programs include the Premier Hospital Quality Incentive Demonstration Project, which tested the extent to which financial bonuses would improve the quality of care provided to Medicare patients, and a Massachusetts-based Medicaid program that offered financial incentives for improving care for pneumonia and prevention of surgical infections. One evaluation of the Premier Hospital Quality project found no evidence of improvement in performance scores for pay-for-performance hospitals compared to control-group hospitals (Werner et al. 2011). A second study found no difference between pay-for-performance hospitals and control hospitals in 30-day mortality for patients with acute myocardial infarction, congestive heart failure, pneumonia, or coronary artery bypass graft surgery (Jha, Orav, and Epstein 2011). An evaluation of the Massachusetts Medicaid hospital-based pay-for-performance program similarly found no evidence of improvement in quality (Ryan and Blustein 2011; Ryan, Blustein, and Casalino 2012).

Two of the strongest US-based studies of pay-for-performance in the physician sector evaluated the quality incentive programs introduced in 2002 by PacifiCare Health Plan, a large network HMO, to medical groups in California. Rosenthal and colleagues (2005) measured physician responses for three preventive-care services—cervical cancer screening, mammography, and haemoglobin A1c tests—and found that rates improved modestly for cervical cancer screening (an increase of 3.6 percentage points, or 10% over baseline) but not for mammography and the hemoglobin A1c test. A follow-up study (Mullen, Frank, and Rosenthal 2010) that examined the effect of PacifiCare's quality incentive program and another large pay-for-performance program, by the Integrated Healthcare Association, produced mixed results: a positive effect only for cervical cancer screening, and no effect for mammography, the hemoglobin A1c test, or asthma medication. Overall, the study concluded that the P4P scheme did not meaningfully improve quality.

In 2004, the UK National Health Service (NHS) introduced pay-for-performance as a central element of its Quality Outcomes Framework (QOF). The QOF was a complex initiative that included quality indicators with respect to clinical care for defined chronic diseases and specified services; practice organization and management; and patient experience. It also included support for computerized information technology and initiatives to promote team-based care. A number of studies have evaluated the impact of the QOF on quality of care (e.g., Campbell et al. 2007, 2009; Doran et al. 2006; Millett et al. 2007; Serumaga et al. 2011; Steel et al. 2007; Vaghela and Thornhill 2009), and two recent reviews (Doran and Roland 2010; Gillam, Siriwardena, and Steel 2012) summarize the evidence to date.

The QOF improved certain aspects of processes of care. Practices have become more systematic and active in identifying and reviewing patients with conditions that were subject to the physician incentives, in developing protocols, and in renewing appointment systems. Computer systems now provide prompts during consultations if a target applies. While this is a positive development in many respects, it has also prompted complaints that framework-related computer alerts compete with patients presenting problems for the attention of the GP; that quantifiable aspects of care subject to incentives under the framework are prioritized over less quantifiable aspects of care (Doran and Roland 2010); and that these and related changes risk creating a kind of "tick-box medicine" (McDonald, White, and Marmor 2009).

Quality of care, as measured by compliance with the clinical quality indicators, appears to have improved modestly during the first year in some areas but to have then plateaued, with little or no continued increase after the second year. A number of analysts (e.g., Campbell et al. 2009) argue that the positive early results may largely reflect non-financial quality initiatives begun prior to the introduction of the incentives, or even contemporaneous other investments in complementary resources such as electronic medical record systems. The QOF appears to have narrowed the gap in performance between practices in the most deprived and least deprived regions within the United Kingdom. The evidence that improvements in care processes led to improvements in outcomes is mixed. Improved control of epilepsy and diabetes is associated with fewer emergency admissions for complications, but improved performance with respect to coronary heart disease indicators did not lower hospital admission rates.

Both of the recent reviews (Doran and Roland 2010; Gillam, Siriwardena, and Steel 2012) conclude that the impact of the QOF framework in terms of quality has been modest at best, and they caution policymakers about expanding the program further or introducing similar schemes.

Impact of pay-for-performance on costs

Only a few studies have examined the impact of pay-for-performance on system costs, and even then the assessment of costs was secondary to the assessment of their effectiveness and was often incomplete. A recent systematic review of studies that attempted to assess the efficiency of pay-for-performance, broadening the criteria to include studies that were not formal economic evaluations, yielded nine studies (Emmert et al. 2012). Further, their combination of mixed findings and poor methodological design (e.g., a number of them did not have control groups or include administration costs) led to the conclusion that we do not have sufficient evidence at this time to make any conclusions regarding the efficiency of pay-for-performance. A common observation about bonus-based pay-for-performance is that the cost per unit of change achieved can be high because a large share of bonus payments goes towards providers who already meet the target standards—for example, Rosenthal et al. (2005) found that 75% of all payments went to providers who met the performance targets at baseline—providing them with a windfall gain while doing nothing to improve quality, and raising substantially the cost of inducing change among physicians below the target.[6] At this time, however, the evidence base is simply too limited to draw any strong conclusions about the impact of pay-for-performance on system costs.

Can pay-for-performance drive quality improvement and help bend the cost curve?

In summary, current evidence indicates that pay-for-performance schemes that target incentive payments on particular aspects of care are, at best, of mixed effectiveness for improving quality. They induce increased provision in only some services some of the time, and when they do, the responses are of modest size. We do not have a good understanding of why providers do not respond. Advocates argue that these disappointing results reflect poor design of pay-for-performance schemes, and in particular that the bonus incentives in many plans have often been too small.[7] Larger payments may elicit larger responses—though this does not follow automatically (Ariely et al. 2009)—but they would also make the programs more costly. The evidence of generally poor effectiveness alone should caution policymakers that pay-for-performance cannot be the foundation for efforts to improve quality while controlling costs.[8]

---

6 Although a small number of hospital-based schemes have used penalties, pay-for-performance for physicians almost universally entails the payment of bonuses to those who meet targets rather than the imposition of penalties on those who fail to meet performance targets. The evidence from behavioural economics and psychology in many contexts reveals that people are more sensitive to losses than to gains (Kahneman 2011), suggesting that penalties would be more effective in changing behaviour. Further, a penalty scheme sends the signal that the current payment system presupposes the delivery of high-quality care, providing full payment to those who meet reasonable standards of care and penalizing only those who fall short. Finally, a penalty scheme has obvious fiscal appeal.

7 While the bonuses in many schemes have been relatively small, the UK QOF payments were large. Between 2002–03 and 2005–06, the average income of a GP who was also a senior practice partner increased nearly 60%, or by about £41,600 ($66,600). By 2005–06 more than one-quarter of average GP income stemmed from payments received under the QOF. The bigger problem for QOF may have been that the performance thresholds were set too low.

8 Such is the appeal of such incentives, however, that the Institute of Medicine, after observing that "most studies [of pay-for-performance] have failed to demonstrate any significant effects on processes of care" (2007), nonetheless recommended the introduction of financial incentives for quality. Cited in McDonald et al. 2009.

We would argue, however, that the effectiveness of such incentive schemes is not even their central deficiency. Even if they were effective, such pay-for-performance incentives cannot be the foundation for a serious, comprehensive effort to improve quality. As conventionally conceived, pay-for-performance links bonus payments to achieving specific quality targets, most commonly associated with the delivery of a specific service and less commonly with a specific health outcome. The set of services to which such bonuses can be tied, consequently, is small (it is notable that the same small set of services appears repeatedly across pay-for-performance schemes internationally). A large proportion of what constitutes high-quality care cannot be equated with a specific action or the delivery of a specific service to which a bonus payment can be tied. Again, even if the set of such services were large, such pay-for-performance would require a parallel system of hundreds of individual bonus indicators and associated payments—essentially a confusing, administratively cumbersome parallel fee schedule. Finally, such schemes have questionable long-run properties.

Attempts to revise quality thresholds over time are resisted by the medical profession. In 2009 the UK National Institute for Health and Care Excellence (NICE) recommended increasing maximum levels for the threshold scheme, but GPs rejected this during negotiations with the government over a new contract, so thresholds were kept below most practices' level of performance, removing the financial incentive for further quality improvement. Removing bonuses for services once quality has improved can cause performance to fall below pre-incentive levels. In the United Kingdom, for example, influenza immunization rates for asthmatics fell after the corresponding indicator was removed from the framework in 2006–07. This finding is consistent with Kaiser Permanente's experience with the introduction and removal of performance incentives for retinopathy, cervical screening, and diabetes blood sugar control. While the introduction of financial incentives was associated with modest improvements in rates of provision for each, subsequent removal of the incentives caused the rates of provision of retinopathy and cervical screening to fall below the pre-incentive baseline levels (Lester et al. 2010). Such effects are consistent with a concern that, over time, the use of such incentives can erode internal, intrinsic professional motivation (Bowles and Polania-Reyes 2012; Giacomini et al. 1996).

Funding schemes, cost, and quality

The generally negative findings regarding the effectiveness of targeted incentives embodied in pay-for-performance schemes should not obscure the broader truth that *incentives matter*. Funding schemes create financial incentives, and decades of research on fee-for-service, capitation, and other payment mechanisms confirm that these incentives shape provider behaviour, system costs, and (though it is less well documented) quality (Gosden et al. 2000; Rosen 1989). Providers consistently (though not always) respond in predictable ways to the incentives embodied in these basic payment mechanisms. In those instances when they do not respond as expected, consideration of institutional context or some other factor often reveals why.[9]

Improving quality of care and cost control requires careful attention to the incentives within a funding scheme. The financial incentives in a funding scheme should first and foremost not get in the way of good performance, and ideally they should reinforce complementary non-financial approaches to improve performance. Many policy analyses of the impact of fee-for-service on quality, for example, emphasize more the problem that fee-for-service inhibits providers from practising in a way known to represent better quality than that providers lack incentive to provide high quality. The first order of business, therefore, should be the removal of such incentives so that providers committed to providing high-quality care are not penalized for doing so. With this in mind, it is useful to consider the incentives of basic funding methods and their impacts on costs and quality.

Impact of funding methods on costs and quality

Payment method and health-care costs

A provider's incentive to control costs varies directly with the extent to which the payment received is set prospectively, before services are provided. Prospectiveness gives a provider incentive to produce services in the least costly way and to use services efficiently to produce health among his or her patients, since no additional payment is received for additional activity. In contrast, under retrospective payment the amount of funding received depends on the volume of services provided, creating incentive to provide more services, since additional activity attracts additional payment.

---

9 For example, capitation is often promoted as providing incentive for physicians to care about the health of their enrollees and to therefore provide more preventive care than physicians paid by fee-for-service. Evidence documents that capitation-funded providers do not do so. Why? Because in a world of highly mobile patients, it makes no financial sense for a physician to incur costs today to prevent illness that will occur long in the future, when the patient is unlikely to still be enrolled in his or her practice.

Among the traditional funding methods, prospectiveness increases as we go from fee-for-service to case-based payment, capitation, and fully prospective global budget. Fee-for-service (FFS) is highly retrospective because a provider receives payment for each additional service provided—the basis for the widespread concern that fee-for-service leads to overprovision of services. Case-based funding, which is used most extensively in the hospital sector, is more prospective because the payment for an episode of care is set ahead of time and does not vary with the amount of services provided within an episode of care. The provider, therefore, has incentive to reduce the costs associated with treating a given case (but, among other things, also has incentive to increase the number of cases treated, since each case attracts additional payment). Capitation extends prospectiveness by fixing the amount a provider receives to assume responsibility for the care of an individual during a defined period of time. The provider therefore has incentive to minimize costs associated with all services covered by the capitation payment. Capitation is used most commonly to fund primary care only, but it can be used for a wide range of physician, hospital, and other services. The more services that are included in the capitation rate, the greater the provider's incentive to control costs across service areas and the less the provider's ability to shift costs off the budget. Finally, fully prospective global budgets, which are used most commonly for hospitals, set the total funding at the start of the funding period.

While prospectiveness encourages greater cost-consciousness, it also creates incentive for providers to skimp on care, to selectively attract individuals whose costs can be expected to fall below the prospectively set payment, and to shift costs from the settings paid prospectively to settings paid retrospectively. Case-based funding, for example, encourages a hospital to admit less severely ill patients within a diagnostic category and to discharge patients as soon as possible (perhaps too quickly) to alternative settings. And capitation encourages physicians to enrol lower-risk patients within a risk category, and when used in primary care, it encourages physicians to (over) refer patients to specialists. Blended funding methods that mix prospective and retrospective payment in a single funding scheme, such as a base of capitation with partial fee-for-service, mitigate the unwanted incentives of each, ideally leading to an optimal balance of incentives with respect to service provision and risk selection (Newhouse 1996).

Evidence from a wide variety of settings confirms that, in general, prospective payment leads to greater cost control, while more retrospective payment leads to higher costs. A review of costs under capitation in the context of managed care (Hellinger 1996) found significantly lower spending and utilization under capitation. Similarly, the RAND health insurance experiment found two striking results: that annual spending on patients assigned to a capitation-funded HMO was 28% lower, and that days in the hospital were 41% fewer than patients assigned to a FFS plan with a 0% co-insurance rate (Newhouse 1993). In both cases it would be incorrect to attribute all of the cost differences to capitation per se, since more differed than just payment, but this evidence is consistent with a large body of research. Physicians paid by fee-for-service order substantially more tests, elective procedures, and consultations than physicians paid by capitation; they also hospitalize their patients more (Goodson 2001; Miller 2009). Finally, a randomized controlled trial of funding found that physicians paid by fee-for-service provided more services than physicians paid by salary, and more services than recommended by clinical guidelines (Hickson, Altemeier, and Perrin 1987).

Although the evidence clearly indicates that prospective payment provides greater cost control, if poorly designed, even a prospective payment scheme can be inflationary. Expenditures are the product of quantity and price, and analyses of alternative payment methods generally take prices as given. Unless a funder pays careful attention to prices, any funding scheme can generate cost increases.[10] This can play out in a number of ways. Ontario, for instance, has in recent years been a leader among provinces at integrating capitation payment into blended funding for primary care, but it has also experienced large growth in physician expenditures (Henry et al. 2012). The reasons are many, but one factor has been a strategy to entice physicians into reformed primary-care practices by making such practices financially attractive, through generous payments for activities beyond those reimbursed by traditional fee-for-service. Funders also commonly set capitation rates in a manner that links them to expenditures in the FFS sector, thereby transmitting the inflationary pressures of fee-for-service into the capitation sector.[11] Finally, a prospective global budget can be

---

10 One might ask as well about the relationship between price and quality. Payment rates below a minimum level, such as for the cost of providing a service, likely have a detrimental effect on quality, but there is no evidence or reason to believe that increasing payment rates above certain reasonable levels leads to higher quality.

11 Because capitation payment requires a provider to both deliver services and bear financial risk, the capitation payment rate has to reflect both of these activities through the inclusion of a risk premium. Hence, the per patient capitation rate should exceed the pure expected costs of the services themselves. While this raises the costs slightly, the funder benefits because it has transferred financial risk to the provider, so the funder can establish fully predictable costs for services included in the capitation rate.

inflationary if it is in reality soft, so that each time a funded institution runs a deficit, the funder provides incremental funding—a phenomenon familiar to Canadians.

Other factors beyond price-setting can generate inflationary tendencies, even within largely prospective payment systems. A funding scheme that offers providers a free choice among multiple payment methods (e.g., fee-for-service or capitation) induces non-random selection that can lead to higher costs. If offered the choice between fee-for-service and capitation, physicians with high-cost practice styles will tend to choose fee-for-service, while physicians with low-cost practice styles will tend to choose capitation, leading to overall costs higher than within a pure fee-for-service system. Separate payment streams across sectors create opportunities for cost-shifting and potentially increased costs. As noted, capitation-funded physicians have incentive to lower the threshold for referral to specialists, thereby shifting costs from their capitated budget onto the fee-for-service budget, while hospitals in the United States responded to case-based payment by discharging patients earlier to skilled nursing facilities (reimbursed retrospectively).

The key message from both theoretical and empirical analyses of alternative funding methods is that putting providers at financial risk for their actions (even if only partially) through funding models that include a larger component of prospective payment provides greater cost control, but that policymakers must pay careful attention to system design to avoid unintended adverse consequences for both quality and cost control.

Payment method and quality of care

Analyses of the incentives embedded within alternative funding methods offer few clear predictions regarding their comparative impact on quality of care, and the limited empirical literature investigating the relationship between funding method and quality offers mixed findings. Because traditional payment mechanisms do not explicitly link payment to quality, they have little direct impact on quality; any such impact works indirectly through mediating factors. The payment method, for example, influences not only the volume and mix of services, as we have emphasized, but also how a practice organizes the production of services. Because the capitation payment received does not depend on who delivers a service or even what specific service is provided, capitation provides greater scope for innovative delivery arrangements that integrate both non-physician providers and selected specialist providers (e.g., psychiatrists) to provide greater access to specialized services such as nutrition and mental health care. Because payment does not depend on the delivery of a service for which a fee code exists, capitated practices can more easily use technologies such as phone or email consultations to interact with patients. And because capitated practices have well-defined enrolled practice populations, they are better able to create disease registries or contact identifiable groups of patients. None of these (or related) features guarantee higher quality, but they do support a wider range of quality-focused activities.

The greatest quality-related concern with prospective payment is its possible detrimental effect on quality of care caused by skimping—providing less care than that associated with high-quality treatment. A review of the evidence regarding the impact of capitation and case-based funding on quality concluded that the evidence for such a negative impact is "not compelling" (Christianson et al. 2007). There are several possible reasons. The prospective incentives studied were designed for the most part to reduce utilization of services, and the link between service reduction and quality in the studies is not clear, especially when utilization may have been excessive prior to introduction of different payment arrangements. In addition, the literature reports results for a wide range of quality and outcome measures, making it difficult to detect patterns in the findings. And although the use of multiple indicators of quality and patient outcomes, as was the case in many studies, enables a richer interpretation of findings, when results across indicators conflict, no clear overall picture of the impact of a payment method emerges.

Directions in payment reform to support improved quality and cost control

Public and private insurers around the world are experimenting with novel funding arrangements designed to simultaneously improve quality and control costs. In the United States, passage of the *Patient Protection and Affordable Care Act* has spurred numerous demonstration projects, pilot programs, and other initiatives in innovative payment arrangements (McClellan 2011). The principal aim of much funding reform is to control costs and improve quality by increasing coordination across providers within the health-care system. Many of the commonly cited well-performing health systems—Kaiser Permanente, Group Health of Puget Sound, and Virginia Mason, for example—are unified, fully integrated systems that coordinate care through all parts of their systems. The hope is that better-designed funding methods can induce such coordination even in the absence of full organizational integration. A corollary to this is greater appreciation that effective policy requires integrating the design of the funding scheme and the delivery organization so that they jointly reinforce each other towards achieving key system goals. This contrasts with historical approaches, which viewed the design of funding schemes and of delivery organizations as almost independent activities, whereby different funding methods could in principle be mixed and matched with different delivery models. The push towards full capitation during the 1990s in the context of managed care, which was in part aimed at achieving greater integration, is viewed as a failed experiment (McClellan 2011). Providers and patients (perhaps encouraged by providers) alike rebelled against managed care, with both its "interference" in clinical practice and its restrictions on patient choices. Further, many health plans were unable to manage the full financial risk transferred to them.

The new funding methods therefore emphasize blended approaches that combine traditional funding mechanisms in novel ways, transferring some but not all of the financial risk to providers and linking payment to both cost savings and quality. This basic idea manifests itself in many ways—for example, gain-sharing between physicians and hospitals, or condition-specific capitation (Miller 2009)—but the two most prominent approaches are bundled payment and shared-savings models. We therefore focus on these. Each builds on a different element of the current system. Bundled payment builds on extensive experience internationally with case-based funding for inpatient hospital services; it extends the payment bundle to include services delivered by a number of providers and organizations across a full episode of illness. Shared-savings models build on the predominance of fee-for-service payment among physicians; they impose over a patient population a form of global budget that includes both physician and hospital services. Each model in its own way attempts to force coordination of care across providers by bringing them under a single funding stream.

Bundled payment represents a case- or episode-based method of payment that, as noted, combines payment for care across multiple providers and settings, often with explicit links to quality and performance standards. The intent is to create incentive to reduce costs (in part through better coordination) across the providers and services in the bundle, while the linkage to quality measures is intended to guard against skimping on care.

Many health-care systems internationally have extensive experience with case-based funding methods in the inpatient hospital sector (Busse et al. 2012; Sutherland 2011), and case-based funding has been used to a lesser extent outside hospitals. Bundled payment, however, is far more challenging to develop than traditional case-based funding methods. The payment must cover a more diverse set of services, provided by multiple providers, to a more heterogeneous patient population, and, ideally, all linked to explicit quality standards. US-based public and private payers have the greatest experience creating bundled payments, although in 2010 the Netherlands introduced bundled payment for three conditions—coronary pulmonary heart disease, diabetes, and cardiovascular risk management—as part of a three-year experiment (Mosca, personal communication; Struijs and Baan 2011).

Evidence regarding the effectiveness of bundled payment is limited. An early US Medicare demonstration project in the 1990s found that bundled payment for cardiac bypass surgery reduced expenditures on bypass surgery by 10% and had little or no effect on patient outcomes (Nelson 2012). The Medicare program is currently completing an evaluation of the Bundled Payment Acute Care Episode Demonstration Project, which ran from 2009 to 2013; in 2013 it launched the Bundled Payments for Care Improvement Initiative, which will test four alternative bundled payment arrangements for hospital inpatient and post-acute care services within an episode of illness. In the private sector the most prominent trial of bundled payment is Geisinger's ProvenCare program. Geisinger is a fully integrated health-care plan that first offered bundled payment for bypass surgery and has since expanded it to include selected other surgeries, such as hip replacement and cataract removal. In its first year, Geisinger's bundled payment for cardiac surgery led to reductions in adverse events, including a 10% drop in readmissions; shorter average length of stay; and reduced hospital charges. More recent data presented by Geisinger executives suggest a 44% readmission reduction over 18 months (Mechanic and Altman 2009).

Perhaps the most ambitious effort to develop bundled payment is the US-based PROMETHEUS (Provider Payment Reform for Outcomes, Margins, Evidence, Transparency, Hassle Reduction, Excellence, Understandability, and Sustainability) payment model (de Brantes, Rosenthal, and Painter 2009; Hussey, Ridgely, and Rosenthal 2011). PROMETHEUS is designed to pay for all of the care required to treat a defined clinical episode, based on recommendations derived from clinical guidelines and experts. The payment rates for these bundles are called "evidence-informed case rates." It has thus far defined 21 bundles that include chronic medical conditions such as diabetes, acute medical conditions such as acute myocardial infarction, and procedures such as hip replacement. It distinguishes two sources of variation in the total cost of care: variation caused by random factors not controllable by the provider and variation related to "care production" under the control of the provider. PROMETHEUS transfers financial risk for controllable costs to the provider, while insurers retain responsibility for financial risk due to random factors. The program has required investing in robust quality measures, creating new arrangements among providers for assigning accountability, defining episodes, identifying "potentially avoidable costs," and developing data systems to meet the large demands on data. These challenges have proved formidable. In the case of the PROMETHEUS pilot, as of mid-2011, after three years of work, none of the pilot sites had actually executed a bundled payment.

The shared-savings approach, in contrast, defines an annual global budget for the care of a defined population. If at the end of the year actual costs are less than the budget, the savings can be shared between the funder and the providers. The providers, however, get the savings only if their care meets defined quality standards. At the heart of this approach are accountable care organizations (ACOs), networks of physicians, and other providers that provide a full continuum of care for a group of patients (Berenson 2012). Providers in the ACO are paid by fee-for-service; the global budget is based on the historical costs of providing care to the individuals associated with ACO primary-care providers.[12] In one version of shared savings, providers bear no upside risks: if expenditures come in below the budget, the funder shares the savings with the ACO, but if expenditures exceed the budget, the funder bears the full cost. In a second version, the ACO bears both upside and downside risk: in addition to sharing savings, if the ACO exceeds the budget, it bears responsibility for a share of the excess. There is also considerable variation in how the savings/overruns are shared between the ACO and the funder. Finally, many shared-savings models try to distinguish "legitimate" increases in costs from those argued to represent unnecessary or inappropriate care, which are the responsibility of the ACO. The ACO is liable only for that portion for which it is held responsible. But the basic approach essentially sets up two funding tracks: the first track is traditional payments based on the volume and intensity of services produced (or whatever existing payment system is in place) and the second is based on overall cost reductions with

---

12 Importantly, there is no roster of enrollees. Patients are free to seek care from any provider they wish (inside or outside the ACO). Patients (and their costs and quality indicators) are assigned to an ACO provider based on the patient's patterns of usage. At the end of the year, an ACO provider is assigned those patients who received a plurality of their primary-care services from him or her. Note also that the budget is based purely on historical expenditures for an associated patient, whether those costs are high or low compared to similar patients who seek services from other providers.

improvements in quality. The goal is to provide financial incentives for providers to work together to deliver better care at a lower cost at the person level, in a manner that is not possible through fee-for-service or bundled payments (McClellan et al. 2010).

Currently there is no evidence regarding the effectiveness of these types of ACO-based shared-savings models in either generating cost savings or improving quality. The Center for Medicaid and Medicare Services is currently testing alternative ACO shared-savings models within the Medicare program, and their use by private health plans is growing (Berenson 2012). The most relevant evidence at present is from the Medicare Physician Group Practice demonstration project, which involved nine multi-specialty group practices and one physician–hospital organization; they were eligible to retain a portion of the savings they generated for Medicare, relative to a projected spending target, and they could increase their share of savings depending on how well they performed on a set of 32 quality measures. The results of this demonstration project were mixed. Of the ten large medical groups participating in the demonstration, three received no financial bonus at all. Of those that did earn a bonus, the average annual amount was $5.4 million, ranging from a few hundred thousand dollars to about $16 million. Only two participants reduced health spending enough to receive bonuses in all five years. The bottom line is that the Physician Group Practice demonstration did not meaningfully reduce spending growth ($121 per beneficiary over five years for Medicare), although each of the physician organizations was able to meet performance benchmarks for the majority of the quality measures.

Conclusion

This review leads to the somewhat paradoxical conclusion that although targeted incentives in the form of conventional pay-for-performance are ineffective in improving quality and controlling costs, incentives do matter, so funding reform is an essential part of the overall reforms needed to improve quality in our health-care system while reining in rising costs. We focus on implications of this for research on the use of financial incentives and on approaches to funding reform.

A key research implication is that we need to understand better why providers respond to financial incentives the way they do (or don't). Research on their responses has to go beyond simply documenting the magnitude of any such response to probe provider motivation and how aspects of the context influence provider responses. As highly functioning professionals with considerable autonomy, strong professional norms, and complex responsibilities, it shouldn't be surprising that physician responses to pay-for-performance are more nuanced and variable than are the responses of low-skilled workers, for whom such incentives appear to elicit large and predictable responses.

A key policy implication is that funding reform should be viewed as an enabler rather than the primary driver of change. Achieving a high-quality, low-cost system will require better information, more and better measurement, greater accountability, and stronger integration and coordination. Hence, funding reform must be combined with and support a full range of initiatives—organizational, regulatory, managerial, informational—that mutually reinforce one another in creating a culture of quality improvement and cost-consciousness.

Internationally, efforts to use funding to support improved quality and reduced costs focus on creating funding streams that create accountability across providers, care settings, and sectors. Many of the most serious quality and cost problems arise from fragmentation of care and lack of continuity across parts of the system. This is particularly true for the most challenging complex patients with multiple chronic conditions, an ever-growing share of patients. Prominent features of the emerging funding approaches include blended funding, which puts providers at some but not full financial risk for the costs of the services they provide, and explicit linkages between cost reduction and quality improvement. In some cases these linkages are designed primarily to prevent skimping—in a sense, they are defensive. But in others, quality improvement is a primary objective of the reform. Though much experimentation is underway regarding the design of such payment systems, currently little evidence exists on the effectiveness of these approaches with respect to either cost control or quality improvement. So while there is broad agreement about the general approach and the goals, there is no strongly prescriptive evidence to guide specific aspects of the design of funding systems.

What are the implications for Canada? The two foci of funding reform in Canada have been primary care and hospitals. In primary care, provinces are moving away from full fee-for-service payment towards blended approaches that incorporate a mixture of capitation, partial fee-for-service, programmatic funding, and other minor elements. The shift towards capitation-based blended funding should continue, as it has at least two desirable features: It provides much greater scope for alternative practice organizations that incorporate non-physician providers, novel care process, and a greater focus on the health and needs of a defined, rostered patient population. While this shift will not, in and of itself, necessarily lead to quality improvements (indeed, the evidence suggests that it alone will not), it lays a foundation on which other initiatives can be built. Further, given the dramatic growth in medical school enrolment over the past decade and the pending growth in physician supply, controlling costs for physician services demands a much smaller role for open-ended fee-for-service payment.

Funding reform in the Canadian hospital sector has emphasized a shift from global budgets to case-based payment for inpatient care (under the label "activity-based payment"). The precise goals of this shift are not always well articulated, but they include increased hospital throughput, decreased average length of stay, increased admissions, increased efficiency in the production of hospital-based care, and reduced costs. While the evidence of its impact on volume and length of stay is strong, evidence in terms of productive efficiency is equivocal, and evidence of its impact on costs suggests that the opposite is more likely (for a discussion of these issues, see Sutherland 2011 and Sutherland et al. 2011).[13]

Neither of these reforms will create the kinds of accountability and coordination across providers that characterize trends in funding reform outside of Canada. But they do represent a shift in this direction. Pushed further and combined with complementary non-financial quality initiatives, such funding reform can move us closer to realizing the vision of improved quality within a fiscally sustainable system.

References

Appleby, J., V. Raleigh, F. Frosini, G. Bevan, H. Gao, and T. Lyscom. 2011. *Variations in Health Care: The Good, the Bad and the Inexplicable.* London: King's Fund.

Ariely, D., U. Gneezy, G. Loewenstein, and N. Mazar. 2009. "Large Stakes and Big Mistakes." *Review of Economic Studies* 76, no. 2: 451–69.

Armour, B., M. Pitts, R. Maclean, et al. 2001. "The Effect of Explicit Financial Incentives on Physician Behavior." *Archives of Internal Medicine* 161, no. 10: 1261–66. http://dx.doi.org/10.1001/archinte.161.10.1261.

Berenson, R. 2012. "Health Policy Brief: Next Steps for ACOs." *Health Affairs*, January 31.

Berwick, D., and A. Hackbarth. 2012. "Eliminating Waste in U.S. Health Care." *Journal of the American Medical Association* 307, no. 14: 1513–16.

Bowles, S., and S. Polania-Reyes. 2012. "Economic Incentives and Social Preferences: Substitutes or Complements?" *Journal of Economic Literature* 50, no. 2: 368–425. http://dx.doi.org/10.1257/jel.50.2.368.

Busse, R., A. Geissler, W. Quentin, and M. Wiley. 2012. *Diagnosis-Related Groups in Europe: Moving Towards Transparency, Efficiency and Quality in Hospitals.* Berkshire, UK: Open University Press.

---

13 Even if a funding model creates greater incentive for efficiency in the production of hospital services, the larger source of inefficiency is in the use of hospital services (i.e., in appropriate care), which activity-based funding addresses in only a limited way.

Campbell, S., D. Reeves, E. Kontopantelis, E. Middleton, B. Sibbald, and M. Roland. 2007. "Quality of Primary Care in England with the Introduction of Pay for Performance." *New England Journal of Medicine* 357, no. 2: 181–90. http://dx.doi .org/10.1056/NEJMsr065990.

Campbell, S. M., D. Reeves, E. Kontopantelis, B. Sibbald, and D. M. Roland. 2009. "Effects of Pay for Performance on the Quality of Primary Care in England." *New England Journal of Medicine* 361, no. 4: 368–78. http://dx.doi.org/10.1056/ NEJMsa0807651.

Canadian Medical Association. 2010. *Health Care Transformation in Canada: Change That Works, Care That Lasts.* Ottawa: Canadian Medical Association.

Christianson, J., S. Leatherman, and K. Sutherland. 2007. *Financial Incentives, Health-care Providers and Quality Improvements: A Review of the Evidence.* London: Health Foundation.

de Brantes, F., M. Rosenthal, and M. Painter. 2009. "Building a Bridge from Fragmentation to Accountability: The Prometheus Payment Model." *New England Journal of Medicine* 361, no. 11: 1033–36.

Doran, T., C. Fullwood, H. Gravelle, et al. 2006. "Pay-for-Performance Programs in Family Practices in the United Kingdom." *New England Journal of Medicine* 355, no. 18: 375–84. http://dx.doi.org/10.1056/NEJMsa055505.

Doran, T., and M. Roland. 2010. "Lessons from Major Initiatives to Improve Primary Care in the United Kingdom." *Health Affairs* 29, no. 5: 1023–29. http://dx.doi.org/ 10.1377/hlthaff.2010.0069.

Drummond, D., and D. Burleton. 2010. *Charting a Path to Sustainable Health Care in Ontario: 10 Proposals to Restrain Cost Growth without Compromising Quality of Care.* TD Economics Special Report, May 27. Toronto: TD Bank Financial Group.

Emmert, M., F. Eijkenaar, H. Kemter, A. S. Esslinger, and O. Schoffski. 2012. "Economic Evaluation of Pay-for-Performance in Health Care: A Systematic Review." *European Journal of Health Economics* 13, no. 6: 755–67. http://dx.doi .org/10.1007/s10198-011-0329-8.

Falk, W., M. Mendelsohn, and J. Hjartarson. 2011. *Fiscal Sustainability and the Transformation of Canada's Health Care System.* Toronto: Mowat Centre and School of Public Policy and Governance at the University of Toronto.

Fisher, E. A., J. P. Bynum, and J. S. Skinner. 2009. "Slowing the Growth of Health Care Costs: Lessons from Regional Variation." *New England Journal of Medicine* 360, no. 9: 849–52.

Giacomini, M., J. Hurley, J. Lomas, V. Bhatia, and L. Goldsmith. 1996. "The Many Meanings of Money: A Health Policy Analysis Framework for Understanding Financial Incentives." Working paper no. 96–6. Hamilton, ON: McMaster University Centre for Health Economics and Policy Analysis.

Gillam, S., A. Siriwardena, and N. Steel. 2012. "Pay-for-Performance in the United Kingdom: Impact of the Quality and Outcomes Framework—A Systematic Review." *Annals of Family Medicine* 10, no. 5: 461–68. http://dx.doi.org/10.1370/ afm.1377.

Giuffrida, A., T. Gosden, F. Forland, et al. 2000. "Target Payments in Primary Care: Effects on Professional Practice and Health Care Outcomes." *Cochrane Database of Systematic Reviews* 3. http://dx.doi.org/10.1002/14651858.CD000531.

Goodson, J. D. 2001. "The Future of Capitation: The Physician Role in Managing Change in Practice." *Journal of General Internal Medicine* 16, no. 4: 250–56. http:// dx.doi.org/10.1046/j.1525-1497.2001.016004250.x.

Gosden, T., F. Forland, I. S. Kristiansen, M. Sutton, B. Leese, A. Giuffrida, M. Sergison, and L. Pedersen. 2000. "Capitation, Salary, Fee-for-Service and Mixed Systems of Payment: Effects on the Behaviour of Primary Care Physicians." *Cochrane Database of Systemic Reviews* 3.

Hellinger, F. J. 1996. "The Impact of Financial Incentives on Physician Behavior in Managed Care Plans: A Review of the Evidence." *Medical Care Research and Review* 53, no. 3: 294–314. http://dx.doi.org/10.1177/107755879605300305.

Henry, D., S. Schultz, R. Glazier, R. S. Bhatia, I. Dhalla, and A. Laupacis. 2012. *Payments to Ontario Physicians from Ministry of Health and Long-Term Care Sources 1992/93 to 2009/10*. Toronto: Institute for Clinical Evaluative Sciences.

Hickson, G. B., W. A. Altemeier, and J. M. Perrin. 1987. "Physician Reimbursement by Salary or Fee-for-Service: Effect on Physician Practice Behaviour in a Randomized Prospective Study." *Pediatrics* 80, no. 3: 344–50.

Hurley, J. 2010. *Health Economics*. Toronto: McGraw-Hill Ryerson.

Hurley, J., P. DeCicca, J. Li, and G. Buckley. 2011. "The Response of Ontario Primary Care Physicians to Pay-for-Performance Incentives." Working paper no. 11–2. Hamilton, ON: McMaster University Centre for Health Economics and Policy Analysis.

Hussey, P. S., M. S. Ridgely, and M. Rosenthal. 2011. "Implementing New Payment Models: The PROMETHEUS Bundled Payment Experiment—Slow Start Shows Problems in Implementing New Payment Models." *Health Affairs* 30, no. 11: 2116–24. http://dx.doi.org/10.1377/hlthaff.2011.0784.

Institute of Medicine. 2001. *Crossing the Quality Chasm: A New Health System for the 21st Century*. Washington, DC: National Academy Press.

Institute of Medicine. 2012. *Best Care at Lower Cost: The Path to Continuously Learning Health Care in America*. Washington, DC: National Academies Press.

James, J. 2012. "Health Policy Brief: Pay-for-Performance." *Health Affairs*, October 11.

Jha, A. K., E. J. Orav, and A. Epstein. 2011. "Low-Quality, High-Cost Hospitals, Mainly in South, Care for Sharply Higher Shares of Elderly Black, Hispanic, and Medicaid Patients." *Health Affairs* 30, 10: 1904–11. http://dx.doi.org/10.1377/hlthaff.2011.0027.

Kahneman, D. 2011. *Thinking, Fast and Slow*. New York: Farrar, Strauss and Giroux.

Kantarevic, J., and B. Kralj. 2013. "Link Between Pay for Performance Incentives and Physician Payment Mechanisms: Evidence from the Diabetes Management Incentive in Ontario." *Health Economics* 22, no. 12: 1417–39. http://dx.doi.org/10.1002/hec.2890.

Kiran, T., J. C. Victor, A. Kopp, B. R. Shah, and R. H. Glazier. 2012. "The Relationship between Financial Incentives and Quality of Diabetes Care in Ontario, Canada." *Diabetes Care* 35, no. 5: 1046–55. http://dx.doi.org/10.2337/dc11-1402.

Lester, H., J. Schmittdiel, J. Selby, B. Fireman, S. Campbell, J. Lee, A. Whippy, and P. Madvig. 2010. "The Impact of Removing Financial Incentives from Clinical Quality Indicators: Longitudinal Analysis of Four Kaiser Permanente Indicators." *British Medical Journal* 340 (May 11): c1898–c1902. http://dx.doi.org/10.1136/bmj.c1898.

McClellan, M. 2011. "Reforming Payments to Health Care Providers: The Key to Slowing Health Care Cost Growth while Improving Quality?" *Journal of Economic Perspectives* 25, no. 2: 69–92.

McClellan, M., A. McKethan, J. Lewis, J. Roski, and E. Fisher. 2010. "A National Strategy to Put Accountable Care into Practice." *Health Affairs* 29, no. 5: 982–90. http://dx.doi.org/10.1377/hlthaff.2010.0194.

McDonald, R., J. White, and T. Marmor. 2009. "Paying for Performance in Primary Medical Care: Learning about and Learning from 'Success' and 'Failure' in England and California." *Journal of Health Politics, Policy and Law* 34, no. 5: 747–76. http://dx.doi.org/10.1215/03616878-2009-024.

McGlynn, E. A. 1998. *Assessing the Appropriateness of Care: How Much Is Too Much?* Santa Monica, CA: Rand Corporation.

McGlynn, E., et al. 2003. "The Quality of Health Care Delivered to Adults in the United States." *New England Journal of Medicine* 348, no. 26: 2635–45. http://dx.doi.org/10.1056/NEJMsa022615.

McKethan, A., M. Shepard, S. L. Kocot, N. Brennan, M. Morrison, and N. Nguyen. 2009. *Improving Quality and Value in the U.S. Health Care System.* Washington, DC: Bipartisan Policy Center.

Mechanic, R., and S. Altman. 2009. "Payment Reform Options: Episode Payment Is a Good Place to Start." *Health Affairs* 28, no. 2: w262–w271. http://dx.doi.org/10.1377/hlthaff.28.2.w262.

Miller, H. 2009. "From Volume to Value: Better Ways to Pay for Health Care." *Health Affairs* 28, no. 5: 1418–28. http://dx.doi.org/10.1377/hlthaff.28.5.1418.

Millett, C., J. Gray, S. Saxena, G. Netuveli, and A. Majeed. 2007. "Impact of a Pay-for-Performance Incentive on Support for Smoking Cessation and on Smoking Prevalence among People with Diabetes." *Canadian Medical Association Journal* 176, no. 12: 1705–10. http://dx.doi.org/10.1503/cmaj.061556.

Mullen, K. J., R. G. Frank, and M. B. Rosenthal. 2010. "Can You Get What You Pay For? Pay-for-Performance and the Quality of Healthcare Providers." *Rand Journal of Economics* 41, no. 1: 64–91. http://dx.doi.org/10.1111/j.1756-2171.2009.00090.x.

Nelson, L. 2012. *Lessons from Medicare's Demonstration Projects on Value-Based Payment.* Working Paper 2012–02. Washington, DC: Congressional Budget Office.

Newhouse, J. P. 1996. "Reimbursing Health Plans and Health Providers: Efficiency in Production versus Selection." *Journal of Economic Literature* 34, no. 3: 1236–63.

Newhouse, J., and Health Insurance Experiment Group. 1993. *Free for All? Lessons from the RAND Health Insurance Experiment.* Cambridge, MA: Harvard University Press.

Øvretveit, J. 2009. *Does Improving Quality Save Money? A Review of Evidence of Which Improvements to Quality Reduce Costs to Health Service Providers.* London: Health Foundation.

Rosen, B. 1989. "Professional Reimbursement and Professional Behavior: Emerging Issues and Research Challenges." *Social Science and Medicine* 29, no. 3: 455–62. http://dx.doi.org/10.1016/0277-9536(89)90294-3.

Rosenthal, M., R. Frank, Z. Li, and A. Epstein. 2005. "Early Experience with Pay for Performance: From Concept to Practice." *Journal of the American Medical Association* 294, no. 14: 1788–93. http://dx.doi.org/10.1001/jama.294.14.1788.

Rosenthal, M. B., B. E. Landon, S-L. T. Normand, R. G. Frank, and A. M. Epstein. 2006. "Pay for Performance in Commercial HMOs." *New England Journal of Medicine* 355, no. 18: 1895–1902.

Ryan, A., and J. Blustein. 2011. "The Effect of the MassHealth Hospital Pay-for-Performance Program on Quality." *Health Services Research* 46, no. 3: 712–28. http://dx.doi.org/10.1111/j.1475-6773.2010.01224.x.

Ryan, A., J. Blustein, and L. Casalino. 2012. "Medicare's Flagship Test of Pay-for-Performance Did Not Spur More Rapid Quality Improvement among Low-Performing Hospitals." *Health Affairs* 31, no. 4: 797–805.

Scott, A., P. Sivey, D. Ait-Ouakrim, L. Willenberg, L. Naccarella, J. Furler, and D. Young. 2011. "The Effect of Financial Incentives on the Quality of Health Care Provided by Primary Care Physicians." *Cochrane Database of Systematic Reviews* 9. http://dx.doi.org/10.1002/14651858.CD008451.pub2.

Serumaga, B., D. Ross-Degnan, A. Avery, R. Elliot, S. R. Majumdar, F. Zhang, and S. Soumerai. 2011. "Effect of Pay for Performance on the Management and Outcomes of Hypertension in the United Kingdom: Interrupted Time Series Study." *British Medical Journal* 342 (25 January): d108. http://dx.doi.org/10.1136/bmj.d108.

Steel, N., S. Maisey, A. Clark, R. Fleetcroft, and A. Howe. 2007. "Quality of Clinical Primary Care and Targeted Incentive Payments: An Observational Study." *British Journal of General Practice* 57, no. 359: 449–54.

Struijs, J. N., and C. A. Baan. 2011. "Integrating Care through Bundled Payment: Lessons from the Netherlands." *New England Journal of Medicine* 364, no. 11: 990–91. http://dx.doi.org/10.1056/NEJMp1011849.

Sutherland, J. 2011. *Hospital Payment Policy in Canada: Options for the Future.* Ottawa: Canadian Health Services Research Foundation.

Sutherland, J., M. Barer, R. Evans, and R. T. Crump. 2011. "Will Paying the Piper Change the Tune?" *Health Policy* 6, no. 4: 14–21. http://dx.doi.org/10.12927/hcpol.2011.22391.

Town, R., R. Kane, P. Johnson, and M. Butler. 2005. "Economic Incentives and Physicians' Delivery of Preventive Care." *American Journal of Preventive Medicine* 28, no. 2: 234–40.

Vaghela, P., M. Ashworth, P. Schofield, and M. Gulliford. 2009. "Population Intermediate Outcomes of Diabetes under Pay-for-Performance Incentives in England from 2004 to 2008." *Diabetes Care* 32, no. 3: 427–29. http://dx.doi.org/10.2337/dc08-1999.

Werner, R., J. Kolstad, E. Stuart, and D. Polsky. 2011. "The Effect of Pay-for-Performance in Hospitals: Lessons for Quality Improvement." *Health Affairs* 30, no. 4: 690–98. http://dx.doi.org/10.1377/hlthaff.2010.1277.

Wright, C. J., G. K. Chambers, and Y. Robens-Paradise. 2002. "Evaluation of Indications for and Outcomes of Elective Surgery." *Canadian Medical Association Journal* 167, no. 5: 461–66.

three

Tax Burdens and Aging

JOHN RICHARDS AND COLIN BUSBY

Introduction

Canada is a relatively young country; its over-64 population share is less than in all but two other G8 countries (see Figure 3.1). However, it is aging, and doing so at an accelerating rate. While the over-64 share increased merely three percentage points between 1990 and 2010, based on our projection (details discussed below), it will rise another nine points by 2030 (see Figure 3.2). In addition to rising health expenditures associated with an aging population, a second demographic trend with adverse fiscal implications is a declining population share in the active working age years (18–64). For this cohort, which pays the overwhelming majority of taxes, we project an eight-point decline in population share between 2010 and 2030. The problem has a regional dimension, because provinces are not aging at a uniform rate. However, we do not consider this disparity beyond noting the sizeable range of provincial over-64 population shares. It extends from Alberta, at 11.1%, to Nova Scotia, at 16.6%—the share in the latter is half again as large as that in the former.

The purpose of this chapter is to assess the extent of the financial problem posed by an aging population and, viewed from "the top"—at the level of central government agencies—what might be done about it. In terms of equity and efficiency, the case for a single-payer health insurance system is strong. It enables governments to overcome a variety of market failures associated with health services and potentially to undertake major decisions on a reasonably cost-effective basis. Relevant examples include major infrastructure decisions (e.g., opening and closing of hospitals, adoption of diagnostic technology), major decisions surrounding insurance scope (e.g., whether in Canada we extend pharmaceutical insurance coverage), and major compensation decisions affecting health-care workers (via collective bargaining with unions and professional associations representing groups of health-care workers). A single-payer system also enables central agencies to reorganize health-care structures by, for example, delegating decisions

Figure 3.1 Over-64 share of population, G8 countries and provinces, 2011

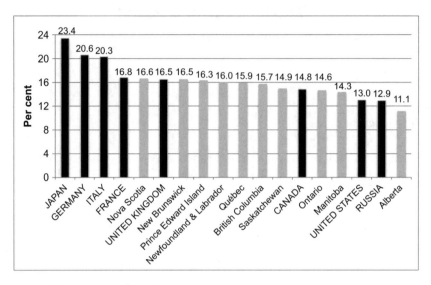

Source: Statistics Canada 2012.

Figure 3.2 Distribution of youth, working-age, and elderly cohorts, selected years, 1990–2050

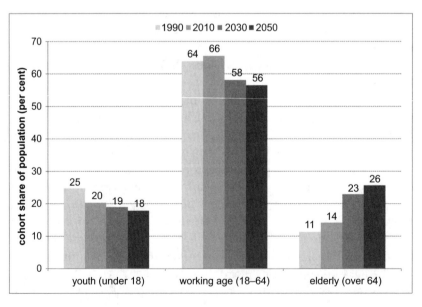

Source: Statistics Canada 2012.

to appointed bodies, such as the trusts operating within the UK National Health Service. But—and this is a major qualification—the success of a single-payer system ultimately rests on the quality of the managerial and political decisions undertaken. There are powerful pressures on government to avoid cost-effective decisions that impose costs on significant interests.

In Canada, discretionary decisions governing public health spending are primarily the prerogative of the 10 provincial governments—subject to the loose constraints imposed by the *Canada Health Act* and potentially by the courts.[1] Ottawa is the equivalent of a small province inasmuch as it finances the health care of residents in the northern territories, on-reserve registered Indians, and to some extent registered Indians living off-reserve. Via equalization and the Canada Health Transfer, Ottawa finances a quarter of provincial health-care spending.[2] Provinces finance the residual via own-source taxation.

The fiscal history of public health-care budgeting over the past four decades can be divided into three periods (see Figure 3.3). The first, from the introduction of provincial single-payer systems until the early 1990s, was characterized by "fiscal drift." During this period neither Ottawa nor the provinces paid sufficient attention to fiscal discipline in the administration of their respective social programs. To the extent that they addressed the emerging fiscal dilemmas, governing elites indulged in bouts of mutual recrimination. The provinces protested that Ottawa erected national standards but unilaterally restricted its cost-sharing as the federal debt worsened. Ottawa replied that the provinces were violating the spirit of cost-sharing agreements by irresponsible expansion of provincial social programs that could be cost-shared with Ottawa.

By the early 1990s, Canada had become one of the most seriously indebted of OECD member countries. There followed a half-decade of "fiscal crisis" during which politicians of both orders brought an end to two decades during which aggregate Canadian public finances had been in continuous deficit. Dramatically they demonstrated an ability to "bend

---

1 *Chaoulli* is an important precedent for potential future court interventions imposing constraints on provincial health insurance systems. See Morley (2006) and Poschmann (2006).

2 Equalization ensures that "have-not" provinces can generate a predefined threshold level of per capita revenue provided they undertake an average taxing effort on accessible tax bases. Equalization is an unconditional transfer, but, since provinces devote nearly half of their program spending to health care, it is fair to conclude that nearly half of equalization transfers are devoted to provincial health budgets. Adding half of equalization payments to the explicit federal transfer targeted for provincial health expenditures implies that Ottawa finances approximately one-quarter of total provincial spending on this file. For the 2012–13 fiscal year, this estimate of federal transfers was approximately $35 billion (Canada 2012, 243).

Figure 3.3 Annual per cent change in public health expenditures, Canada, 1975–1976 to 2009–2010 (nominal dollars)

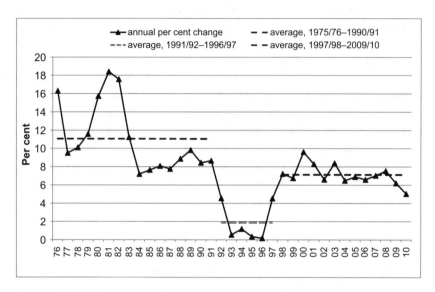

Source: CIHI 2011.

the health-care cost curve." While public opinion was deeply divided over many of the decisions taken, a majority favoured fiscal restraint, including restraint in health-care budgets. Federal and provincial governments that undertook this exercise were rewarded with subsequent re-election.

One provincial government that cut spending growth but nonetheless secured re-election was Québec under the Parti Québécois. In a recent interview, Lucien Bouchard (2012), premier in the second half of the 1990s, responded to the question "What is the political accomplishment of which you are most proud?" His response: "As Premier of Québec, my greatest accomplishment was elimination of the provincial deficit. It was incredibly difficult … we were approaching the abyss, with Québec debt about to be relegated to junk bond status and the province paying ominously high interest rates." Another question: "What was your greatest error?" Bouchard: "I often think of the program to retire nurses."[3]

---

3 The French original is as follows: *L'actualité*: "De quoi êtes-vous le plus fier dans votre carrière politique?" *Bouchard*: "Comme premier ministre du Québec, c'est l'atteinte du déficit zéro. C'était incroyablement difficile … Personne ne semble se rappeler qu'on a mis fin à la décote des finances du Québec, alors qu'on s'approchait de l'abîme, des obligations de pacotille et des taux d'emprunt épouvantables …" *L'actualité*: "Quelle a été votre plus grande erreur?" *Bouchard*: "Je pense souvent aux mises à la retraite des infirmières …"

Bouchard's responses nicely illustrate two points. As a result of underestimation of the importance of fiscal discipline before the 1990s, preserving a single-payer health insurance system in the 1990s required "incredibly difficult" political decisions made in the context of fiscal crisis. Some of those decisions were eminently justifiable in terms of cost-effectiveness. Senior politicians and health administrators had long understood the rationale—in terms of maximizing health benefits from a fixed budget—for closing many hospitals that were too small to provide sophisticated services or were located in communities with declining populations. These hospitals had remained open for decades because of local lobbying. The second point is that, in retrospect, other decisions made in haste proved not to be cost-effective. Québec was not alone in offering inducements to nurses to encourage early retirement and then subsequently regretting the loss of skilled health workers.

Among OECD countries, Canada stands out for the success of its fiscal rehabilitation in the 1990s. However, following the half-decade of fiscal crisis, Canadian provinces entered a third period, characterized by a return to fiscal drift. Perhaps the decline in spending increases in 2010 and 2011 implies a new attention to fiscal discipline, but it is too soon to know.

Others have undertaken similar projection exercises to ours (Drummond 2011; Fortin 2011; Ragan 2012; Robson 2010). What we add to the discussion is the conduct of sensitivity analysis on "service intensity," a variable that should become an important parameter in public discussion of health budgeting. In summary, we disentangle the impact of three variables: two demographic factors that are driving increases in the ratio of public health expenditure to GDP and a third, per capita service intensity:

- *Shift in age distribution of the population.* We have projected the age distribution of the Canadian population under a set of conventional assumptions with respect to fertility, life expectancy, and immigration (both interprovincial and international). (See Table 3.1 for more detail.) Aging of the population distribution generates two effects, both serving to increase public health spending expressed as a share of GDP:
    - *Expenditure effect:* This effect arises from the larger population share of high-needs elderly patients.
    - *GDP effect:* Aging of the population reduces the share of the population in the active labour force cohort (ages 18–64). We assume real GDP per person in this cohort to grow at a constant rate over the projection. The smaller the active labour-force share of the population, the lower the projected per capita GDP.

Table 3.1 Detailed projection assumptions

Service Intensity

Annual real rate of increase, 1998–2009	2.26%
Health service inflation, average annual 1997–2011 change in current government expenditure implicit price index	2.59%

Population Projection

Total fertility rate	1.5 children per woman
Life expectancy progressively rises to reach by 2050 ...	for women 87.5 years for men 82.5 years
Immigration, number and age-sex distribution	unchanged relative to 1996–2011 average

Economic Growth

Annual real increase in productivity per capita among working-age cohort	1.37%

- *Service intensity.* Service intensity in a reference year refers to the average per capita level of spending in that year. Change in service intensity refers to change in per capita spending, holding the population distribution constant. If per capita spending in each age cohort remains constant, then any subsequent change in per capita health spending reflects change in the population distribution, not a change in service intensity. (Prior to the new millennium, population aging was of minor importance; hence changes in per capita spending were due essentially to changes in service intensity.) Service intensity may rise for many reasons: introduction of new medical technologies; increase in compensation for health-care providers at a rate above the assumed inflation rate; increase in ratio of health-care workers per capita; expansion of health insurance scope; and so on. In the projections we allow this parameter to vary.

Changes in the public health expenditure ratio due to shifts in population distribution are largely independent of public policy—although not entirely. If a province successfully attracts immigrants in working-age cohorts, that will increase the working-age share and lower the over-64 share, which has been the Alberta experience. If a province designs programs to attract retirees, this will encourage age-sensitive interprovincial migration—which presumably explains why British Columbia has the highest over-65 population share among provinces west of Québec.

Projection results

Figure 3.4 illustrates projected provincial health spending as a share of GDP under alternative rates of increase in service intensity. In Figure 3.4a the annual per capita change in real service intensity calculated for the years 1998–2009 (2.3%) persists to 2050. Provincial health spending rises from 7.7% of GDP in 2012 to 21.8%. If, hypothetically, the share of all age cohorts remained unchanged relative to the base year 2012 distribution, the increase would be from 7.7% to 13.0%. The first row of 2050 results in Table 3.2 decomposes the aging effect—8.8 percentage points (21.8%–13.0%)—into two components: an increase in average per capita spending and a decline in projected per capita GDP. Projections four decades hence are surrounded by so much uncertainty that any point estimate is of limited interest. Projections two decades hence, to 2030, are somewhat more tangible. Table 3.2 reports both.

It is highly unlikely that provincial governments over the next four decades will extrapolate recent rates of service intensity increase. Halving the rate of increase (to 1.1% annually in real terms) generates a somewhat more

Figure 3.4a Provincial health spending to GDP projection. Scenario 1: real service intensity growth rate = 1998–2009 average intensity growth rate

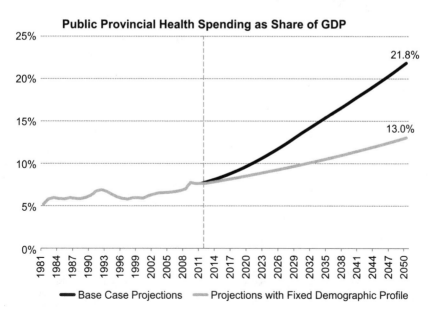

Figure 3.4b Provincial health spending to GDP projection. Scenario 2: real service intensity growth rate = 50 per cent x 1998–2009 average intensity growth rate

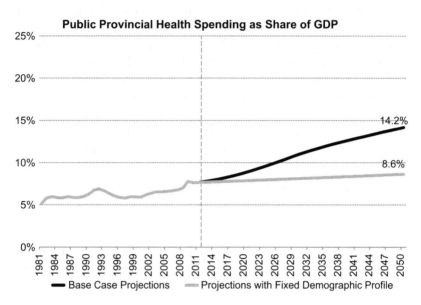

Public Provincial Health Spending as Share of GDP

Figure 3.4c Provincial health spending to GDP projection. Scenario 3: real service intensity growth rate = 25 per cent x 1998–2009 average intensity growth rate

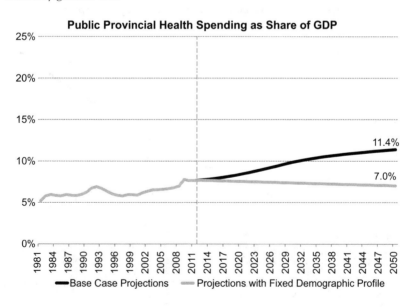

Public Provincial Health Spending as Share of GDP

Table 3.2 Projected effect in 2030 and 2050 of aging on provincial health-care spending as share of GDP, relative to a "no aging" scenario with population distribution anchored on 2012

	Total effect	Increase in Spending/GDP Ratio Due to Higher Average per Capita Spending	Increase in Spending/GDP Ratio Due to Decline in Active Labour Force as Share of Population
Percentage Points of Projected 2030 GDP			
Scenario 1 (real intensity growth rate = 2.3%)	3.7	2.3	1.4
Scenario 2 (real intensity growth rate = 1.1%)	2.9	1.8	1.1
Scenario 3 (real intensity growth rate = 0.6%)	2.5	1.5	1.0
Percentage Points of Projected 2050 GDP			
Scenario 1 (real intensity growth rate = 2.3%)	8.8	6.3	2.5
Scenario 2 (real intensity growth rate = 1.1%)	5.5	3.9	1.6
Scenario 3 (real intensity growth rate = 0.6%)	4.4	3.0	1.3

manageable increase to 14.2% of GDP (Figure 3.4b). If provinces reduce recent rates of intensity increase by three-quarters (to an annual increase of 0.6% in real terms), provincial spending in the absence of population aging would decline (Figure 3.4c). However, even under this scenario of a severe constraint on rate of growth of service intensity, an aging distribution induces rising provincial spending relative to GDP: from 7.7% of 2012 GDP to slightly under 10% of 2030 GDP and slightly over 11% of 2050 GDP.

Not all analysts are persuaded that population aging poses a significant problem for public financing of single-payer health programming in Canada. For example, Morgan and Cunningham (2011), in their analysis of data for British Columbia between 1996 and 2006, find only a negligible impact on per capita health spending due to population aging. However, qualifications need to be made in comparing their analysis with projections such as ours. First, their data cover only a third of total health costs as estimated by the Canadian Institute for Health Information (CIHI).[4] More important, any analysis based on data for the previous two decades, 1990–2010, is a poor guide to fiscal implications for the next two decades, 2010–30. Several parameters in our projection are subject to debate, but two demographic near certainties will generate major fiscal problems for Canadian public finances between 2010 and 2030: (1) the rise in the over-64 share of the population will be much greater than the 1990–2010 rise, and (2) the active labour force cohort will decline as a share of total population, whereas it rose in the previous two decades (refer back to Figure 3.2.)

From a peak in the mid-1990s to 2012, Canada reduced its taxing effort by nearly seven percentage points of GDP. As a result, Canada fell from the middle of the second quartile among OECD member states, ranked by taxing effort, to near the bottom quartile. Over the past two decades, US taxing effort remained within a much narrower range; accordingly, Canada approximately halved the gap in taxing effort between the two countries (see Figure 3.5). Given these trends, there may be a political willingness

Figure 3.5 Government tax plus non-tax revenues as share of GDP, quartiles for OECD member states, Canada, and United States, 1992–2012

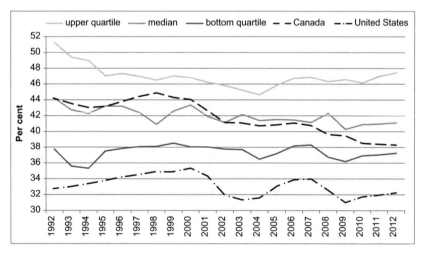

Source: OECD 2012b.

---

4 Morgan and Cunningham include total (public and private) pharmaceutical expenditures and public medical and public hospital expenditures. On a per capita basis, these items comprised approximately one-third of total health costs assessed by CIHI for the year 2006.

among provincial electorates to somewhat accommodate public health-care spending for elderly cohorts by increasing their taxing effort. An increase of three percentage points of GDP would return Canada to the present median among OECD countries.

Is there any significance to the median as constraint on future Canadian taxing efforts? The World Values Survey (2011) affords tentative evidence to the effect that Canadians—and residents of other majority anglophone countries—are among the more adamant of those in OECD member states not wanting government to "do more" than at present. In the survey's 2005–08 round, respondents were asked to indicate the extent of their agreement or disagreement with these propositions: "People should take more responsibility to provide for themselves," and "The government should take more responsibility to ensure that everyone is provided for." Respondents could express complete agreement with the statement (scored at 10), compete agreement with the contrary position (scored at 1), or degrees of (dis)agreement with each by choosing a number between 1 and 10. Among 17 OECD member states, average national scores ranged from 3.5 to 6.4 and were strongly correlated with average taxing effort in those countries over the decade 1999–2008. As might be expected, scores shift towards people taking more responsibility at higher rates of taxing effort and, *mutatis mutandis*, towards the opposite proposition at lower rates of taxing effort. The anglophone countries (United States, Britain, Australia, New Zealand, and Canada) and Switzerland were outliers. For any given taxing effort, residents of these countries were more inclined to conclude that people should be taking more personal responsibility.

Arguably, the direction of causation should be inverted in the medium term; public opinion imposes a floor and a ceiling on the ability of democratically elected governments either to tax and spend or to not tax and not spend. Canada's average response is 6.0 on the 10-point scale. Based on a simple regression across the 17 countries, this response is 1.3 points higher than expected, given its taxing effort—because Canada belongs to the anglophone subset. A three-percentage-point increase in taxing effort would increase Canada's average score in a future survey from its present value to 6.2, placing it close to the apparent ceiling of public tolerance for government's "taking more responsibility."[5]

---

5 The OLS results are as follows: $y = 2.38 + 1.26x_1 + 0.06x_2$, where y is the predicted national score, x_1 takes the value 1 for anglophone countries (United States, Britain, Australia, New Zealand, Canada) and 0 elsewhere; and x_2 is average revenue/GDP over the decade 1999–2008. The adjusted R^2 is 0.44; both regressors are significant at 0.025. See also Richards (2011).

Limitations of the projection

A first limitation of the projection is the assumption of a uniform annual increase in service intensity across all age cohorts over the four decades. Such an assumption serves to highlight the interaction of population aging and rising service intensity but ignores the potential to spend more among some age cohorts with the intent of reducing spending at other ages.

A second limitation is to ignore potential cost-effective policy initiatives that reallocate health-care funding between public and private sources. For example, Ottawa may at some point take responsibility for a national pharmaceutical insurance program—a component of health costs heavily skewed towards over-64 cohorts. To do so need not affect provincial spending but would modestly increase total public health spending. The core of present provincial health spending is for medical and hospital services. Since the introduction of universal single-payer programs in the 1960s, pharmaceuticals have become a far more significant dimension of care. The provinces have responded with ad hoc catastrophic drug insurance programs that are both inequitable and inefficient relative to provincial management of core medical and hospital programs. Many, including Morgan and colleagues (see Chapter 5), have argued the case for a national formulary-based program that, subject to modest user fees, insures all prescribed drugs deemed medically necessary.[6] A national program creates the potential, with a modest increase in public spending, to reduce total (public plus private) spending on pharmaceuticals. Admittedly, the United Kingdom is among the lowest of OECD member states in terms of drug use, and Canada may not want or be able to replicate the UK experience. Were Canada to realize UK pharmaceutical spending/GDP ratios, we would lower total pharmaceutical expenditures by 0.8 percentage points of 2012 GDP—a 0.9 point decline in private spending combined with a 0.1 point increase in public spending.[7] (See Table 3.3)

A third limitation is that we make no evaluation of the implications for quality and equity of health services arising from tighter control on service intensity increases. Probably the result will be some shift to private

---

6 For example, Steve Morgan et al. (2013) have recently written a monograph surveying policy options with respect to pharmacare. In 2004 the provinces proposed that Ottawa assume responsibility for such a program. Ottawa rejected the proposal and instead offered an essentially unconditional extension of the Canada Health Transfer. Greg Marchildon (2006) criticized Ottawa for rejecting the provincial proposal.

7 These are small fractions of GDP. Realize, however, that 1% of the 2012 Canadian GDP is $18 billion, approximately equal to annual provincial health expenditures in British Columbia.

Table 3.3 Canada, United Kingdom, and OECD, selected comparative health statistics, 2009

	Canada	United Kingdom	OECD Average
Population Health			
Population share age 65 and older (% of total, 2011)	14.8	16.5	
Life expectancy at birth (years)	80.7	80.4	79.5
Life expectancy among men age 65 (years)	18.1	18.1	17.2
Life expectancy among women age 65 (years)	21.3	20.8	20.5
Potential years of life lost among men under age 70 (years/100,000)	4,168	3,988	4,689
Potential years of life lost among women under age 70 (years/100,000)	2,554	2,479	2,419
Infant mortality rate (deaths/1,000 live births)	5.1	4.6	4.4
Smoking (% of population age 15 and older who smoke daily)	16.2	21.5	22.1
Health Personnel			
Doctors (doctors/1,000)	2.4	2.7	3.1
Nurses (nurses/1,000)	9.4	9.7	8.4
Health Financing			
Remuneration relative to average national wage: (a) salaried, (b) self-employed			
General practitioners	(b) 3.1	(a) 1.9, (b) 3.6	
Specialist doctors	(b) 4.7	(a) 2.6	
Nurses	(a) 1.2	(a) 1.1	
Total health expenditure (% of GDP)	11.4	9.8	9.6
Public share of total (% of total)	71	84	72
Out-of-pocket (private, non-insured; % of total)	15	10	
Private insurance and other (% of total)	14	6	
Total pharmaceutical spending (% of GDP)	1.81	1.02	1.50
Public (% of GDP)	.76	.86	.90
Private (% of GDP)	1.06	.16	.60

Note: Statistics refer to 2009 except as noted.
Sources: OECD 2012a; Statistics Canada 2012.

health care.[8] However, there is no obvious optimum public–private share. At 71%, the current Canadian public share of spending is very close to the OECD average. More crucial than preserving this ratio is the quality of public-sector management of the health sector, maintenance of high ethical standards among care providers, and attention to incentives within the public health sector that offset adverse selection and moral hazard—among both patients and care providers.

Policy analysis and conclusion

Our first recommendation is modest: that political and administrative elites discuss aggregate public health spending in terms of an appropriate cap to place on growth of service intensity (as we have defined it) and be prepared to define budgets in terms of such a cap. There is no unambiguously optimal value for health-care spending as share of GDP. Debating the allocation of public funds among competing uses lies at the heart of politics in any high-income society, in which a universal health insurance system is inevitably the most important single spending envelope.

Robson (2010) has suggested that provinces raise taxing efforts now and set aside a surplus to be drawn down during future years of maximum health-care cost.[9] He draws a parallel between the implications of demography for future health-care spending and the Canada/Québec Pension Plan. Given prevailing payroll tax rates in the early 1990s, trends in productivity increases, and demographic projections, the C/QPP fund would have been exhausted sometime in the present decade (the 2010s). Without radical restructuring, the C/QPP would have become essentially a second, pay-as-you-go equivalent of Old Age Security, with only a tenuous link to individual contributions. To reduce the absolute payroll tax increase required to fund future entitlements, a mid-1990s reform pre-emptively doubled the payroll tax and thereby

---

8 Since Canada adopted a single-payer form of health insurance, the one sustained episode of restraint was the mid-1990s crisis. Between 1975–76 and 1990–91, the average public and private rates of increase in health expenditures were similar (11.7% private, 11.1% public); between 1997–98 and 2009–10 they were also similar (7.0% private, 7.1% public). Between 1991–92 and 1996–97 the average rate of public health-care spending fell to 1.9%. Allowing for population increase and inflation, per capita service intensity declined in the mid 1990s. The decline was partially offset by private spending. The rate of growth of the latter also declined in this interval, to an average 5.7% annual increase. Since 1997 the public share has been stable at approximately 70%, close to the OECD average (CIHI 2012, 12).

9 Robson's projection assumed a fixed 2% annual increase in per capita service intensity.

replenished the C/QPP fund available for future decades of maximum payout. Were provinces to pre-fund health care on an equivalent basis to the C/QPP, it would require an increase in taxing effort of four percentage points of GDP.

Canadian governments may agree to increase taxing effort somewhat over this decade—not that they would or should devote all incremental revenue to health-care spending. And they may agree to discuss health budgets in terms of capping the rate of increase of service intensity. It is highly unlikely that they will follow the C/QPP precedent.

If we are looking for "good but unlikely to be adopted anytime soon" ideas to manage health-care costs, a more interesting strategy is to examine what some other countries with universal health insurance are doing. As Blomqvist and Busby (2012a, 2012b) insist in two recent policy monographs, in virtually all dimensions Canada has better outcomes than does the United States—but that is a very low benchmark. More meaningful, they suggest, is to compare Canada with certain other countries such as the United Kingdom. Although it is not the only health system worthy of serving as a benchmark, here we consider relevant features of the UK health system. Like Canada, the United Kingdom has evolved a single-payer system whereby the state finances the great majority of health services via general revenue and constrains the ability of care providers to work in both the private and public sectors simultaneously. Inasmuch as the United Kingdom enables private purchase of core medical services—provided patients pay the full cost of such care, over and above their general tax liability—the constraint on patients is lower than in Canada.[10]

The United Kingdom achieves broadly similar population health outcomes to Canada's while spending considerably less as a share of GDP (11.4% in Canada, 9.8% in the UK in 2011).[11] In terms of life expectancy at birth and containing tobacco addiction, Canada performs slightly better than the United Kingdom; in terms of infant mortality and potential years of life lost among those under age 70, Canada fares slightly worse. The United Kingdom and Canada maintain similar ratios

---

10 The basic alternative to a single-payer system is "managed competition," which requires all residents to buy health insurance from one among multiple insurance plans that offer patients at least the regulated minimum coverage and satisfy other regulations intended to limit adverse selection and moral hazard. In addition to the United Kingdom, Blomqvist and Busby draw lessons for Canada from the Netherlands, a country whose insurance system is based on "managed competition."

11 The difference, 1.6% of GDP, is nearly twice British Columbia's 2012–13 health ministry budget.

of core professional personnel (doctors and nurses) relative to population (see Table 3.3).

The Canadian system is decentralized inasmuch as each province enjoys great autonomy in health program design. At its birth in 1948, the UK National Health Service (NHS) was run out of Whitehall as a hierarchical organization not unlike the army. Over the past quarter-century, UK governments both Labour and Conservative have decentralized the NHS via creation of multiple "trusts," defined in terms of region and health function.[12] These are led by boards with broad discretion over major financial decisions pertaining to hospitals and remuneration of doctors and other NHS employees. These institutional reforms have been far more extensive than any undertaken by their Canadian counterparts.

Several institutional features of the NHS should be of interest to Canadian governments contemplating cost-effective health policy innovations:

- *Capitation as dominant means of compensating primary-care providers:*
  Whereas most Canadian general practitioners (GPs) receive
  their income via fee-for-service, their UK equivalents receive a
  negotiated amount per patient on the GP's roster, the amount
  varying by age, gender, and other patient characteristics. Neither
  mode of compensation should be evaluated as a means to reduce
  GP incomes, and both generate certain perverse incentives
  among care providers.[13] An underappreciated virtue of capitation
  is the relative ease of introducing new health professions into
  the delivery of primary health care. As Blomqvist and Busby
  (2012b, 5) note, "the bulk of activity in the health system has
  shifted away from acute care to the monitoring and treatment of
  chronic illnesses." Clinical pharmacists and nurse practitioners
  can play a valuable role in cost-effective delivery of primary care.
  In the Canadian context, their employment in this context has
  been limited, in large part because of the difficulty of designing a

---

12 The UK government is presently undertaking further restructuring of the NHS. Primary-care trusts will give way to somewhat differently configured "clinical commissioning groups." Maynard (see Chapter 17) may well be right in his skepticism as to the benefits promised by this latest reconfiguration of the NHS.

13 Note that among self-employed GPs, those in the United Kingdom realize an average income slightly higher (relative to the national average wage) than do their Canadian counterparts—3.6 versus 3.1 (see Table 3.3).

suitable mechanism for their remuneration within a fee-for-service environment.

- *Salary as primary means of compensating specialist doctors:* In the United Kingdom most specialists are employees of hospitals, their salaries negotiated by the relevant hospital trust. Hospital managers are obliged to include the cost of specialists among the costs of other necessary inputs in the course of budgeting. The result has been UK specialist incomes similar to (relative to the respective average national wage) those of most other OECD countries. Not so in Canada, however, where nearly all specialists are self-employed, as are GPs. As illustrated in Table 3.3, Canadian specialists have negotiated relative incomes much higher than those of salaried UK specialists, in part because the cost of specialists is not internal to hospital budgeting.[14]

- *Integration of pharmaceuticals as a component of universal health insurance and integration of pharmaceutical with hospital and medical programming:* In terms of annual expenditures, the three major envelopes of Canadian health-care spending are hospitals, pharmaceuticals, and physician compensation—in that order. Steve Morgan and colleagues make a powerful case in this volume and elsewhere (Morgan et al. 2013), to the effect that cost control in this envelope (of both public and private spending) is impossible without "pharmacare," by which they mean that "financing for pharmaceuticals would be integrated with other health care financing such that health system managers and health care providers have the incentive to engage in prudent expenditure management, including evidence-based formulary restrictions, tough-but-fair price negotiations, and financial risk-sharing with the health professionals who make critical prescribing decisions" (Chapter 5). Were Canada able to repeat the NHS experience, it would entail a modest increase in public health-care spending but a marked reduction in total (public plus private) spending (see Table 3.3). As is the case for most categories of health-care spending, over-64 cohorts consume disproportionately more pharmaceuticals than younger cohorts. Hence pharmacare can be considered a pre-emptive initiative to contain the health-care costs of aging.

---

14 Relative to average national wage, Canadian specialist incomes are the third highest among 23 OECD member countries with available data (OECD 2012a, 67).

- *Extensive use of internal markets:* Internal markets require that public agencies (until 2013 described as "trusts" in the UK context) purchase services from other public agencies. Not without controversy, UK governments have made extensive use of this principle in designing NHS reforms. For example, primary-care trusts pay a fraction of deemed hospital costs to the relevant hospital trust for patients hospitalized by the GPs working under the trust. The intent there is to provide an incentive to constrain GP resort to hospitalization.

In conclusion, there is no guarantee that Canadians will elect governments, in either Ottawa or the provinces, willing to experiment with institutional reform of public health administration on a scale that has taken place in the United Kingdom. However, if we do not address the fiscal implications of an aging population in an orderly manner, the result will probably be a replay, at some point over the next decade, of disorderly imposition of spending caps analogous to those imposed in the 1990s.

References

Blomqvist, A., and C. Busby. 2012a. "Better Value for Money in Healthcare: European Lessons for Canada." Commentary no. 339. Toronto: C. D. Howe Institute. http://dx.doi.org/10.2139/ssrn.2021330.

———. 2012b. "How to Pay Family Doctors: Why 'Pay per Patient' Is Better Than Fee for Service." Commentary no. 365. Toronto: C. D. Howe Institute.

Bouchard, L. 2012. "Confidences d'un ex: entrevue avec Lucien Bouchard." *L'actualité*, 1 October, 44–46.

Canada. 2012. *Economic Action Plan*. Ottawa: Ministry of Finance.

CIHI (Canadian Institute for Health Information). 2012. National Health Expenditure Trends: 1975–2011. Ottawa: CIHI.

Drummond, D. 2011. "Therapy or Surgery? A Prescription for Canada's Health System." Benefactor's lecture. Toronto: C. D. Howe Institute.

Fortin, P. 2011. "Staying the Course: Quebec's Fiscal Balance Challenge." Commentary no. 325. Toronto: C. D. Howe Institute. http://dx.doi.org/10.2139/ssrn.1808146.

Marchildon, G. 2006. "Federal Pharmacare: Prescription for an Ailing Federation?" *Inroads* 18: 94–108.

Morgan, S., and C. Cunningham. 2011. "Population Aging and the Determinants of Healthcare Expenditures: The Case of Hospital, Medical and Pharmaceutical Care in British Columbia, 1996 to 2006." *Healthcare Policy* 7, no. 1: 67–79.

Morgan, S., J. Daw, and M. Law. 2013. "Rethinking Pharmacare in Canada." Commentary no. 384. Toronto: C. D. Howe Institute.

Morley, G. 2006. "Judges: Canada's New Aristocracy—An Interview with Allan Blakeney." *Inroads* 18: 30–47.

OECD (Organisation for Economic Co-operation and Development). 2012a. *Health at a Glance, 2011*. Paris: OECD.

———. 2012b. "Economic Outlook." Accessed 10 October 2012. http://www.oecd .org/eco/outlook/economicoutlookannextables.htm

Poschmann, F. 2006. "The Courts Are Doing Their Job: A Discussion with Patrick Monahan." *Inroads* 18: 48–55.

Ragan, C. 2012. *Canada's Looming Fiscal Squeeze*. Rev. ed. Ottawa: Macdonald-Laurier Institute.

Richards, J. 2011. "Idle Speculation: Prefunding the Boomers' 'Frail Elderly' Care and Legitimizing a Carbon Tax." In *New Directions for Intelligent Government in Canada: Papers in Honour of Ian Stewart*, edited by F. Gorbet and A. Sharpe, 227–48. Ottawa: Centre for the Study of Living Standards.

Robson, W. 2010. "The Glacier Grinds Closer: How Demographics Will Change Canada's Fiscal Landscape." E-brief 106. Toronto: C. D. Howe Institute.

Statistics Canada. 2012. *The Canadian Population in 2011: Age and Sex*. Cat. no. 98–311–X2011001. Ottawa: Statistics Canada.

World Values Survey. 2011. World Values Survey Wave 5 (2005–2008) Official Aggregate v. 20140429. www.worldvaluessurvey.org.

PART II
Pan-Canadian Cost Drivers and Political Considerations

four

Common Provincial Determinants and Cost Drivers

LIVIO DI MATTEO AND J. C. HERB EMERY

Introduction

The sustainability of public financing for health-care issues will define the next quarter-century of Canadian public policy, given that health spending is rising faster than economic growth (Di Matteo 2010; Marchildon, McIntosh, and Forest 2004). The sustainability issue has been addressed in several recent studies (Dodge and Dion 2011; TD Bank Financial Group 2010), but with some exceptions they have focused mainly on aggregate health spending.[1] Rising government expenditures for health care in Canada may be sustainable, but governments and taxpayers are particularly sensitive to the fact that health care is an expensive service. Whether it is for reasons of fiscal sustainability or simply for reducing the tax burden, governments in Canada are interested in restraining the growth of health-care expenditures, especially given that greater spending is not always associated with improved health outcomes. This study contributes to the analysis of sustainability by examining the determinants and drivers of provincial government health spending. Some recent trends in government health expenditure are reviewed to establish context for the issue. Then estimates of the determinants of health expenditure by category, using regression analysis, are constructed to provide additional insight on expenditure drivers. Finally, a policy analysis is provided of what it might take to bend the cost curve.

The past decade has seen particularly rapid rates of increase in provincial government health expenditures, but health expenditure growth is a long-term issue. Moreover, when provincial government health spending from 1975 to 2009 is examined by expenditure category, the evidence reveals that some categories have risen much faster than others. Drugs, capital spending and other health expenditures such as home care have been growing at faster annual rates than the core of Canadian "medicare"

---

1 One major exception is a recent report by the Canadian Health Services Research Foundation (Constant et al. 2011) that notes that the fastest-growing areas of health spending are capital, drugs, and public health. See also CIHI 2011.

and the areas subject to single-payer funding discipline, which in turn have not been growing much faster than many measures of the resource base. Sustainability and bending the cost curve are nonetheless still an issue given the large share of government health expenditure occupied by hospital and physician spending and the greater growth in new categories and areas of health spending.

Regression analysis reveals some diversity across categories in terms of the key determinants and drivers of real per capita provincial government spending by category. For example, when it comes to an aging population, increases in physician spending are driven especially by the proportion of population aged 70 to 74 and 85 plus. Hospital spending, on the other hand, declines with respect to the population share aged 75 to 79 and 85 years plus. Ultimately, many of these determinants and cost drivers are linked to the price of health-care services. Bending the cost curve will require strategies to shift to lower cost inputs and, ultimately, determine ways for greater productivity of medical service providers to result in lower prices of health-care services.

Trends and context in provincial government health expenditure

Real per capita provincial government health spending over the period 1975 to 2009 shows rising expenditures, with spending acceleration after 1996; this has generated some alarming predictions, especially when simple growth rates are extrapolated into the future. For example, a report by the TD Bank Financial Group (2010) argued that in Ontario, if public-sector health expenditure continues to grow at 6.5% per year, then health will consume about 80% of the provincial government budget by 2030, compared to 46% today. Another report, for Alberta (Di Matteo and Di Matteo 2009), argued that by 2030 Alberta government health expenditures could account for as little as 32% and as much as 87% of government revenues.

In 1975, average real per capita provincial government health expenditure (in 1997 dollars) was $1,149; it reached $2,718 by 2009, with some substantial differences across provinces both in real per capita amount of spending and expenditure growth rates. Growth rates are highest in the Atlantic provinces of Newfoundland and Labrador, New Brunswick, and Nova Scotia, at over 3%. They are lowest in Ontario, British Columbia, and Québec.

Examining the growth in total provincial government health spending does not take into account differences in the composition of spending over time, as expenditure categories have grown at different rates. Health expenditure data are available by category for the period since 1975; when

Figure 4.1 Median average annual growth rates for real per capita provincial revenue sources and provincial government health expenditure categories, 1976–2009

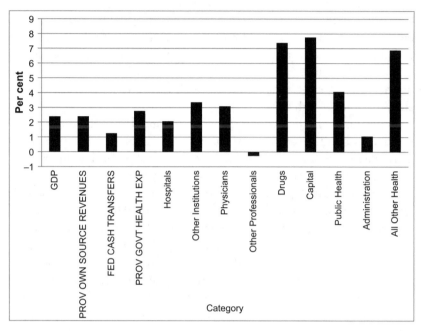

Source: CIHI 2011.

the median of average annual average growth rates across the provinces is calculated for these categories and compared to growth rates in the resource indicators, it shows that some categories of provincial government health spending are keeping pace with resource and revenue growth while others are not (see Figure 4.1).[2]

---

2 Data on provincial government health expenditures come from the Canadian Institute for Health Information, and are provided in nine separate expenditure categories. *Hospitals* expenditures are for public acute- and chronic-care hospitals as well as those specializing in such areas as pediatrics and neurology. *Other Institutions* refers to residential care facilities such as homes for the aged, homes for the physically and mentally handicapped, and facilities to treat drug and alcohol problems. *Physicians* expenditures cover the professional health services provided by physicians; however, physicians on the payrolls of hospitals or public agencies are excluded and instead included in other relevant categories. *Other Professionals* includes dentists, chiropractors, optometrists, private-duty nurses, and physiotherapists. The *Drugs* category includes expenditures on provincial government prescription drug plans. *Capital* expenditures are expenditures on construction, machinery, and equipment for hospitals and

For the period 1975 to 2009, real per capita GDP across Canada's provinces grew at a median annual rate of 2.4%, real per capita provincial government total revenues at 1.7% (with real per capita own-source revenues at a median of 2.4% and federal cash transfers at 1.3%), and real per capita health spending at 2.8%—growth rates in health spending have generally outstripped resource growth.[3] However, the median growth rate for real per capita provincial government hospital spending across the provinces was 2.1%, for Other Institutions it was 3.4%, and for Physicians 3.1%. Drugs, on the other hand, grew at 7.4%, Public Health at 4.1%, Capital at 7.8%, and All Other Health at 6.9%.

While hospital and physician spending appear to be slower growing compared to these other categories, suggesting some success at containing costs and sustaining services, it is also the case that some of this lower growth in spending may be the product of rationing quantity.[4] Concerns about access to family physicians and specialists, emergency department wait times, and wait lists for medical procedures have all arisen since the 1990s. In other words, if the level of access to services had been maintained over time, then it is likely we could have seen much higher spending growth for hospitals and doctors.

What is also intriguing about these median growth rates is the comparison to private-sector spending median growth rates over the same time period (see Figure 4.2). Over the 1975–2009 period, the private share of health spending in Canada grew from 24% to 29%. While median annual average real per capita provincial government health spending grew at 2.8%, private-sector

---

other health institutions. *Public Health* expenditures generally cover measures to prevent the spread of communicable diseases, as well as food, drug, and workplace safety. *Administration* expenditures refers to spending related to the cost of providing health insurance programs as well as the costs of infrastructure to operate health departments; however, the administrative cost of running hospital and drug programs is included under the relevant category of service. Finally, the *All Other Health* expenditure category represents remaining spending on home care, medical transportation, hearing aids, and eyeglasses.

3 These were calculated as the median of the annual averages of the average of annual growth rates for each province for the period 1976–2009. Health spending growth has been characterized by phases, with spending increases since the mid 1990s being particularly pronounced. It should be noted that for the period 1996 to 2009, real per capita GDP across Canada's provinces grew at a median annual rate of 2.5%, provincial government total revenues at 2.6% (with own-source revenues at a median of 2.9% and federal cash transfers at 2.8%), and health spending at 3.7%. All series were deflated with the CIHI Government Expenditure Price Index.

4 It should also be noted that there has been a shift in the provision of services from hospitals, such that there has been a change in the bundle of services accounted for in the hospital category over time. So it may be that 1975 hospital services were less sustainable than the 2009 bundle of services. At the same time, the reduced hospital services have increased spending on "other institutions," in which case it is their combined growth rate that should actually matter.

Figure 4.2 Comparing median average annual per capita growth rates for provincial government and private health expenditures, 1976–2009

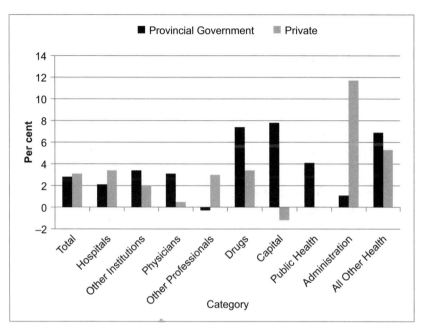

Source: CIHI 2011.

health spending grew at 3.1%. This suggests that rising costs are a feature of both public and private health spending in Canada, implying that the two sectors likely share some common determinants. It is also possible that public spending may be a determinant of or a complement to private spending, and that public-sector expenditure restraint increases private spending as people turn to it for needs unmet by policymaker design. Patients are shifted to non-hospital care settings and non-physician service providers that are part of the mixed public/private–payment part (a.k.a. "private health care") of the health-care system. Across the expenditure categories, private-sector growth rates were higher than those of provincial governments for Hospitals,[5] Other Professionals, and Administration. The gap was particularly notable in the

---

5 Public and private hospitals sell different products. In this case we are likely seeing a response to demand for "enhanced" services—extra fees for privacy, flowers in the room, more attention from attendants. This came out in the debate over Alberta's Bill 11. Since the CHA only requires full public payment for "basic ward care," the enhancements for the "hotel" part of hospital stays can be extra charges. The suggestions were made that private hospitals would be selling a lot of these. See Currie, Donaldson, and Lu 2003.

Figure 4.3 Contribution to median growth rate of provincial government health spending by expenditure category, 1976–2009

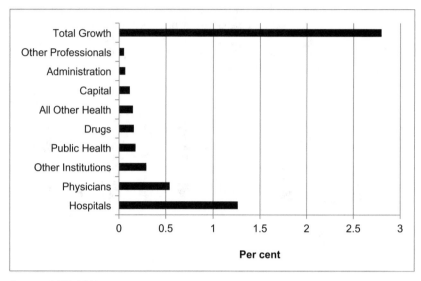

Source: CIHI 2011.

Administration category, where the growth rate was 11.7% for the private sector and 1.1% for provincial governments. Provincial government growth rates were higher than in the private sector for the categories of Other Institutions, Drugs, Capital, and All Other Health.

Growth rate differences across categories have implications for the overall growth in provincial government health spending but must be considered alongside the relative expenditure share of these categories. For example, over the period 1975 to 2009, the share of hospitals in total provincial government health spending—the largest single expenditure category—declined from 55% to 37%, with an average over the entire period of 45%. The next largest category, Physicians, remained relatively stable over the entire period, at an average share of 19%. Together, hospitals and physicians still account for approximately 56% of total provincial government health spending, making them key to any attempts at bending the cost curve, even if their growth rates are below categories such as Drugs and All Other Health.[6] These are core services, making up the universal basket of medically necessary hospital and medical care services. Indeed, Figure 4.3 takes the expenditure shares of the various categories and applies

---

6 As well, these are the only two categories covered by the *Canada Health Act*.

Figure 4.4 Real per capita provincial government hospital expenditure, 1975–2009 (1997 dollars)

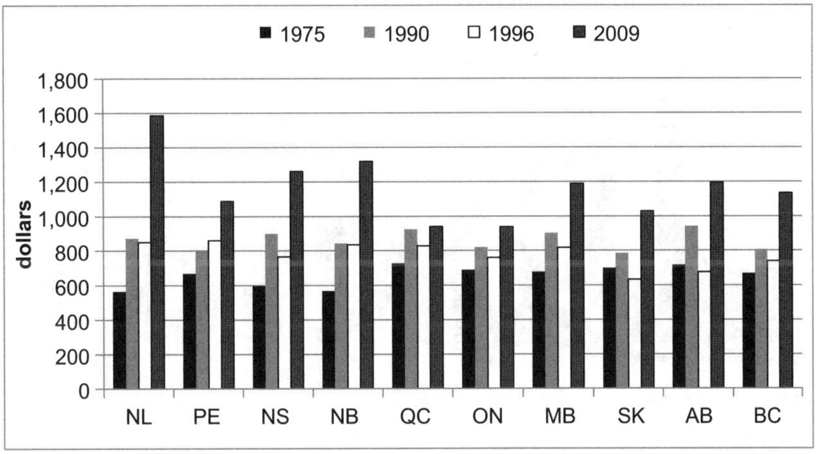

Sources: CIHI 2011; Statistics Canada.

them to the median growth rate for total provincial government health spending to provide an estimate of the contribution of each category to growth. Over the period 1975–2009, hospitals on average contributed 1.17 out of the 2.8 percentage points of growth in total provincial government health spending, with physicians next at 0.5 percentage points.

There are also provincial differences when it comes to expenditure categories. For example, real per capita provincial government hospital expenditures have also gone through three phases—a rising phase from 1975 to the early 1990s, a retrenchment phase from the early to mid 1990s, and a rapid increase phase since the mid-1990s, as Figure 4.4 depicts quite clearly. There are differences in real per capita spending across the provinces and growing divergence in per capita hospital spending after the mid 1990s. Moreover, when you rank the provinces according to growth in spending over the entire period, growth in hospital spending has been the greatest in Newfoundland and Labrador, New Brunswick, and Nova Scotia and least in Saskatchewan, Ontario, and Québec (see Figures 4.5a and 4.5b). In nominal terms, highest-ranked Newfoundland and Labrador now spends approximately $1,000 per capita more on hospitals than lowest-ranked Québec.

Similar patterns are also present across other health expenditure categories, with divergences in levels of per capita spending across the provinces as well as growth rates over time. Newfoundland and Labrador,

Figure 4.5a Ranked per cent growth in real per capita provincial government hospital expenditure, 1975–2009

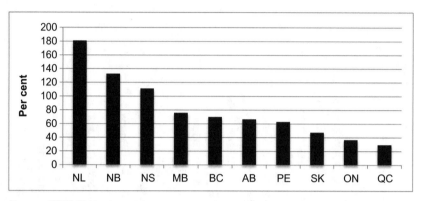

Source: CIHI 2011.

Figure 4.5b Ranked per cent growth in real per capita provincial government hospital expenditure, 2000–2009

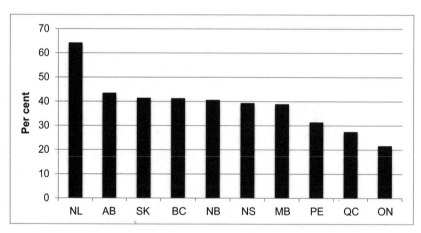

Source: CIHI 2011.

Prince Edward Island, and New Brunswick have seen the largest increases in real per capita physician spending, while Alberta, Québec, and British Columbia have seen the lowest. In the case of drugs, the greatest increases in drug spending have been in Ontario, Prince Edward Island, and Newfoundland and Labrador, while the lowest increases are found in Alberta, Saskatchewan, and British Columbia.

How much of the provincial variations in health-care spending is due to differences across provinces in demographic and environmental factors? How much is due to the different approaches of the provinces to health-care systems when it comes to providing and managing care? For example, in the case of drugs, British Columbia has been a pioneer, first in the implementation of reference-based pricing and then in the implementation of an income-based drug benefit program for seniors, which may explain why real per capita provincial government spending on drugs is lowest in British Columbia. Understanding these drivers of health expenditure categories is ultimately a necessary component of understanding health-care sustainability and bending the cost curve.

Determinants of provincial government health spending by expenditure categories

While descriptive statistics are useful for providing an overview of trends and patterns in the public health expenditure system, understanding the specific determinants and drivers of health expenditure in a manner that controls for confounding factors requires regression estimates. A pooled time-series cross-section regression[7] model is estimated for each provincial government health expenditure category, taking the form

$$(1)\ H_{it} = f(d_{1it}, d_{2it}, \ldots d_{nit}) + e_{it}$$

where H_{it} is real per capita government health expenditures of the ith province at period t and d_1 to d_n represent a vector of social, demographic, economic, and policy variables of the ith province or territory at time t that are determinants of H_{it}, and e_{it} is an error term. These determinants are essentially expenditure drivers; the literature has identified these key drivers to include population growth, physician numbers, population aging, income, inflation, and enrichment factors such as technological change as proxied by time trend (Constant et al. 2011).

The specific variables employed are defined in Table 4.1 and include real per capita GDP; population; time trend[8]; the proportions of population aged 65–69 years, 70–74 years, 75–79 years, 80–84 years, and 85 years and

---

7 The pooled regression is preferable to single-province estimates because pooling allows for a larger sample and more degrees of freedom.

8 A time trend (YEAR) is sometimes used to account for technological change's expenditure impact. If new techniques generate cheaper health procedures, there could be expenditure reductions associated with technological change. Cutler et al. (1998) report that between 1983 and 1994, the real quality-adjusted price of heart attack treatments declined at

Table 4.1 Regression variable definitions

Dependent Variables

Real per capita provincial government health expenditures in 1997 dollars, deflated using the Government Current Expenditure Implicit Price Index

Rpgtothltc	Total
Rpghospc	Hospitals
Rpgothinstc	Other institutions
Rpgphysc	Physicians
Rpgothprofc	Other professionals
Rpgdrugsc	Drugs
Rpgcapitalc	Capital
Rpgpubhltc	Public health
Rpgadminc	Administration
Rpgothltc	All other health

Independent Variables

rgdpc	Real per capita gross domestic product in 1997 dollars, deflated using the Government Current Expenditure Implicit Price Index
rpgfedtransc	Real per capita federal cash transfer revenues in 1997 dollars, deflated using the Government Current Expenditure Implicit Price Index
nfld	1 if Newfoundland, 0 otherwise
pei	1 if PEI, 0 otherwise
ns	1 if Nova Scotia, 0 otherwise
nb	1 if New Brunswick, 0 otherwise
que	1 if Québec, 0 otherwise
ont	1 if Ontario, 0 otherwise
man	1 if Manitoba, 0 otherwise
sask	1 if Saskatchewan, 0 otherwise
alta	1 if Alberta, 0 otherwise
bc	1 if British Columbia, 0 otherwise
prop6569	Proportion of population aged 65 to 69
prop7074	Proportion of population aged 70 to 74
prop7579	Proportion of population aged 75 to 79
prop8084	Proportion of population aged 80 to 84
prop85plus	Proportion of population aged 85 or greater

Table 4.1 (Continued)

Dependent Variables

Totphysc10000	Number of physicians per 10,000 population
Rprovdebtintc	Real per capita provincial government debt interest (1997 dollars)
Rpgownrevc	Real per capita provincial government own-source revenue (1997 dollars)
Pop	Total provincial population
year	Year
privshare	Private share of total health expenditure
epf	1 if Established Programs Financing in effect (1977–95), 0 otherwise
cha	1 if *Canada Health Act* in effect (1984–2009), 0 otherwise
chst	1 if Canada Health and Social Transfer in effect (1996–2004), 0 otherwise
chtcst	1 if separate Canada Health Transfer and Canada Social Transfer in effect (2005–09), 0 otherwise

over[9]; real per capita federal cash transfers[10]; real per capita provincial debt interest[11]; and physicians per 10,000 population.[12]

Another set of dummy variables is specified to capture shifts in federal transfer payment regimes for health care and other programs and the onset of the *Canada Health Act* in 1984.[13] In addition, the private share of health spending is included to capture the effect of changing private shares on real

---

an annual rate of 1.1%. At the same time, with expensive new treatments or increased productivity of physicians, technological change can be associated with rising health expenditures as the quantity of services transacted increases. Given that technological change occurs over time, a time index is a way to control for the effect of technological change on health expenditures, but it is an imperfect one.

9 An aging population is a source of some debate as to its importance as a health-care expenditure driver. For a sample of papers for Canada, see Denton and Spencer (1995), Hogan and Hogan (2002), and Seshamani and Gray (2004). While aging is seen as a factor in rising health expenditures, its contribution has recently been determined to be modest, contributing around one-third of the average expected annual health expenditure increase of 3%. Other factors driving the other two-thirds of the increase in health spending—such as rising care expectations, time to death, rising input prices, and technological change—are thought to be the more important issue. There is also a vast international literature on the importance of an aging population on health expenditure impact that has reached similar conclusions; see Bryant et al. (2004), Getzen (1992), O'Connell (1996), Palangkaraya and Yong (2009), and Spillman and Lubitz (2000).

10 Federal cash transfers are important operating revenue sources for Canada's provincial governments but vary across provinces and time. About half of federal transfers are

per capita government health spending. Inflation is accounted for in all these regressions by using constant purchasing power real data (in 1997 dollars).

Province dummies to capture fixed effects are also included in the regressions. All other things given, some provinces may spend more or less than others, based on differences in historical patterns, health system culture, or tax systems. As well, shares of rural and remote populations also differ across provinces, though using a province dummy is a crude way to capture this particular difference.

The data for these regression variables were obtained from the National Health Expenditure database constructed by the Canadian Institute for Health Information (CIHI) and also from CANSIM/Statistics Canada and the Federal Fiscal Reference Tables. More specific details on the variable sources are available in Di Matteo (2010), Appendix II. The estimations are pooled time-series cross-sections using generalized least squares (GLS), assuming heteroskedastic panels with cross-sectional correlation and panel specific ar(1); the results are presented in Table 4.2. The estimation package is Stata 11 and testing was conducted on the data.

---

specifically marked for health, though general-purpose transfers such as equalization can also be applied to health.

11 Balanced budgets after the mid 1990s opened up a fiscal dividend that enabled provinces to spend more on health even while lowering income and corporate taxes; see Landon et al. (2006). Incorporating the ability to borrow and the price of borrowing to sustain health-spending levels and increases is a challenge to incorporate into a regression model. What may be a key issue is the borrowing capacity (quantity of debt and debt limits) along with the price of borrowing (the borrowing rate). In the early 1990s, provinces such as Saskatchewan seemed to be nearing the limits of their borrowing capacity, requiring sharp reductions in spending (see Mackinnon 2003). Up until the 1990s, debt service could be positively associated with health spending when debt levels were low but negatively associated when debt levels were high and provinces faced borrowing constraints. For an excellent survey of the international health expenditure determinants literature, see Gerdtham and Jonsson (2000). The first generation of such determinants studies often used international data; see Brown (1987), Gerdtham et al. (1992), Leu (1986), and Parkin, McGuire, and Yule (1987). See also Ariste and Carr (2003), Barros (1998), Di Matteo and Di Matteo (1998), Gerdtham et al. (1998), and Hitiris and Posnett (1992).

12 Physicians are the patient gateway into hospital services, diagnostic testing, specialist services, and prescription drug spending, and their decisions have an impact on health expenditures. As well, there is the potential for supplier-induced demand.

13 In 1977, Established Programs Financing (EPF) replaced federal–provincial cost sharing for health with a block grant. Under EPF, provincial governments were still expected to comply with the conditions under the *Hospital Insurance and Diagnostics Act* (1957) and the *Medical Care Act* (1966). In 1984 came the *Canada Health Act* (CHA), which tied receiving federal transfers to basic conditions for running a health-care system. In 1996, EPF and the Canada Assistance Plan, which funded income support, were collapsed into one transfer and the cash portion was reduced by one-third. This new payment was called the Canada Health and Social Transfer (CHST). Finally, in 2005 the CHST was broken up into two transfer payments, the Canada Health Transfer and the Canada Social Transfer.

Table 4.2 Regression results

	Irpgtothltc	z	Irpghospc	z	Irpgothinstc	z	Irpgphysc	z	Irpgothprofc	z
Totphysicianper10000	0.00701	1.83	0.00959	2.15	-0.00326	-0.33	0.02171	4.59	0.00842	0.65
rgdpc	0.00000	4.08	0.00000	2.15	0.00000	-0.39	0.00000	1.90	0.00000	0.29
rpgfedtransc	0.00000	-0.46	-0.00001	-1.37	0.00004	2.51	0.00001	0.78	0.00001	0.27
rpgownrevc	-0.00001	-1.19	0.00000	0.40	0.00001	0.67	-0.00001	-1.53	0.00000	0.14
rprovdebtintc	-0.00005	-2.36	-0.00007	-3.27	0.00004	0.71	-0.00015	-6.18	0.00013	1.90
prop6569	7.18488	3.72	11.84592	5.45	5.64304	1.04	1.78552	0.87	20.89785	3.24
prop7074	-0.99524	-0.38	3.62639	1.17	17.81755	2.62	7.53691	2.55	1.53894	0.18
prop7579	0.54006	0.16	-8.21068	-2.16	25.40185	3.14	5.68828	1.62	-20.51409	-2.00
prop8084	2.40324	0.55	5.46736	1.13	20.08133	1.92	-5.43441	-1.20	-76.91904	-5.42
prop85plus	6.08841	1.34	-4.45834	-0.90	40.81096	3.17	14.27268	2.78	-41.30189	-2.53
nfld	-0.19902	-2.25	-0.15933	-1.60	-0.67527	-3.37	-1.26946	-8.14	0.33800	1.18
pei	-0.27863	-2.83	-0.25424	-2.40	-1.36354	-5.88	-1.35991	-8.36	1.32925	4.23
ns	-0.33556	-3.93	-0.25223	-2.75	-1.50926	-6.04	-1.23689	-8.28	0.87308	3.17
nb	-0.26980	-2.94	-0.20362	-2.07	-1.33941	-6.13	-1.23149	-7.97	0.01762	0.05
que	-0.10065	-2.47	-0.09901	-1.82	-0.20232	-1.82	-0.58684	-8.43	0.32066	2.68
man	-0.23126	-2.89	-0.21613	-2.52	-1.02040	-5.42	-1.16345	-8.12	1.22196	4.97
sask	-0.25148	-2.93	-0.32384	-3.55	-1.34197	-5.79	-1.14450	-7.95	1.94417	7.35
alta	-0.12439	-1.72	-0.16502	-2.07	-0.60304	-3.77	-0.80582	-6.21	1.29475	5.45
bc	-0.15931	-2.45	-0.27192	-3.82	-0.86656	-4.27	-0.28544	-1.68	1.35633	7.02

(Continued)

Table 4.2 (Continued)

	Irpgtothltc	z	Irpghospc	z	Irpgothinstc	z	Irpgphysc	z	Irpgothprofc	z
pop	-0.00002	-2.75	-0.00004	-3.96	-0.00011	-5.54	-0.00009	-5.83	0.00010	3.68
privshare	-0.71491	-7.07	-0.38033	-3.59	-1.38263	-5.83	-0.47612	-4.00	0.31706	1.00
cha	-0.00602	-0.51	0.00279	0.22	-0.03704	-1.34	-0.00374	-0.37	0.01140	0.38
epf	-0.00337	-0.29	-0.02011	-1.65	0.05054	1.91	-0.02996	-3.02	0.06773	2.28
chst	-0.03558	-2.13	-0.06839	-3.91	0.10845	2.77	-0.03738	-2.63	0.00964	0.22
chtcst	-0.03335	-1.58	-0.06045	-2.70	0.10105	2.03	-0.02896	-1.59	-0.04591	-0.82
year	0.02082	11.42	0.01560	7.19	-0.00263	-0.57	0.01948	9.23	0.02463	3.27
_cons	-34.09908	-9.58	-24.48102	-5.81	9.83305	1.10	-32.54137	-7.93	-46.32339	-3.18
Wald chi2(26)	2698.83		1376.93		1338.49		6314.8		608.85	

	Irpgdrugsc	z	Irpgcapitalc	z	Irpgpubhltc	z	Irpgadminc	z	Irpgothhltc	z
totphysicianper10000	-0.00045	-0.05	-0.04651	-1.24	-0.03380	-2.97	0.03241	2.16	0.02181	1.52
rgdpc	0.00000	-0.98	0.00004	3.30	0.00001	2.68	0.00000	0.48	0.00001	1.54
rpgfedtransc	0.00001	0.87	-0.00009	-1.05	0.00003	1.45	0.00006	2.20	-0.00009	-2.91
rpgownrevc	0.00002	2.15	-0.00004	-0.83	0.00001	0.40	0.00004	2.37	-0.00003	-1.49
rprovdebtintc	-0.00013	-2.17	0.00028	1.12	-0.00026	-4.50	-0.00018	-2.08	0.00021	2.68
prop6569	12.25323	2.58	-13.68245	-0.74	-13.55963	-2.61	11.60852	1.49	2.49856	0.36
prop7074	13.87174	2.22	14.04503	0.53	13.78416	1.87	-6.17268	-0.58	-38.17720	-4.01
prop7579	9.43117	1.15	15.36675	0.45	17.59795	1.89	-9.41114	-0.64	14.51925	1.21
prop8084	-22.92250	-2.09	-3.78482	-0.08	-15.21120	-1.25	34.53145	1.94	-60.30646	-3.87

	lrpgdrugsc	z	lrpgcapitalc	z	lrpgpubhltc	z	lrpgadminc	z	lrpgothhltc	z
prop85plus	**-68.45531**	**-5.12**	78.17377	1.63	**51.90290**	**3.73**	**-105.56320**	**-5.14**	-6.82573	-0.42
nfld	0.02336	0.10	**2.89718**	**3.31**	**1.93877**	**9.25**	**-2.18730**	**-5.31**	**-0.98859**	**-2.87**
pei	0.07855	0.33	**2.52316**	**2.94**	**2.02335**	**8.29**	**-0.97597**	**-2.20**	-0.53649	-1.49
ns	**0.53103**	**2.87**	**2.33708**	**3.45**	**1.37822**	**7.07**	**-1.43771**	**-3.41**	**-1.08923**	**-3.54**
nb	0.35635	1.66	**2.83471**	**3.52**	**1.62571**	**7.90**	**-1.63682**	**-4.04**	**-1.10530**	**-2.38**
que	-0.00963	-0.06	**1.14013**	**3.81**	**0.80955**	**8.93**	-0.34910	-1.92	**-0.69871**	**-4.46**
man	0.29506	1.51	0.95281	1.20	**1.87857**	**11.49**	**-1.37321**	**-3.73**	-0.03304	-0.11
sask	**0.79642**	**3.42**	**1.67806**	**2.43**	**2.07934**	**11.41**	**-1.44176**	**-3.72**	-0.13160	-0.43
alta	0.02213	0.10	**2.06625**	**2.72**	**2.10653**	**13.22**	**-1.67473**	**-5.08**	**-0.97586**	**-3.03**
bc	0.21516	1.26	**1.76233**	**3.55**	**1.58392**	**9.95**	**-0.94697**	**-3.23**	0.02332	0.11
pop	0.00005	2.28	**0.00025**	**3.35**	**0.00021**	**11.50**	**-0.00019**	**-4.93**	**-0.00007**	**-2.12**
privshare	**-0.70903**	**-3.16**	**-6.00689**	**-5.71**	**-1.10614**	**-3.20**	-0.19104	-0.51	**1.53168**	**4.00**
cha	0.05006	1.64	-0.05134	-0.54	-0.01289	-0.53	-0.02836	-0.65	0.05413	1.51
epf	0.04006	1.33	-0.09068	-0.97	**0.05659**	**2.33**	**-0.09035**	**-2.05**	**0.07155**	**2.05**
chst	-0.07371	-1.67	**-0.32110**	**-2.34**	0.06095	1.68	-0.07369	-1.16	-0.03379	-0.65
chtcst	-0.09836	-1.78	-0.23316	-1.35	0.07850	1.73	-0.06070	-0.75	-0.10556	-1.62
year	**0.08682**	**12.09**	0.00853	0.35	**0.01971**	**3.36**	**0.04124**	**4.64**	**0.08717**	**11.07**
_cons	**-168.67410**	**-12.15**	-15.01565	-0.32	**-37.13368**	**-3.27**	**-76.90404**	**-4.46**	**-168.13490**	**-11.06**
Wald chi2(26)	3014.3		211.7		5036.02		430.96		2318.73	

*Bold italic denotes significant at the 5% level.

Normality plots of the key variables at the provincial level found real per capita GDP and transfers to be normally distributed, while population and the proportion aged 65 and over were less likely to be so. Levin-Lin-Chu and Harris-Tzavalis[14] unit root tests for panel data, with panel means and time trend both included and excluded, were conducted for the variables in the dataset; the variables exhibited a high degree of stationarity, with the null hypothesis of a unit root being rejected for many of the variables.[15] Box-Cox testing found the linear specification for real per capita total provincial government health spending to be more suitable than log-linear[16]; however, a log-linear specification is estimated to allow interpretation of the coefficients as percentages. Finally, Hausman test statistics supported the use of a fixed-effects versus a random-effects model, and therefore a specification with province dummies was retained.

Key significant determinants (at the 5% level) of real per capita provincial government health expenditures across the expenditure categories include real per capita GDP, time trend, proportions of population aged 65 years and over, total physicians per 10,000 population, private share of total health spending, and provincial debt interest and revenue variables.

Resource base variables such as real per capita GDP, federal transfers, and own-source provincial government revenues are generally positively and significantly associated for several categories. Of particular interest is the negative and significant relationship between real per capita provincial debt interest expenditures and most of the health expenditure categories. This result in particular underscores the importance of the fiscal dividend

---

14 The Levin-Lin-Chu test requires that the ratio of the number of panels to time periods tend to zero asymptotically and does not suit datasets with a large number of panels and relatively few time periods. The Harris-Tzavalis test assumes that the number of panels tends to infinity while the number of time periods is fixed. This dataset has a small number of panels (10) and a fixed number of time periods. It should be noted that panel test outcomes are often difficult to interpret if the null of the unit root is rejected; the best that can often be concluded is that "a significant fraction of the cross-section units is stationary or cointegrated." See Breitung and Pesaran (2005).

15 As well, Westerlund (2007) tests for co-integration in panel data were performed on earlier specifications and the null hypothesis of no co-integration was rejected, meaning that there was co-integration and the regressions were not spurious. These tests were done for each of the expenditure categories but on only six variables (the limit of the Stata module employed): total physicians per 10,000 population, real per capita GDP, population, real per capita federal cash transfers, proportion of population aged over 65 years, and real per capita provincial own-source revenues.

16 Box-Cox testing was conducted by regressing a real per capita health expenditure variable on the model variables. The value of theta was 0.31. As well, a Ramsay-Rest test on the variables used in the Box-Cox test that the model has no omitted variables did not support the presence of omitted variables.

obtained from getting public spending under control in the 1990s, combined with low interest rates and its impact on public spending.

The number of physicians per 10,000 of population is a positive and significant determinant of provincial government health spending for hospital,
physician, and administrative spending and negative and significant for public health spending. Adding one physician per 10,000 of population is associated with a 1% increase in real per capita provincial government spending,
a 2.2% increase in real per capita physician spending, a 3.2% increase in
administrative spending, and a 3.4% decrease in public health spending.

The age variables show some positive impacts on real per capita provincial government health expenditures as the population ages, but those
increases are tied to the share aged 75 years and under. As that demographic bulge moves into the ages over 75, expenditures in many categories
actually start to decline relative to the population below age 65 years of
age.[17] As well, there are some major differences across the specific categories. When it comes to aging, increases in physician spending are driven
especially by the proportions of population aged 70 to 74 and 85 plus.
Hospital spending per capita actually declines with respect to the population aged 75 to 79 and 85 years plus. On the other hand, these age categories are, not surprisingly, especially large drivers of spending for Other
Institutions. Drug spending is positively and significantly related to the
share of population under the age of 75, as provincial drug plans generally
begin to kick in for individual beneficiaries at age 65. There are significant
negative associations with the population shares aged 80 years and over
across several categories.

With respect to provincial fixed effects, all other things given, most
provinces spend less than Ontario when it comes to real per capita total
health spending, hospitals, administration, and physicians. However, for
public health and capital spending, other provinces tend to spend more.
There are no major significant differences among provinces when it comes
to drugs.

Population is negatively and significantly related to real per capita
spending for the bulk of provincial government health spending (total,
Hospitals, Physicians, Other Institutions, Administration, and All Other
Health), suggesting that significant economies of scale are present in
provincial government health spending. Time trend is a positive and

---

17 Much of this reflects costs in the last year of life, and it turns out that younger seniors have
   more effort expended trying to treat them to prevent death. At greater ages, less care is
   provided in the final year of life, in part because of "living directives." For a discussion of
   why this is the case, see Brown and Suresh (2004).

significant driver of several categories, while the private share is a negative and significant driver of several other categories.

Analysis and discussion

The preceding regression results show that there are several significant drivers of provincial government health spending, and several can be viewed as cost-side variables with implications for bending the cost curve. For example, physicians are a positive and significant driver of administrative costs. What can be done to administer physician services in a more cost-effective manner? As well, what can be done, particularly in smaller jurisdictions, to generate the economies of scale usually found in larger-population jurisdictions for some of the major expenditure categories? Population aging varies in its impact as aging progresses, with declines often offsetting increases as the population ages. The exception is other institutional care, where the trend is steadily upward. What can be done in the area of other institutional care to deal with the impact of an aging population?

In some respects, these approaches represent traditional paths to bending the cost curve via administrative controls ostensibly designed to promote greater efficiency. The results for the provincial dummy variables and for the time-trend variable suggest that there are other cost and expenditure determinants whose impact is real but more difficult to explicitly capture in macro-level regression analysis. For example, the positive impact of time trend could be capturing the impact of not only technological change but also rising prices and wages in the health-care sector. Differences across provinces in real per capita spending could be capturing differences in compensation levels from regional labour markets as well as institutional differences or entrenched historical patterns of spending.

Deber (2009) maintains that there are four ways to contain health-care costs:

1. Increase the efficiency of health-care delivery.
2. Increase the administrative controls on the use of these services.
3. Limit the resources available through the health-care system.
4. Increase the financial incentives for patients to limit their use of medical services.

In Canada we have attempted the first three ways through provincial single-payer administration of medically necessary hospital and physician services (stipulated as "insured services" under the *Canada Health Act*), but the fourth has generally been avoided. Indeed, much of the policy debate on how to solve the fiscal challenges in health care in Canada focuses on whether the fourth option is needed or whether all we need to do can be accomplished by the first three approaches. This latter approach is polarizing, as it quickly devolves into a highly ideological debate over whether or not there should be a larger market role in the provision of health care.

However, there is a fifth way to address rising health-care expenditures, and that is to consider how we can reduce prices. While health costs (or expenditures) are ultimately the product of price multiplied by quantity, for the most part in Canada we treat health care as a "fixed-price" system where only controls on quantities are used to control expenditures. There are at least three ways that provincial governments could do this: (1) they could continue to treat prices as fixed but shift care settings and care providers to lower-priced inputs, (2) they could devise mechanisms to make prices sensitive to productivity changes in health care, or (3) they could devise mechanisms to have prices adjust to reflect levels of needs in the population. Of these approaches, the first two are the most likely to bear fruit, given the fact that it is easier to identify where less expensive but high-quality care substitutions can be made or to measure the impact of a productivity gain. Also problematic are identifying the changing needs of a population and objectively measuring the acuity of a condition.

Shifting care to lower-price settings and providers

Some of what makes health care expensive is that Canadian provinces have focused public payment on the most expensive health-care providers—physicians—and the most expensive health-care settings—hospitals. This is in some respects the path-dependent outcome of a historical process that saw public health care first extended to universal hospital services, followed by physician services. Facing a menu of inputs for producing services, Canada selects the highest-price options. It is widely believed that Canadians rely too much on doctors and hospitals, so one avenue for reducing health-care expenditures without reducing quantity of services comes down to reducing the length of stays in hospital and shifting service sites from hospitals to lower-capital-provisioned long-term care or community care facilities or to home care, and from physicians to other qualified health-care providers. In effect, the substitution of person and place in care provision effectively lowers the prices paid by the public payer, which should have the effect of reducing the rise in total public health care expenditures. The potential for expenditure growth restraint in health care is large. Currently Canadians aged 65 and over, many with chronic conditions, account for half of total spending on hospitals and doctors in Canada.

The Canadian population is aging. The proportion of Canadians aged 65 and over is forecast to increase from around 15% today to 25% by 2030. Health spending is much higher for Canadians over age 65, so considerable debate has occurred as to whether population aging will challenge the financial sustainability of Canada's single-payer medicare systems for doctors and hospital services. Remarkably, economists and health-services researchers largely agree as to the apparent modest impact of population aging on the growth of aggregate health spending, though the results in these regressions suggest it may be more significant for institutional care. Most estimates suggest that per capita health spending has risen, and will rise, at only 1% per year. As this growth rate is less than that for the size of the economy (GDP), it follows that population aging is a manageable cost driver for public payers that poses little threat to the sustainability of single-payer Canadian medicare.[18]

It is possible that many of these persons could be treated in the home or in less capital-intensive care settings such as assisted living, receiving care from family or nurses and nurse's aides. For example, where a senior occupying an acute-care bed represents system costs of $1,100 per day in Alberta, the per diem rate in supported-care settings can be as low as $100 per day. Similar differences may exist in other provinces.

Health-care prices should be linked to productivity

What has apparently made health care so expensive has been technological change that allows our system to do more, thereby fuelling the expectations of Canadians that the system can do more for them. What is surprising is that few commentators on health-care costs seem to notice that health care is the only context in which innovation and the rising expectations of the

18 This relatively optimistic assessment of the impact of population aging on health costs is also contested in this volume, by John Richards, who argues the opposite (see Chapter 3). See also Denton and Spencer (1995), Evans et al. (2001), and Hogan and Hogan (2002). This normative assessment of the impact of population aging may be optimistic, since it ignores the possibility that population aging will result in a decreasing labour force and lower output per worker. To offset the negative economic consequences of population aging for economic growth and health-care spending, Canada will need to make productivity gains.

population have been presented as a "problem."[19] In any other sector of the economy, technology and innovation have been the solution to fiscal challenges, and higher expectations of the population are benign since the system can meet them. There has been less recognition that the cost of devices and software may be of lesser importance than the prices of the provider services using the technology.

In Canada we effectively treat health care as a somewhat "fixed-price" system where the fees for services and budgets for facilities are not determined to reflect productivity of the system. This is what makes health care so expensive. New health-care technology cuts the time required for a surgery or a treatment and also increases the volumes of surgeries and treatments. However, it is also true that the gains from new technology can be captured by the service providers instead of the funders. Most strategies of public payers in Canada for dealing with technology have amounted to managing (restraining) the use of new technologies, with a focus on the cost of the technology, rather than ensuring that they capture the benefits of technologies.[20]

What is not appreciated enough in the health policy debate is that health care, medical treatment in particular, may be the only sector of our economy that has this characteristic. The lesson from other sectors is that there is a fifth way that we have not seriously considered—that is, to influence the price of health-care services such that when technology and the skill levels of providers increase the volume of services (productivity increases), the prices of services fall. For example, if one considers the cost of computing power, which has diffused widely, the cost of computing power today is 1/1,000 of its 1970 value. In other words, we have been able to afford more of what computers have to offer because the price of those services fell with the rapid increase in productivity of the sectors using the technology.

---

19 Michael Decter is a prominent exception to this generalization. He has publicly discussed the disconnect between technologically generated advances in productivity in health care and the prices paid to providers. For example, see Karen Howlett, "How the Factory Floor Inspired a New Model for Health Care," *Globe and Mail*, 9 November 2010, http://www.theglobeandmail.com/news/national/time-to-lead/part-4-how-the-factory-floor-inspired-a-new-model-for-health-care/article1315002/ (accessed 26 November 2013). More typical of the literature is the perspective that questions whether the value of the productivity gains in health from technological advances justifies the costs, without reference to the potential for prices to fall. See David M. Cutler and Mark McClellan, "Is Technological Change in Medicine Worth It?" *Health Affairs* 20, no. 5 (2001): 11–29.

20 There is evidence that governments are beginning to realize this. Take the case of Ontario, where fees are being reduced for services such as cataract removal, which have seen dramatic productivity gains over the past decade.

Why have productivity gains not been captured on the cost side when it comes to health care? Provincial governments are aware of the potential to contain costs through changes in the pricing of drugs, through influencing the fee schedules of physicians, and through physician payment reform. The potential to alter prices paid for care is an attraction of private service delivery and competition for service volumes.[21] Provincial governments seeking to reform the pricing of health-care services and products have not had an easy time of it, as their efforts have typically resulted in public disputes with those with strong vested interests in the outcome, such as medical associations, health-care unions, and pharmaceutical wholesalers and retailers.

Conclusion

The comparison of growth rates of expenditures on health care to expected growth in resources as a basis for determining sustainability is an incomplete basis for evaluation. Essentially it is an attempt to determine if we will continue to be able to afford the health-care system we have now. What it cannot account for is whether that is the health-care system we will need. For example, the majority of health-care spending in Canada is for doctors and hospitals, and that spending goes largely to pay for acute-care medical treatment. With the decline of infectious diseases and increasing longevity and other factors, acute-care needs are increasingly competing with chronic disease care needs. Chronic disease management does not need to be carried out in a hospital or by a doctor, so in terms of sustainability of health-care spending relative to which needs are growing, hospitals and doctors should be growing less relative to other spending categories than they currently are. Sustaining the status quo of the current system may result in insufficient allocation (or reallocation) to the system of resources that we increasingly need.

It is also the case that the policy focus should be on total health-care expenditures and not just the public portion of those expenditures. Presumably there is some notionally objective level of health-care needs to be met through the health-care system, of which acute-care medical treatment is an important segment. As sustainability of public expenditures on health care—which is overwhelmingly acute medical care—can be

---

21 See, for example, Ruseski (2009), which discusses competition in Canadian health-care services, and Dranove, Capps, and Dafny (2009), which focuses on cataract services as an application of competitive procurement processes.

promoted by shifting services from domains dominated by public coverage to domains with mixed public/private financing, we need to be cognizant that lower spending by public payers is not clearly a good-news story; all that may be happening is that the burden of covering rising costs has been shifted to other sources of payment. In other words, public expenditures are being controlled by paying less through public sources instead of solving the problem of rising health-care costs.

As we discussed earlier, while median annual average real per capita provincial government health spending grew at 2.8% over the period 1976 to 2009, private-sector health spending grew at 3.1%. If private-sector health spending accounts for 30% of total health spending, then the policy-relevant growth rate of total health spending is closer to 3% per year than 2.8%. On a more detailed level, consider that the median growth rate for real per capita provincial government hospital spending across the provinces was 2.1%. While this may seem like a manageable growth rate for spending, it must be kept in mind that it has been achieved by reducing hospital length of stay and patient use of inpatient services. This must have created a need for outpatient treatments and other services that are part of the mixed payment system and not part of the accounting for hospitals.

Decades of health-care reform initiatives designed to restrain expenditure growth have focused on increasing efficiency through better administrative management, restructuring the delivery system, or simply limiting the flow of resources to the system. In the long term, all these approaches have ultimately failed to restrain growth to the growth rate of the resource base. Moreover, all these approaches have neglected the role of prices in driving up health-care costs. Ultimately, provincial governments will need to focus on the role of health-care "prices" in their efforts to bend the health-care cost curve.

References

Ariste, R., and J. Carr. 2003. "New Considerations on the Empirical Analysis of Health Expenditures in Canada, 1966–1998." Health Policy Research working paper no. 02–06. Ottawa: Health Canada.

Barros, P. P. 1998. "The Black Box of Health Care Expenditure Growth Determinants." *Health Economics* 7, no. 6: 533–44. http://dx.doi.org/10.1002/(SICI)1099 -1050(199809)7:6<533::AID-HEC374>3.0.CO;2-B.

Breitung, J., and M. H. Pesaran. 2005. *Unit Roots and Cointegration in Panels.* Working paper no. 1565. Munich: CESifo.

Brown, M. C. 1987. "Caring for Profit: Economic Dimensions of Canada's Health Industry." Vancouver: Fraser Institute.

Brown, R., and U. Suresh. 2004. "Further Analysis of Future Canadian Health Care Costs." *North American Actuarial Journal* 8, no. 2: 1–10. http://dx.doi.org/10.1080/ 10920277.2004.10596133.

Bryant, J., A. Teasdale, M. Tobias, J. Cheung, and M. McHugh. 2004. "Population Ageing and Government Health Expenditures in New Zealand, 1951–2051." Working paper no. 04/14. Wellington: New Zealand Treasury.

CIHI (Canadian Institute for Health Information). 2011. *Health Care Cost Drivers: The Facts.* Ottawa: CIHI.

Constant, A., S. Peterson, C. D. Mallory, and J. Major. 2011. "Research Synthesis on Cost Drivers in the Health Sector and Proposed Policy Options." Reports on Cost Drivers and Health System Efficiency no. 1. Ottawa: Canadian Health Services Research Foundation.

Currie, G., C. Donaldson, and M. Lu. 2003. "What Does Canada Profit from the For-Profit Debate on Health Care?" *Canadian Public Policy/Analyse de politiques* 29, no. 2: 227–51. http://dx.doi.org/10.2307/3552457.

Cutler, D. M., M. McClellan, J. P. Newhouse, and D. Remler. 1998. "Are Medical Prices Declining? Evidence from Heart Attack Treatments." *Quarterly Journal of Economics* 113, no. 4: 991–1024. http://dx.doi.org/10.1162/003355398555801.

Deber, R. 2009. "Canada." In *Cost Containment and Efficiency in National Health Systems: A Global Comparison*, edited by J. Rapoport, P. Jacobs, and E. Jonsson, 15–40. Weinheim, Germany: Wiley-VCH.

Denton, F. T., and B. G. Spencer. 1995. "Demographic Change and the Cost of Publicly Funded Health Care." *Canadian Journal on Aging* 14, no. 2: 174–92. http://dx.doi.org/10.1017/S0714980800011806.

Di Matteo, L. 2010. "The Sustainability of Public Health Expenditures: Evidence from the Canadian Federation." *European Journal of Health Economics* 11, no. 6: 569–84. http://dx.doi.org/10.1007/s10198-009-0214-x.

Di Matteo, L., and R. Di Matteo. 1998. "Evidence on the Determinants of Canadian Provincial Government Health Expenditures, 1965–1991." *Journal of Health Economics* 17, no. 2: 211–28. http://dx.doi.org/10.1016/S0167-6296(97)00020-9.

———. 2009. "The Fiscal Sustainability of Alberta's Public Health Care System." SPP Research Papers: The Health Series 2, no. 2. Calgary: University of Calgary School of Public Policy.

Dodge, D. A., and R. Dion. 2011. "Chronic Healthcare Spending Disease: A Macro Diagnosis and Prognosis." Commentary no. 327. Toronto: C. D. Howe Institute.

Dranove, D., C. Capps, and L. Dafny. 2009. "A Competitive Process for Procuring Health Services: A Review of Principles with an Application to Cataract Services." SPP Research Papers: The Health Series 2, no. 5. Calgary: University of Calgary School of Public Policy.

Evans, R. G., K. M. McGrail, S. G. Morgan, M. L. Barer, and Clyde Hertzman. 2001. "Apocalypse No: Population Aging and the Future of Health Care Systems." *Canadian Journal on Aging/La Revue canadienne du vieillissement* 20 (Suppl. 1): 160–91. http://dx.doi.org/10.1017/S0714980800015282.

Gerdtham, U. G., and B. Jonsson. 2000. "International Comparisons of Health Expenditure: Theory, Data and Econometric Analysis." In *Handbook of Health Economics*, vol. 1, edited by A. J. Culyer and J. P. Newhouse, 11–53. Elsevier Science. http://dx.doi.org/10.1016/S1574-0064(00)80160-2.

Gerdtham, U. G., B. Jonsson, M. MacFarlan, and H. Oxley. 1998. "The Determinants of Health Expenditure in the OECD Countries: A Pooled Data Analysis." In *Health, the Medical Profession and Regulation: Developments in Health Economics and Public Policy*, vol. 6, edited by P. Zweifel, 113–34. http://dx.doi.org/10.1007/978-1-4615-5681-7_6.

Gerdtham, U. G., J. Sogaard, F. Andersson, and B. Jonsson. 1992. "An Econometric Analysis of Health Care Expenditure: A Cross-Section Study of the OECD Countries." *Journal of Health Economics* 11, no. 1: 63–84. http://dx.doi.org/10.1016/0167-6296(92)90025-V.

Getzen, T. E. 1992. "Population Ageing and the Growth of Health Expenditures." *Journals of Gerontology: Series B, Psychological Sciences and Social Sciences* 47: S98–104.

Hitiris, T., and J. Posnett. 1992. "The Determinants and Effects of Health Expenditure in Developed Countries." *Journal of Health Economics* 11, no. 2: 173–81. http://dx.doi.org/10.1016/0167-6296(92)90033-W.

Hogan, S., and S. Hogan. 2002. "How Will the Ageing of the Population Affect Health Care Needs and Costs in the Foreseeable Future?" Discussion paper no. 25. Ottawa: Commission on the Future of Health Care in Canada.

Landon, S., M. L. McMillan, V. Muralidharan, and M. Parsons. 2006. "Does Health-Care Spending Crowd Out Other Provincial Government Expenditures?" *Canadian Public Policy* 32, no. 2: 121–41. http://dx.doi.org/10.2307/4128724.

Leu, Robert E. 1986. "The Public-Private Mix and International Health Care Costs." In *Public and Private Health Services*, edited A. J. Culyer and B. Jonsson, 41–63. Oxford: Basil Blackwell.

MacKinnon, J. 2003. *Minding the Public Purse: The Fiscal Crisis, Political Trade-Offs, and Canada's Future.* Montreal: McGill-Queen's University Press.

Marchildon, G. P., T. McIntosh, and P. G. Forest, eds. 2004. *The Fiscal Sustainability of Health Care in Canada: The Romanow Papers*, vol. 1. Toronto: University of Toronto Press.

O'Connell, J. 1996. "The Relationship between Health Expenditures and the Age Structure of the Population in OECD Countries." *Health Economics* 5, no. 6: 573–78. http://dx.doi.org/10.1002/(SICI)1099-1050(199611)5:6<573::AID-HEC231>3.0.CO;2-L.

Palangkaraya, A., and J. Yong. 2009. "Population Ageing and Its Implications on Aggregate Health Care Demand: Empirical Evidence from 22 OECD Countries." *International Journal of Health Care Finance Economics* 9, no. 4: 391–402. http://dx.doi.org/10.1007/s10754-009-9057-3.

Parkin, D., A. McGuire, and B. Yule. 1987. "Aggregate Health Care Expenditures and National Income: Is Health Care a Luxury Good?" *Journal of Health Economics* 6, no. 2: 109–27. http://dx.doi.org/10.1016/0167-6296(87)90002-6.

Ruseski, J. .2009. "Competition in Canadian Health Care Service Provision: Good, Bad or Indifferent." SPP Research Papers, The Health Series 2, no. 4. Calgary: University of Calgary School of Public Policy.

Seshamani, M., and M. Gray. 2004. "A Longitudinal Study of the Effects of Age and Time to Death on Hospital Costs." *Journal of Health Economics* 23, no. 2: 217–35. http://dx.doi.org/10.1016/j.jhealeco.2003.08.004.

Spillman, B. C., and J. Lubitz. 2000. "The Effect of Longevity on Spending for Acute and Long-Term Care." *New England Journal of Medicine* 342, no. 19: 1409–15. http://dx.doi.org/10.1056/NEJM200005113421906.

TD Bank Financial Group. 2010. *Charting a Path to Sustainable Health Care in Ontario: 10 Proposals to Restrain Cost Growth without Compromising Quality of Care.* TD Economics Special Reports. Toronto: TD Canada Trust.

Zweifel, P., S. Felder, and M. Meiers. 1999. "Ageing of Population and Health Care Expenditure: A Red Herring?" *Health Economics* 8, no. 6: 485–96. http://dx.doi.org/10.1002/(SICI)1099-1050(199909)8:6<485::AID-HEC461>3.0.CO;2-4.

five
Pharmaceuticals

STEVEN G. MORGAN, JAMIE R. DAW, AND PAIGE A. THOMSON

Introduction

The rate at which pharmaceutical expenditure is growing—the pharmaceutical cost curve—is a preoccupation of many researchers, policymakers, and stakeholders. This is partly because, on average, prescription drug costs grew more rapidly than any other major component of Canadian health-care spending in the 1980s, 1990s, and 2000s. Indeed, until very recently, upward was the only direction in which the pharmaceutical cost curve was being bent in Canada. This is also partly because, despite being the second largest component of health-care spending in Canada (at over $32 billion per year), pharmaceuticals used outside hospitals are not an insured service under the *Canada Health Act*. Therefore pharmaceuticals are financed by many payers in Canada, which raises administrative costs and disperses the responsibility (and potentially the ability) to control costs to a variety of public and private payers, the latter of which may have lower incentives to control drug spending. The result of this system is that many Canadians—both insured and uninsured—are bearing considerable financial burdens associated with necessary medicines.

Some of the determinants of Canadian pharmaceutical expenditure growth are global in nature, such as the growth in the number of drugs available to treat an increasing variety of conditions. However, in an international comparison, Canada stands out as a case of exceptionally high and uncontrolled drug spending, suggesting that other countries have been more successful in controlling spending through a variety of policies. Thus we suggest that the pharmaceutical cost curve is perhaps more malleable than Canadians realize. In this chapter we review evidence on the drivers of pharmaceutical cost growth and the policies that have been used in various attempts to contain those costs. We conclude that one of the major obstacles to bending the pharmaceutical cost curve in Canada is our multi-payer, non-universal system of prescription drug financing—in short, no cost control without pharmacare.

A macro view of drug cost growth

The nature of pharmaceutical cost drivers can be understood by looking at historical trends in drug spending and drug development. Figure 5.1 illustrates a long-term view of prescription drug spending in Canada. The figure illustrates inflation-adjusted (2011 dollars) wholesales of medicinal products per capita from 1931 to 1975 and inflation-adjusted retail spending per capita on prescription drugs from 1975 through to 2011.

Figure 5.2 illustrates five-year moving averages of the number of new drugs approved for sale in the United States from 1946–50 through to 2006–10. To illustrate the relative novelty of new drugs approved over time, the drugs are placed into one of three mutually exclusive categories: the "first-of-kind" drugs to be approved within chemical or biologic subgroups; "early follow-ons," approved within 10 years of respective first-of-kinds; and "late follow-ons," approved 10 or more years after respective first-of-kinds (Morgan, Cunningham, and Law 2012). This provides a long view of innovation and competition in drug

Figure 5.1 Inflation-adjusted prescription drug spending per Canadian, 1931–2011 (2011 dollars)

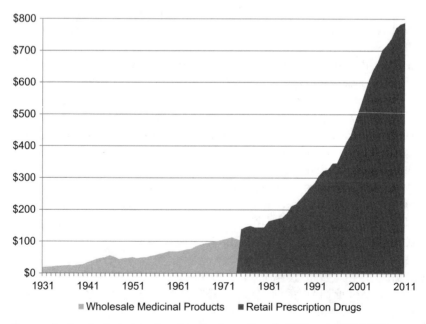

Source: Authors' calculations, based on Statistics Canada 1983 and CIHI 2012b.

Figure 5.2 Five-year averages of all therapeutic new molecular entities (NMEs) approved by US Food and Drug Administration, by level of novelty, 1946–1950 to 2006–2010

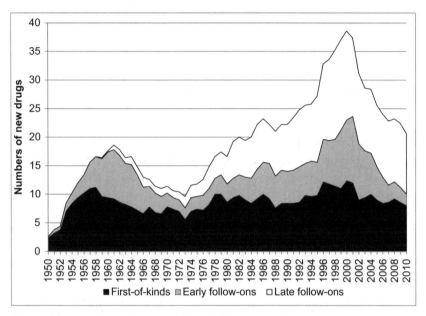

Source: Morgan, Cunningham, and Law 2012.

development—both major, largely exogenous forces affecting prescription drug costs.

Important periods of rapid pharmaceutical cost growth have coincided with periods of significant drug development. For example, drug spending in Canada grew rapidly during the postwar therapeutic revolution of the 1950s and 1960s. During this time, a wide range of new anti-infectives, cardiovasculars, and neurologicals came to market (Temin 1980). This was followed by a lull in drug development during the 1970s that coincided with a reduced rate of drug spending growth in Canada. Drug development was driven forward again in the late 1970s through the 1980s by the paradigm of "rational drug design"—many new drugs were "designed" by using a better understanding of the structure of biologic targets they might interact with (Hopkins et al. 2007; Mowery 2004; Nightingale 2000; Temin 1980). New classes of blockbuster drugs—high-selling drugs generating more than US$1 billion in sales—were created in this era, including still dominant classes of cardiovascular, gastrointestinal, and neurological drugs. Evidence from these decades demonstrates how rapid increases in drug spending follow drug development trends.

Then, rather than entering a bust cycle in the 1990s, as might have been predicted from earlier boom-and-bust cycles of drug development, the total numbers of drug approvals increased sharply. Only this time the major category of drugs to be approved was that of "follow-on" drugs—drugs with marginal therapeutic advantage entering established categories, sometimes more than a decade after their comparable predecessors. Again drug cost escalation in the 1990s and early 2000s grew dramatically. Moreover, evidence suggests that much of this growth was due to increased use of the newer follow-on drugs (or "me too" drugs) that were brought to market in that era (Morgan et al. 2005). As we will explain, the literature on cost drivers is consistent with this hypothesis. To the extent that this is true, it suggests that appropriate policy levers could have controlled related costs.

The micro determinants of cost growth

Studies of prescription drug cost growth generally consider the effects of four broad categories of cost drivers: (1) population aging (and health needs, if measurable); (2) the volume of prescription drugs used by a population (age-adjusted, if possible); (3) the choice of drugs selected for a given course of treatment; and (4) the prices paid for the specific drugs dispensed (including costs of dispensing, where relevant). Canadian findings on the relative impact of these cost drivers during the 1990s and early 2000s are reasonably consistent. The most recent comprehensive data for Canada comes from the second edition of the *Canadian Rx Atlas* (Morgan et al. 2008). Overall findings from those reports are listed in Table 5.1.

Per capita spending on prescription drugs in Canada grew at an inflation-adjusted rate of 6% per year between 1998 and 2007. Population aging contributed just 0.9 percentage points to the annual growth rate over the period, leaving 5.1 percentage points to be explained by other factors. This modest contribution of aging to prescription drug expenditures is consistent with literature on both aging and general health-care expenditures and pharmaceutical costs in Canada and abroad (Evans et al. 2001; Morgan and Cunningham 2011; Van Tielen, Peys, and Genaert 1998).

The increased volume of prescription drugs purchased by Canadians was the most significant driver of age-standardized prescription drug spending in Canada between 1998 and 2007, contributing 3.3 percentage points to the

Table 5.1 Magnitude and sources of growth in inflation-adjusted per capita spending in Canada, 1998–2007 (2007 dollars)

Per capita expenditure in 1998	$324
Per capita expenditure in 2007	$578
Average annual growth rate	6.0%
Growth rate due to population aging	0.9%
Age-standardized growth rate	5.1%
Volume of therapy	3.3%
Cost impact of therapeutic choices	2.0%
Price changes, including generic savings	− 0.3%

Source: Morgan et al. 2008.

annual growth in inflation-adjusted per capita drug expenditures (Morgan et al. 2008). Volume was a major driver both of overall costs and for most leading therapeutic categories of treatment. Moreover, although national data do not allow for such detailed analyses, data from British Columbia indicate that patients are being prescribed drugs from an increasing number of drug categories, and, in particular, they are receiving more and more days of therapy per category of treatment (Morgan 2006). While part of this trend may be the result of the increased burden of chronic disease, it is also the case that definitions of chronic disease have changed over this period, with falling thresholds for treating risk factors such as high cholesterol, hypertension, and depression. Thus costs have not been driven up only by the fact that Canadians are treating health conditions more often with prescription drugs; costs have also been driven up by the fact that Canadians are increasingly being diagnosed with chronic conditions that are being treated with prescription drugs. These micro trends are consistent with patterns of drug development, which saw dramatic increases in the availability of first-of-kind and follow-on drugs for chronic disease in the 1980s and 1990s.

Changes in the types of drugs selected for treatment constituted the second largest driver of prescription drug spending trends in Canada overall, and for most major therapeutic categories (Morgan et al. 2008). Decisions about which drugs to select for a given course of treatment contributed 2.0 percentage points to the annual growth in inflation-adjusted per capita age-standardized drug expenditures in Canada between 1998 and 2007.

Changes in the type of drug selected from within therapeutic categories played a particularly important role in the 1990s, when new "blockbuster" drugs were entering established therapeutic categories and securing sometimes significant market share despite being premium-priced in relation to comparable drugs. For example, a study of prescription drug expenditure in British Columbia found that 80% of expenditure growth from 1996 to 2002 was due to the use of new drugs that were brought to market during that period but deemed comparable to medicines brought to market before 1990 (Morgan et al. 2005). Those new "me-too" drugs were on average four times more expensive than older generic alternatives within the same therapeutic classes.

Though for some brand and generic drugs in Canada, sticker prices went up between 1998 and 2007, savings from increased generic availability and use counteracted that pressure on cost by reducing the effective price paid per drug prescribed. In fact, the increased availability and use of generics in Canada generated savings equivalent to 0.6% per year on inflation-adjusted per capita prescription drug expenditures during this period (Morgan et al. 2008). It is notable that savings of that magnitude were generated at a time when Canadian prices for generic drugs were relatively high—roughly 70% of the equivalent brand-name drug. As discussed below, restraints on generic drug pricing introduced in recent years have made generics an even more potent cost saver in Canada. While perhaps long overdue, such generic pricing policy changes have come just in time to capitalize on a wave of blockbuster drugs that are coming off patent worldwide.

Provincial variation

The extent of variation in prescription drug spending levels and trends across Canada provides a rough indication of the extent to which prescription drug expenditure may be modified by changes in policy and practice. Figure 5.3 illustrates total private and public expenditure on prescription drugs for each province from 1990 to 2011. The figure presents the spending levels in terms of inflation-adjusted (2011) dollars per capita so that magnitudes of difference over time and across provinces can be easily interpreted. The differences are striking.

There is a west-to-east gradient in total prescription drug spending per capita, with British Columbia being consistently among the lowest-spending provinces and Nova Scotia, New Brunswick, Québec, and Newfoundland and Labrador being the highest-spending provinces. Moreover, while there have always been differences in per capita

Figure 5.3 Inflation-adjusted per capita spending by province, 1990–2011 (2011 dollars)

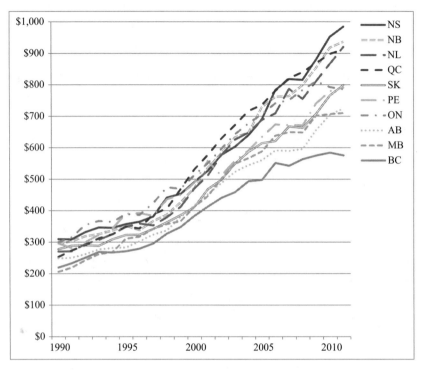

Source: Authors' calculations, based on CIHI 2012b.

expenditures on prescription drugs across provinces, these differences have grown in recent years. Differences between the highest and lowest levels of prescription drug spending per capita in the provinces were roughly 40% before 2005; the coefficient of variation across provinces was roughly 11% before that period. In the past five years, however, that difference has grown to 71%, and the average coefficient of variation across provinces is now 15%. To put those numbers in perspective, provincial variation in medical services (the closest complement to outpatient prescription drug use) is declining, with differences between the highest- and lowest-spending provinces falling from approximately 80% in the 1990s to approximately 45% today; coefficients of variation fell from 22% to 11% over the same period.

Some of Canada's interprovincial variation in spending on prescription drugs can be explained by differences in the ages of provincial populations.

Table 5.2 Overall cost (private and public expenditure) of age-standardized deviation from national average for spending on prescription drugs in 2007, by province and source of deviation from average (millions of dollars)

	Total Cost of Age-Standardized Deviation from National Per Capita Average	Cost of Age-Standardized Difference in Volume of Drug Use	Value of Age-Standardized Difference in Cost of Therapeutic Choices	Value of Age-Standardized Difference in Drug Prices, Including Generic Savings
QC	595	308	40	247
ON	140	274	9	– 142
NB	49	63	– 18	5
NS	41	87	– 35	– 11
NL	8	34	– 30	4
PE	1	4	– 4	1
MB	– 52	– 49	– 14	11
AB	– 89	6	– 70	– 24
SK	– 92	– 68	– 29	6
BC	– 701	– 455	– 208	– 38

Source: Morgan et al. 2008.

However, the most recent age-standardized assessment of per capita spending, in 2007, found that significant variations persisted after age standardization (Morgan et al. 2008). As illustrated in Table 5.2, the aggregate impacts of variations in age-standardized cost drivers were dramatic for some provinces. For example, holding age constant, if cost drivers in Québec were the same as the national average, total spending on prescription drugs in that province would be $595 million lower than was actually the case in 2007. Most of this difference ($308 million) was a result of higher age-standardized volumes of prescription drugs purchased per capita. Higher prices—due to less generic drug use and higher pharmacists' fees paid per unit—also explained much of this variation ($247 million). Similarly, if all cost drivers in British Columbia were the same as the national average on an age-standardized basis, total spending on prescription drugs in that province would be $701 million higher than was the case in 2007. Most of the difference is a result of British Columbia residents purchasing fewer prescription drugs holding age constant ($455 million) and selection of lower-cost treatment options within therapeutic categories ($208 million).

International comparisons

Evidence of age-standardized variations across provinces suggests that policy and practice may have a significant effect on prescription drug spending levels in Canada. These data do not, however, clearly indicate whether provinces such as Québec are overspending or provinces such as British Columbia are underspending. However comparisons to average prescription drug spending internationally give a reasonably clear answer to those questions.

Figure 5.4 illustrates trends in per capita spending on pharmaceuticals for a selection of Organisation for Economic Co-operation and Development (OECD) countries. Data are illustrated in inflation-adjusted (2010) Canadian dollars per capita so that differences across countries and over time can be easily interpreted. The countries selected include the seven comparator countries used by Canada's Patented Medicine Prices Review Board, plus Australia and New Zealand; the latter two are frequently used as comparators to Canada for pharmaceutical policy purposes.

Figure 5.4 Inflation-adjusted per capita spending on pharmaceuticals, selected OECD countries (2010 PPP Canadian dollars)

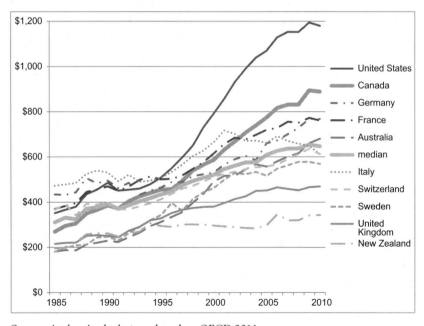

Source: Authors' calculations, based on OECD 2011.

Figure 5.4 clearly shows that the United States has become a major outlier in terms of pharmaceutical spending. It is also notable, however, that apart from the United States, no other country in the OECD (including all of those not shown in Figure 5.4) currently spends more per capita on pharmaceuticals than Canada.

Canada was not always a high spender on pharmaceuticals. Through to 1996, per capita drug spending in Canada was roughly equal to the median level of spending among comparable countries. But starting in the late 1990s, pharmaceutical spending in Canada outpaced the spending of most comparable countries except for the United States. These trends have major financial implications for Canada. Our pharmaceutical spending is now 37% above the median for comparator countries—that's $242 per capita or $8.2 billion in annual spending that we may or may not "need" to be paying.

Supply-side cost control

Cost control in Canada has largely focused on supply-side measures that aim to either directly control supply prices or foster forms of supply-side competition that result in lower prices. Because policy institutions play an important role in the nature of policy instruments chosen over time and the effects of those instruments, we review supply-side cost-control mechanisms in a quasi-chronological order. We begin with generic availability, use, and pricing because such factors were an important part of early cost-control efforts and have become critical again today. We then review international reference pricing policies because those tools underpinned federal price regulations implemented in 1987. Therapeutic reference pricing follows as the tool that was widely talked about (but very narrowly applied) in the 1990s. Finally we discuss the use of negotiated rebates as a condition of formulary listing, because such practices went from almost never being used in Canada before 2000 to routinely being used in some (but certainly not all) provinces.

Generic availability, use, and pricing

Policies that aim to produce savings from generic medicines must achieve three outcomes: prescribing of drugs for which generics are available, dispensing of generics when available, and competitive generic prices. In light of evidence for what the federal government viewed to be excessively high drug pricing in the 1950s and 1960s, Canada passed a compulsory licensing

Figure 5.5 Brand shares of total sales in multi-source diuretic drug markets under BC PharmaCare's Low Cost Alternative (LAC) program for seniors, 1986–1995

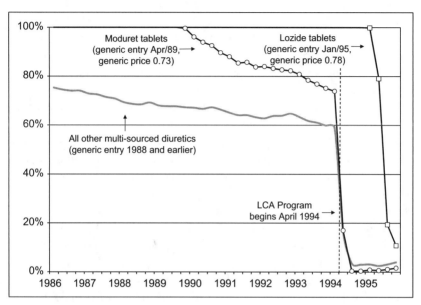

Source: Morgan 2000.

provision for drug patents in 1969 that would allow generics to compete with patented drugs (Lexchin 1993). In the 1970s, many provinces began efforts to promote savings with legislation to permit generic substitutions when drugs were prescribed by brand name (as most prescriptions were written, then and now). Such laws made substitutions possible but did not address the lack of financial incentives for pharmacists and patients to consider generic substitutions. If a patient was fully insured and the pharmacist was paid markups in proportion to costs, there would be little incentive for generic use (Gorecki 1992; Grootendorst et al. 1996).

In the late 1980s and early 1990s, provinces began to use generic reference pricing policies to encourage patients to request generics when available. Under such policies, patients would be required to pay the difference between generic drug prices and brand-name drug prices if a generic was available. British Columbia implemented such a policy, called the Low Cost Alternative Program, in 1994. Evidence of its impact is provided in Figure 5.5, which plots the share of market held by brand-name versions of diuretic drugs with generic competition at the time. The grey line in

Figure 5.5 represents the sales-weighted average market share held by the 10 brand-name diuretics that were subject to generic competition on or before 1988. Despite years of generic availability, these brands had lost only 40% of their markets to generics by the first quarter of 1994. Within two quarters of the Low Cost Alternative Program's being in effect, however, these brands held only 3% of their markets. Similar rates of generic penetration occurred in other drug markets, including the two other diuretic drug markets illustrated in Figure 5.5.

Now, decades later, in a post–compulsory licensing world with relatively effective generic substitution policies in place in most provinces, governments must place stronger emphasis on securing low generic prices. It has historically been accepted that generics can be listed in provincial formularies if they offer a discount in the range of 30% to 35% of their equivalent brand. Prior to elimination of the compulsory licensing provisions of Canada's *Patent Act*—when Canada was the only country among its peers to have generic versions of patented drugs—a 30% discount on still-patented drugs was likely an acceptable discount. Regrettably, however, the policy of listing any generic drug offering only 30% to 35% off brand-name prices appears to have limited retail price competition for generic drugs in Canada. Studies have shown that generic prices in Canada are high relative to comparator jurisdictions—in some cases on the magnitude of tenfold higher then generic prices abroad (Morgan et al. 2007; Patented Medicine Prices Review Board 2006).

The potential to generate savings from generic competition is currently higher now than it has ever been before, because drugs that represent an unprecedented share of the pharmaceutical market are coming off patent. For example, it is estimated that approximately one-third of drugs used in 2009 will be available in generic form by 2014 (Canadian Generic Pharmaceutical Association 2012; CIHI 2012a). In Canada, drugs that will "go generic" by 2014 have a combined wholesale volume of more than $8 billion (CIHI 2012a).

Led by Ontario, provinces have responded to the new opportunities for generic savings by passing legislation to limit generic prices. The mandated discounts required range from 60% in New Brunswick and Newfoundland and Labrador to 75% in Québec and Ontario (Benefit Partners 2012). Several provinces have required that the legislated discounts apply to both public and private payers alike, which significantly increases the impact of the policies, given that no provincial government pays for more than half of drug purchases in any province. Ontario's case is notable because it was the first to introduce these policies, in 1993; it has required the deepest discounts to date; and it mandates that discounts apply to all purchasers in the province. It is estimated that Ontario's policy reduced expenditure on generics in 2010 by between \$181 million and \$194 million over six months (Law, Ystma, and Morgan 2011). If this level were applied nationally—and noting that several of the best-selling drugs in Canada have recently lost patent protection—a policy such as Ontario's would likely reduce Canadian drug spending by \$2 billion or more.

Despite these successes, there is room for provincial governments to drive down generic prices even further. Even with the lowest price cap in the country, Ontario has still been shown to overpay for most generic medicines relative to some comparator countries that use competitive tendering to determine generic drug prices (Law 2012). Regrettably, competitive tendering processes would be difficult to operationalize in Canada's non-universal, multi-payer drug financing system, which significantly increases tendering administration costs, fragments purchasing power, and does not offer sufficient incentives to firms. However, systems for collaboration across provinces and payers may be possible. It is also possible that provincial governments might secure sufficient savings from tendering processes to justify the extension of universal public coverage for the generics tendered. There are several drugs for which prices could be secured at a sufficiently low price to render such a program cost-saving for the public sector, despite providing universal coverage—a rare opportunity for governments to simultaneously save health dollars while providing equitable access (Law and Morgan 2011).

International reference pricing

When Canada eliminated compulsory licensing as a requirement of the Canada–US free trade agreement, concerns about increased prices for brand-name pharmaceuticals led to establishment of the Patented Medicine Prices Review Board (PMPRB) in 1987 (Lexchin 1993). The PMPRB does not set prices but rather exercises its authority over drug prices through a statutory framework based at its core on international reference pricing. Though the PMPRB's system of price tests is complicated, maximum allowable ex-factory prices for patented medicines in Canada are ultimately derived from (manufacturer-reported) ex-factory prices in seven other countries: France, Germany, Italy, Sweden, Switzerland, the United Kingdom, and the United States (Patented Medicine Prices Review Board 2012).

International reference pricing (IRP) policies are not unique to Canada. As of 2010, such policies were employed in 23 of the 27 member states of the European Union (Leopold et al. 2012). While the few studies examining IRP policies in European jurisdictions have demonstrated some success in achieving lower prices (Leopold et al. 2012), the effectiveness of international reference pricing is contingent on the choice of comparator countries and the extent to which international pricing is transparent. The selection of comparator countries used by the PMPRB has been criticized given the exclusion of comparators with low drug prices, such as Australia, and the inclusion of countries that tend to have among the highest drug prices in the industrialized world, including Germany, Switzerland, and the United States (Lexchin 1997). Furthermore, the 1998 Auditor General's review of the PMPRB found that the only foreign country selling approximately 20% of the medicines under review was the United States (Office of the Auditor General of Canada 1998).

Even with a broader base of comparator countries, a major threat to the utility of international reference pricing is the industry's reaction to the extent to which the tool is used. The OECD and the World Bank have both observed that the widespread use of external reference pricing is resulting in harmonization of official list prices for pharmaceuticals and increased use of confidential negotiations as a means for manufacturers to price-discriminate across markets and payers (Docteur, Paris, and Moise 2008; Seiter 2010). Thus the list prices of drugs in an increasing number of comparator countries do not reflect the real price paid—a result of confidential price rebates from manufacturers to health-care payers. These trends potentially undermine the utility of Canada's patented medicine price tests and leave under- and uninsured Canadians at a significant disadvantage, given that provincial governments are increasingly negotiating their own confidential rebates on what are increasingly viewed as inflated list prices.

Therapeutic reference pricing

Therapeutic referencing pricing policies were, at least until recent years, widely used by drug plans internationally. These policies can vary, but all are based in the first instance on defining groups of drugs that are sufficiently therapeutically similar that they can be considered interchangeable at the population level—that is, groups for which no drug has systematic advantages over others that can be identified before a patient tries the medicine. Once such therapeutic categories are defined, the policies can take two broad forms.

The first type of referencing pricing policy is statutory price limits based on the cost of alternatives within categories. Countries such as Germany and Australia effectively use prices charged for drugs within therapeutic categories to set limits for new drugs that seek to be on the formulary. The reference price for a category can be defined by a single reference drug or by formulae that account for variations in product strengths and forms available within the class. A drug must be priced at or below the therapeutic class reference price—which may fall over time as the prices of medicines within the class fall, as is the case when older versions of a drug are subject to generic competition.

Evidence from Australia suggests that the use of therapeutic referencing to set allowable prices may have been successful in fostering domestic price competition in the past (Morgan, McMahon, and Greyson 2008; Roughead, Lopert, and Sansom 2007). However, with the wave of patent expiries that occurred over the past decade, the Australian government was pressured to prevent generic competition from lowering the reference price of newer, supposedly innovative but comparable products (Morgan, McMahon, and Greyson 2008; Searles et al. 2007). Moreover, the same global pricing pressures that are limiting the effectiveness of international reference pricing are also limiting the effect of these transparent systems of therapeutic reference pricing. For example, for a manufacturer to meet the limit imposed by a therapeutic reference in Australia, it may have to post a price below its international list price, which would result in significant pressure to offer that price in other countries. Thus Australia and other countries are increasingly using negotiated rebates as a mechanism for securing desired prices—rebates that some believe are undermining the transparency and accountability of the previous pricing system (Robertson, Walkom, and Henry 2009).

The second broad form of reference pricing allows for price differentials within therapeutic categories but requires that patients pay some or all of the price difference when they are prescribed high-cost alternatives (Morgan, Hanley, and Greyson 2009). Cost sharing defined by therapeutic reference pricing as it has been applied in Canada simply involves reimbursement of all medicines within a therapeutic group at the reference price (e.g., the price of a low-cost alternative within the class). Patients who receive a drug within the category that is priced above the reference are required to pay the difference. Though reference pricing has been widely discussed in Canada, our experience with this policy is essentially limited to the handful of drug classes to which the government of British Columbia applied reference pricing in the late 1990s. Research evaluating this policy suggests that reference pricing policies were effective in inducing patients to switch to the reference drug, resulting in a larger market share for the reference medicine and reduced drug-plan expenditures (Grootendorst et al. 2002; Morgan, Hanley, and Greyson 2009; Schneeweiss et al. 2002, 2004). Increased physician visits were also observed after the policy change, likely a result of patients visiting physicians to switch medicines. Yet even accounting for this increase, the policies remained cost-saving (Grootendorst et al. 2002; Schneeweiss et al. 2004). While reference price policies can in theory have the adverse effect of prompting patients to stop treatment altogether rather than switch, research does not suggest that this effect occurred to a significant extent in British Columbia (Schneeweiss et al. 2002, 2004).

The introduction of therapeutic reference pricing in British Columbia in the 1990s was highly politicized, facing opposition from manufacturers, health-care providers, and patients (Kent 2000). This perhaps partly explains why it was not adopted by other provinces and never expanded to additional therapeutic categories beyond the five originally introduced. In addition, while the policy was effective in inducing patients to switch to the reference medicine, it did not act to engender price competition within therapeutic classes. One of the reasons for this, of course, was that if a manufacturer lowered its price to match the reference price in British Columbia, it would have been required to pass on similar price reductions to other provinces, including Québec, which has legislation requiring that firms provide its drug plans with the best available prices in Canada.

Tiered formularies, a different form of therapeutic reference pricing, are widely used in the United States. Under a tiered formulary, patients face higher copayments for drugs that cost the drug plan more; for example, they might pay $5 for low-cost generics in a class, $15 for "preferred brands" (with whom the insurer has negotiated a rebate), and $25 for other, higher-cost brands on the formulary. As of 2007, 91% of American workers with employer-sponsored drug coverage faced at least two cost-sharing tiers for prescription drugs, and 75% faced at least three tiers (Claxton et al. 2007). A key element of these policies is that drug plans negotiate discounts from manufacturers in return for a preferred status on the tiered formulary. This creates a form of competitive tendering that, though less transparent than the competition that might have occurred under reference pricing as applied in British Columbia, is more effective in terms of reducing prices (Danzon and Ketcham 2003). It should be noted, however, that tiered copayments (like the flat copayments described below) are associated with increased patient expenditures and access barriers (Huskamp et al. 2005; Morgan, Hanley, and Greyson 2009; Motheral and Fairman 2001).

Product listing agreements

As mentioned above, the widespread use of international reference pricing has resulted in manufacturers' reluctance to provide transparent price discounts on new medicines in any one jurisdiction, lest that discount affect the list prices in other jurisdictions. Instead, manufacturers post inflated list prices on which confidential rebates are negotiated with individual payers. These negotiated deals—referred to as "product listing agreements" (PLAs) in the Canadian context—allow manufacturers to price-discriminate across payers. They are increasingly common in both the Canadian and international landscapes (Adamski et al. 2010; Carlson et al. 2010).

Confidential purchasing agreements have been used by Canadian hospitals for decades as a means to secure lower prices for pharmaceuticals; however, few (if any) such deals were signed in the community setting until quite recently (Gorecki 1992; Morgan, Barer, and Agnew 2003; Paris and Docteur 2007). Moreover, a recent study found a marked variation in PLA use among Canadian provinces that sets up policy tensions regarding inter- and intra-provincial price equity (Morgan et al., 2013). The largest funder of medicines in Canada, the Ontario government, uses PLAs routinely as part of its drug coverage process, while smaller jurisdictions use them infrequently or not at all. While it is likely that payers with significant purchasing power can generate savings and budgetary stability through product listing agreements, the combined cost of negotiations and correlation between plan size and negotiating power puts smaller jurisdictions at a disadvantage. And, as mentioned above, under- and uninsured Canadians face inflated list prices without the benefit of receiving the confidential rebates from the manufacturer.

Though the confidential nature of these agreements is a significant barrier to further study, much research is needed to determine whether product listing agreements are resulting in the outcomes desired by health-care payers. If they are effective at achieving desired goals such as lower prices or budget certainty, the next question is how best to implement them in the Canadian context, such that patients are protected from inflated prices, manufacturers have incentive to provide the best possible deals, and small jurisdictions are given the same opportunity for savings as larger ones. Once again, our non-universal, multi-payer system of drug financing in Canada inhibits best possible outcomes. Indeed, single-payer systems with universal coverage have the potential to reap the maximum benefits of product listing agreement negotiations while avoiding price inequities and administrative inefficiency. The solution appears to be stitching the gaps in pharmacare coverage to ensure that patients are protected from inflated prices and to increase price equity and collective purchasing power.

Demand-side interventions

Demand-side cost-control tools aim to decrease drug plan expenditures by incentivizing patients or prescribers to improve the appropriateness or cost-effectiveness of medicine use. In Canada, demand-side interventions have been targeted primarily at the patient, in the form of policies that require patient financial contributions towards medicines purchased. We review the most common of the tools—copayments and co-insurance—used in the majority of public and private drug benefit plans available to Canadians. We also discuss demand-side interventions that give prescribers incentives to consider the costs of treatments by way of various risk-sharing arrangements. Finally, we discuss efforts to influence prescribing by way of physician-targeted educational efforts.

Copayments and co-insurance

Copayments and co-insurance are direct payments made by the patient, as a fixed-dollar amount per prescription or a fixed percentage of the price of the prescription, respectively. They apply equally to all prescriptions dispensed, regardless of the cost of the medicine, its relative therapeutic advantage, and whether it is brand-name or generic. Both policies are designed to encourage the rational consumption of medicines by patients. Copayments provide no price signal to the patient and thus are aimed primarily at decreasing the use of nonessential medicines. Co-insurance has a similar purpose but is also designed to incent patients to choose cheaper medicines, as medicines with a lower price will also result in a lower direct patient payment. The goal of the insurer in using both of these tools is common: to reduce insurer burden by incenting more appropriate medicine use or, more crudely, by simply shifting costs to the patient. However, a wealth of evidence on these tools suggests that they result in deleterious consequences for patients and can end up costing more health system dollars than they save.

Evidence has debunked the assumption that patients are able to respond to copayments by distinguishing between essential and nonessential medicines. Rather, copayments and co-insurance act to decrease all drug use, both essential and not. This is of particular concern among low-income populations, for whom financial contributions even as low as one or two dollars have been found to deter use (Gemmill, Thomson, and Mossialos 2008; Goldman, Joyce, and Zheng 2007; Tamblyn et al. 2001). Co-insurance also requires the patient to determine which medicines are the lowest-cost substitutes, even though they often don't have the necessary information on price or therapeutic substitutability to do so. In practice it is physicians, not patients, who decide which medicine the patient will use. Thus, by targeting the actor with arguably the least information to make rational decisions about medicine use, copayments and co-insurance do little to improve the appropriateness of medicine use, resulting only in increased patient financial burden. While these policies do decrease drug plan expenditures, the savings do not compensate for the costs associated with non-adherence to needed medicines. In fact, the evidence is clear that copayments and co-insurance reduce essential medicine use, increase the use of other medical services covered by the public system, and ultimately lead to a net increase in health system costs (Dormuth et al. 2009; Hux and Fielding 1999; Morgan, Barer, and Agnew 2003; Tamblyn et al. 2001). Yet in Canada since the 1990s, both of these policies have remained ubiquitous among public and private drug plans alike.

Physician-based incentives

As the actors within the health system most informed on rational medicine use, prescribers and not patients may be the most appropriate target for demand-side financial incentives. Some countries have used various forms of financial incentives to induce physicians to reduce prescribing costs. Evidence suggests that these policies can be effective (Sturm et al. 2007). For example, in Germany physicians have been subject to regional spending caps (1993–2001) and practice-level caps since 2002 (Busse and Riesberg 2004; Delnoij and Brenner 2000; Mossialos and Oliver 2005; Soumerai and Ross-Degnan 1997). The policies have been proven to reduce prescribing volume and the prescribing of high-cost medicines. Their impacts have not, however, been sustained, in part because political pressures have resulted in relatively major pharmaceutical reforms, including modifications to the budget caps, over time (Busse and Riesberg 2004). Risk-sharing policies targeted at prescribers in the United Kingdom have moved in the opposite direction from those in Germany. In the UK, risk sharing has shifted from practice-level fundholding with hard budget caps towards more regional approaches with soft budget caps on individual practices (Mossialos and Oliver 2005).

There is little experience with physician-targeted financial interventions in Canada. However, Canadian jurisdictions have applied a wide variety of physician-targeted educational interventions. There is also a relatively substantial body of evidence on the various forms of interventions to improve physician prescribing that have been used. Overall findings indicate that academic detailing (sending educators to physicians' practices) and audit and feedback processes have positive impacts on prescribing quality, which would often result in reduced pharmaceutical costs (Ostini et al. 2009). Regrettably, however, the impact of educational activities is not often sustained; unlike independent educational efforts, industry-sponsored sources of information arrive on an ongoing basis through myriad channels, including physician detailing, advertising, and drug sampling.

Conclusion

Canada has a drug expenditure problem. We have observed dramatic increases in spending levels over the past 20 years and persistent wide variations in spending across Canadian provinces. In comparison to all other countries but the United States, it would appear that Canada is overspending on medicines rather than underspending. Worse yet, much of our expenditure problem emerged over a period during which many people (including many readers of this book) thought Canada was getting tough on drug costs by way of a combination of federal regulation and provincial formulary management, including the widely discussed reference pricing policies of British Columbia.

The unusually rapid growth in Canadian drug costs during the 1990s and early 2000s (relative to all countries but the United States) gives rise to some evidence-based hypotheses about what enables effective cost control. In particular, Canada and the United States are the only two countries that lack some system of universal coverage for pharmaceuticals. Non-universal, multi-payer systems for drug financing may not create the same incentives to control pharmaceutical costs as systems with universal coverage. This is partly because in multi-payer systems it is always possible to simply offload costs onto patients or other payers, meaning that the proverbial buck stops with nobody—except perhaps individual patients, who face increasing financial burdens associated with the costs of medicines or private drug insurance.

Multi-payer systems may also fragment the market in ways that reduce the effectiveness of expenditure-control mechanisms. The fragmentation of prescription drug financing in Canada has, for example, limited the extent to which evidence-based formulary restrictions actually change prescribing practices and drug pricing. Too few people are affected by any one formulary to dramatically alter the incentives of prescribers and manufacturers. Fragmentation has also limited the extent to which prescribers and the public realize that prescription drugs are inputs into a broader health-care system, the costs and benefits of which must be considered against other components of that system (Brougham, Metcalfe, and McNee 2002).

These historical problems with fragmentation are likely to become worse as the global system of prescription drug pricing changes. To the extent that historical reliance on cross-national comparisons—by many countries around the world, including Canada—is leading drug manufacturers to restrict variations in list prices and to price-discriminate by way of confidential rebates to institutional payers (Docteur, Paris, and Moise 2008; Seiter 2010), managers of drug benefits will be increasingly responsible for managing prices through reimbursement contracts. Fragmentation of the financing system—even if it were universal—reduces the negotiating power of drug plans, increases administrative costs, and generates intra-national price disparities. The net effect of this is that Canada as a whole will be left paying inflated prices and that some payers within Canada will be systematically discriminated against, including small provinces, smaller insurance groups, and the under- or uninsured.

Virtually all evidence-based arguments about how to bend the pharmaceutical cost curve lead to the same conclusion: there can be no cost control without pharmacare. To manage this component of the health-care system appropriately requires incentives and opportunities that are present only when the system of financing is universal. Ideally, financing for pharmaceuticals would be integrated with other health-care financing such that health system managers and health-care providers would have the incentive to engage in prudent expenditure management, including evidence-based formulary restrictions, tough-but-fair price negotiations, and financial risk-sharing with the health professionals who make critical prescribing decisions.

References

Adamski, J., B. Godman, G. Ofierska-Sujkowska, B. Osińska, H. Herholz, K. Wendykowska, O. Laius, S. Jan, C. Sermet, C. Zara, et al. 2010. "Risk Sharing Arrangements for Pharmaceuticals: Potential Considerations and Recommendations for European Payers." *BMC Health Services Research* 10, no. 1: 153. http://dx.doi.org/10.1186/1472-6963-10-153.

Benefit Partners. 2012. "Generic Drug Pricing Reforms." Accessed 20 September 2012. http://www.benefitpartners.com/images/publications/2012/April%205,%20 2012%20-%20Generic%20drug%20pricing%20reforms.pdf.

Brougham, M., S. Metcalfe, and W. McNee. 2002. "Our Advice? Get a Budget!" *Healthcare Papers* 3, no. 1: 83–85, 87–94. http://dx.doi.org/10.12927/hcpap..16915.

Busse, R., and A. Riesberg. 2004. *Health Care Systems in Transition: Germany.* Copenhagen: WHO Regional Office for Europe.

Canadian Generic Pharmaceutical Association. 2012. "The Role of the Generic Pharmaceutical Industry in Canadian Health Care, 2012." Accessed 18 September 2012. http://www.canadiangenerics.ca/en/advocacy/health_care_savings_f.asp.

Carlson, J. J., S. D. Sullivan, L. P. Garrison, P. J. Neumann, and D. L. Veenstra. 2010. "Linking Payment to Health Outcomes: A Taxonomy and Examination of Performance-Based Reimbursement Schemes between Healthcare Payers and Manufacturers." *Health Policy* 96, no. 3: 179–90. http://dx.doi.org/10.1016/j.healthpol.2010.02.005.

Claxton, G., B. DiJulio, B. Finder, E. Becker, S. Hawkins, J. Pickreign, H. Whitmore, and J. Gabel. 2007. "Employer Health Benefits: 2007 Annual Survey." In *Kaiser/HRET Employer Health Benefits Survey*. Chicago: Kaiser Family Foundation.

CIHI (Canadian Institute for Health Information). *Drivers of Prescription Drug Spending in Canada*. 2012a. Ottawa: CIHI. http://www.cihi.ca/CIHI-ext-portal/pdf/internet/drug_spend_drivers_en.

———. 2012b. *Drug Expenditure in Canada, 1985–2011*. Ottawa: CIHI.

Danzon, P. M., and J. D. Ketcham. 2003. "Reference Pricing of Pharmaceuticals for Medicare: Evidence from Germany, the Netherlands and New Zealand." NBER Working Paper no. 10007. Washington, DC: National Bureau of Economic Research.

Delnoij, D., and G. Brenner. 2000. "Importing Budget Systems from Other Countries: What Can We Learn from the German Drug Budget and the British GP Fundholding?" *Health Policy* 52, no. 3: 157–69. http://dx.doi.org/10.1016/s0168-8510(00)00074-9.

Docteur, E., V. Paris, and P. Moise. 2008. *Pharmaceutical Pricing Policies in a Global Market*. Paris: Organisation for Economic Co-operation and Development.

Dormuth, C. R., P. Neumann, M. Maclure, R. J. Glynn, and S. Schneeweiss. 2009. "Effects of Prescription Coinsurance and Income-Based Deductibles on Net Health Plan Spending for Older Users of Inhaled Medications." *Medical Care* 47, no. 5: 508–16. http://dx.doi.org/10.1097/MLR.0b013e318190d482.

Evans, R. G., K. M. McGrail, S. G. Morgan, M. L. Barer, and C. Hertzman. 2001. "Apocalypse No: Population Aging and the Future of Health Care Systems." *Canadian Journal on Aging* 20 (Suppl. 1): 160–91.

Gemmill, M. C., S. Thomson, and E. Mossialos. 2008. "What Impact Do Prescription Drug Charges Have on Efficiency and Equity? Evidence from High-Income Countries." *International Journal for Equity in Health* 7, no. 1: 12. http://dx.doi.org/10.1186/1475-9276-7-12.

Goldman, D. P., G. F. Joyce, and Y. Zheng. 2007. "Prescription Drug Cost Sharing: Associations with Medication and Medical Utilization and Spending and Health." *Journal of the American Medical Association* 298, no. 1: 61–69. http://dx.doi.org/10.1001/jama.298.1.61.

Gorecki, P. K. 1992. *Controlling Drug Expenditures in Canada: The Ontario Experience*. Ottawa: Economic Council of Canada.

Grootendorst, P. V., L. R. Dolovich, A. M. Holbrook, A. R. Levy, and B. J. O'Brien. 2002. *The Impact of Reference Pricing of Cardiovascular Drugs on Health Care Costs and Health Outcomes: Evidence from British Columbia*. Vol. 2, *Technical Report*. Social and Economic Dimensions of an Aging Population research paper no. 71. Hamilton, ON: McMaster University.

Grootendorst, P., L. Goldsmith, J. Hurley, B. O'Brien, and L. Dolovich. 1996. "Financial Incentives to Dispense Low Cost Drugs: A Case Study of British Columbia Pharmacare." Centre for Health Economics and Policy Analysis working paper no. 1996-08. Hamilton, ON: McMaster University.

Hopkins, M. M., P. A. Martin, P. Nightingale, A. Kraft, and S. Mahdi. 2007. "The Myth of the Biotech Revolution: An Assessment of Technological, Clinical and

Organisational Change." *Research Policy* 36, no. 4: 566–89. http://dx.doi.org/10.1016/j.respol.2007.02.013.

Huskamp, H. A., P. A. Deverka, A. M. Epstein, R. S. Epstein, K. A. McGuigan, A. C. Muriel, and R. G. Frank. 2005. "Impact of 3-Tier Formularies on Drug Treatment of Attention-Deficit/Hyperactivity Disorder in Children." *Archives of General Psychiatry* 62, no. 4: 435–41. http://dx.doi.org/10.1001/archpsyc.62.4.435.

Hux, J. E., and D. A. Fielding. 1999. *The Ontario Drug Benefit Program Copayment: Its Impact on Access for Ontario Seniors and Charges to the Program—A Background Document.* Toronto: Institute for Clinical Evaluative Science in Ontario.

Kent, H. 2000. "BC's Reference-Based Pricing Stirs Controversy." *Canadian Medical Association Journal* 162, no. 8: 1190.

Law, M. R. 2013. "Money Left on the Table: Generic Drug Prices in Canada." *Health Policy* 8, no. 3: 25.

Law, M. R., and S. G. Morgan. 2011. "Purchasing Prescription Drugs in Canada: Hang Together or Hang Separately." *Health Policy* 6, no. 4: 22–26.

Law, M. R., A. Ystma, and S. G. Morgan. 2011. "The Short-Term Impact of Ontario's Generic Pricing Reforms." *PLoS ONE* 6, no. 7: e23030. http://dx.doi.org/10.1371/journal.pone.0023030.

Leopold, C., S. Vogler, A. K. Mantel-Teeuwisse, K. de Joncheere, H. G. M. Leufkens, and R. Laing. 2012. "Differences in External Price Referencing in Europe: A Descriptive Overview." *Health Policy* 104, no. 1: 50–60. http://dx.doi.org/10.1016/j.healthpol.2011.09.008.

Lexchin, J. 1993. "Pharmaceuticals, Patents, and Politics: Canada and Bill C-22." *International Journal of Health Services* 23, no. 1: 147–60. http://dx.doi.org/10.2190/UCWG-YBR3-X3L0-NWYT.

———. 1997. "After Compulsory Licensing: Coming Issues in Canadian Pharmaceutical Policy and Politics." *Health Policy* 40, no. 1: 69–80. http://dx.doi.org/10.1016/S0168-8510(96)00886-X.

———. 2006. "Prescription Drug Expenditures and Population Demographics." *Health Services Research* 41, no. 2: 411–28. http://dx.doi.org/10.1111/j.1475-6773.2005.00495.x.

Morgan, S., M. Barer, and J. Agnew. 2003. "Whither Seniors' Pharmacare: Lessons from (and for) Canada." *Health Affairs* 22, no. 3: 49–59. http://dx.doi.org/10.1377/hlthaff.22.3.49.

Morgan, S. G., K. L. Bassett, J. M. Wright, R. G. Evans, M. L. Barer, P. A. Caetano, and C. D. Black. 2005. ""Breakthrough" Drugs and Growth in Expenditure on Prescription Drugs in Canada." *British Medical Journal* 331, no. 7520: 815–16. http://dx.doi.org/10.1136/bmj.38582.703866.AE.

Morgan, S., and C. Cunningham. 2011. "Population Aging and the Determinants of Healthcare Expenditures: The Case of Hospital, Medical and Pharmaceutical Care in British Columbia, 1996 to 2006." *Health Policy* 7, no. 1: 68–79.

Morgan, S. G., C. M. Cunningham, and M. R Law. 2012. "Drug Development: Innovation or Imitation Deficit?" *British Medical Journal* 345: e5880. http://dx.doi.org/10.1136/bmj.e5880.

Morgan, S. G., G. Hanley, and D. Greyson. 2009. "Comparison of Tiered Formularies and Reference Pricing Policies: A Systematic Review." *Open Medicine* 3, no. 3: 131–39.

Morgan, S., G. Hanley, M. McMahon, and M. Barer. 2007. "Influencing Drug Prices through Formulary-Based Policies: Lessons from New Zealand." *Health Policy* 3, no. 1: 1–20.

Morgan, S., M. McMahon, and D. Greyson. 2008. "Balancing Health and Industrial Policy Objectives in the Pharmaceutical Sector: Lessons from Australia." *Health Policy* 87, no. 2: 133–45. http://dx.doi.org/10.1016/j.healthpol.2008.01.003.

Morgan, S., C. Raymond, D. Mooney, and D. Martin. 2008. *The Canadian Rx Atlas.* 2nd ed. Vancouver: Centre for Health Services and Policy Research.

Mossialos, E., and A. Oliver. 2005. "An Overview of Pharmaceutical Policy in Four Countries: France, Germany, the Netherlands and the United Kingdom." *International Journal of Health Planning and Management* 20, no. 4: 291–306. http://dx.doi .org/10.1002/hpm.816.

Motheral, B., and K. A. Fairman. 2001. "Effect of a Three-Tier Prescription Copay on Pharmaceutical and Other Medical Utilization." *Medical Care* 39, no. 12: 1293–304. http://dx.doi.org/10.1097/00005650-200112000-00005.

Mowery, D. C. 2004. *Ivory Tower and Industrial Innovation: University-Industry Technology Transfer before and after the Bayh-Dole Act in the United States, Innovation and Technology in the World Economy.* Stanford, CA: Business Books.

Nightingale, P. 2000. "Economies of Scale in Experimentation: Knowledge and Technology in Pharmaceutical R&D." *Industrial and Corporate Change* 9, no. 2: 315–59. http://dx.doi.org/10.1093/icc/9.2.315.

Office of the Auditor General of Canada. 1998. "Patented Medicines Prices Review Board." http://www.oag-bvg.gc.ca/internet/English/parl_oag_199809_17_e_9323 .html. Accessed 20 September 2012.

Organisation for Economic Co-operation and Development (OECD). 2011. "Frequently Requested Data." *OECD Health Data 2011.* Accessed 27 April 2012. http://www .oecd.org/redirect/document/16/0,3746,en_2649_33929_2085200_1_1_1_1,00 .html.

Ostini, R., D. Hegney, C. Jackson, M. Williamson, J. M. Mackson, K. Gurman, W. Hall, and S. E. Tett. 2009. "Systematic Review of Interventions to Improve Prescribing." *Annals of Pharmacotherapy* 43, no. 3: 502–13. http://dx.doi.org/10.1345/aph.1L488.

Paris, V., and E. Docteur. 2007. *Pharmaceutical Pricing and Reimbursement Policies in Canada.* OECD Health Working Papers no. 24. Paris: Organisation for Economic Co-operation and Development. http://dx.doi.org/10.2139/ssrn.1329308.

Patented Medicine Prices Review Board (PMPRB). 2006. *Non-patented Prescription Drug Prices Reporting: Canadian and Foreign Price Trends.* Ottawa: PMPRB.

———. 2012. *Application of Price Tests for New Drug Products.* Accessed 20 September 2012. http://www.pmprb-cepmb.gc.ca/english/view.asp?x=1206&mid=990.

Robertson, J., E. J. Walkom, and D. A. Henry. 2009. "Transparency in Pricing Arrangements for Medicines Listed on the Australian Pharmaceutical Benefits Scheme." *Australian Health Review* 33, no. 2: 192–99. http://dx.doi.org/10.1071/AH090192.

Roughead, E. E., R. Lopert, and L. N. Sansom. 2007. "Prices for Innovative Pharmaceutical Products that Provide Health Gain: A Comparison between Australia and the United States." *Value in Health* 10, no. 6: 514–20. http://dx.doi .org/10.1111/j.1524-4733.2007.00206.x.

Schneeweiss, S., C. Dormuth, P. Grootendorst, S. B. Soumerai, and M. Maclure. 2004. "Net Health Plan Savings from Reference Pricing for Angiotensin-Converting Enzyme Inhibitors in Elderly British Columbia Residents." *Medical Care* 42, no. 7: 653–60. http://dx.doi.org/10.1097/01.mlr.0000129497.10930.a2.

Schneeweiss, S., S. B. Soumerai, R. J. Glynn, M. Maclure, C. Dormuth, and A. M. Walker. 2002. "Impact of Reference-Based Pricing for Angiotensin-Converting Enzyme Inhibitors on Drug Utilization." *Canadian Medical Association Journal* 166, no. 6: 737–45.

Searles, A., S. Jefferys, E. Doran, and D. A. Henry. 2007. "Reference Pricing, Generic Drugs and Proposed Changes to the Pharmaceutical Benefits Scheme." *Medical Journal of Australia* 187, no. 4: 236–39.

Seiter, A. 2010. *A Practical Approach to Pharmaceutical Policy*. Washington, DC: World Bank. http://dx.doi.org/10.1596/978-0-8213-8386-5.

Soumerai, S. B., and D. Ross-Degnan. 1997. "Prescribing Budgets: Economic, Clinical, and Ethical Perspectives." *Australian Prescriber* 20: 28–29.

Statistics Canada. 1983. "Quantity and Value of Shipments of Selected Manufactured Commodities (Series R621-770)." *Historical Statistics of Canada*. Cat. no. 11-516-X. Ottawa: Statistics Canada. http://www.statcan.gc.ca/pub/11-516-x/sectionr/4147443-eng.htm#5.

Sturm, H., A. Austvoll-Dahlgren, M. Aaserud, A. D. Oxman, C. Ramsay, A. Vernby, and J. P. Kosters. 2007. "Pharmaceutical Policies: Effects of Financial Incentives for Prescribers." *Cochrane Database of Systematic Reviews* 3: CD006731. http://dx.doi.org/10.1002/14651858.CD006731.

Tamblyn, R., R. Laprise, J. A. Hanley, M. Abrahamowicz, S. Scott, N. Mayo, J. Hurley, R. Grad, E. Latimer, R. Perreault, et al. 2001. "Adverse Events Associated with Prescription Drug Cost-Sharing among Poor and Elderly Persons." *Journal of the American Medical Association* 285, no. 4: 421–29. http://dx.doi.org/10.1001/jama.285.4.421.

Temin, P. 1980. *Taking Your Medicine: Drug Regulation in the United States*. Cambridge, MA: Harvard University Press.

Van Tielen, R., F. Peys, and J. Genaert. 1998. "The Demographic Impact on Ambulatory Pharmaceutical Expenditure in Belgium." *Health Policy* 45, no. 1: 1–14. http://dx.doi.org/10.1016/S0168-8510(98)00026-8.

six

Paying the Health Workforce

PHIL LEONARD AND ARTHUR SWEETMAN

Introduction

Health human resources are central to health service delivery and to discussions of costs and their containment in health care. Concerns regarding the rate of growth of health-care spending and the wage bill of health professionals have been on the policy agenda since the dawn of Canadian medicare.[1] If health care is a "normal" or even a "luxury" good (as opposed to what economists term an "inferior" good), then purchasing more as society grows wealthier is to be expected, and health care may—within limits—sustainably grow as a share of total national expenditures. Since the bulk of Canadian health care is publicly funded, this implies both that tax revenue will grow over time and that government expenditures will increase as a share of GDP. The extremely high level of public-sector debt, however, suggests that we may have reached an upper bound on taxpayer willingness to pay.

Two factors are central drivers of the current push to reduce costs. First, governments' fiscal capacity is diminished. In the absence of change, the 2012 Parliamentary Budget Officer's *Fiscal Sustainability Report* paints a dismal picture, using a formal definition of sustainability whereby government debt cannot grow faster than the economy in the long run. Constraint in public health-care spending is also seen as urgent by Di Matteo and Di Matteo (2012), and Dodge and Dion (2011)—especially given government debt levels.

A second driver is population aging. This has not had much impact on health-care costs and government revenue to this point, since the leading edge of the Baby Boom turned 65 only around 2011. Looking forward, while each year's additional health costs and tax revenue reductions due to aging are individually manageable, accumulated over a decade or more they

---

1 Despite different health-care systems, many developed countries face similar challenges with respect to health-care costs, and a variety of approaches are being pursued, as surveyed in the collection edited by Rapoport, Philip, and Jonsson (2009), which includes an interesting paper by Deber (2009) on Canada.

are very appreciable. Further, the changing demographic profile not only increases the per capita need for health services but also implies a substantial change in the nature of the services required. This in turn implies the need for a change in the mix of health professionals.

Apart from the fiscal sustainability motivations for cost containment, an argument for important cost-reducing changes to the deployment of human resources in health care can be made purely on the grounds of efficiency or "good management." That is, as Duckett (2012) summarizes based on a very large research literature, there are value-for-money rationales for pursuing cost containment independent of the aforementioned motivations from outside of the health-care sector. Productivity growth is probably the central long-term motivation, and also the source of the most beneficial improvements, from the "all of society" perspective.[2]

On the positive side, the Canadian Institute for Health Information's *National Health Expenditure Trends* report for 2012 (CIHI 2012b) announced that provincial and territorial government health expenditure was expected to increase by only 2.9% in 2012—the lowest growth since 1997. However, despite the appreciable cost-cutting efforts following the recession of 2008–09, this "low" rate of growth is still above the long-run rate of Canadian GDP growth, which the Parliamentary Budget Officer (2012) reports averaged 2.6% from 1977 to 2011; he projects that it will average only 1.8% from 2012 to 2086. Therefore, the fiscal restraint of the past few years, while clearly successful, can be seen as only the start of a more extensive process. Since the main cost component of public health service delivery is the wage bill of the health workforce, fiscal deficits have important implications for the future of health human resources—and vice versa.

We organize the remainder of the article as follows: First, the second section provides an economic analysis of relevant institutional structures in Canadian health labour markets. The third section outlines three broad approaches to cost containment and provides an initial assessment of each. The fourth section provides a brief introduction to the international context in an effort to understand Canada in a broader framework. Next, the fifth section explores relevant trends in health human resource supply and real per capita expenditures at the provincial level. Physician and

---

2 Some may view a call for increasing productivity as asking workers to work harder. However, this is clearly not consistent with the evidence, which suggests that long-run productivity growth is about working "smarter," not harder. That is, it concerns the introduction and use of technology, the organization and operation of the health-care system, and the institutional structure of society. Sweetman (2002) is an introduction to some relevant issues.

nurse labour market annual earnings are the focus of the sixth section, with trends in the distribution of earnings explored across census years allowing a simultaneous discussion of changes in earnings inequality as well as in mean earnings. Finally, an interpretive discussion and conclusion is presented in the seventh section.

Institutional background and the economic structure of health labour markets

Understanding health labour markets in Canada requires an understanding of the context as described in, for example, Marchildon (2013). As is well known, provincial governments under the Canadian constitution bear almost exclusive responsibility for health care, with provincial medicare programs as the principal form of health insurance. The federal government's main contribution is through its "spending power," whereby it transfers funds to the provinces to support health care and in return imposes certain requirements delineated in the *Canada Health Act*. Under that Act, provincial governments are mandated to be the exclusive funder of "medically necessary" physician and hospital services (i.e., they act as "single payers"). Payment by patients is banned for these services and there is no price competition. This non-competitive product-market structure turns out to have very substantial implications for health labour markets, particularly those for physicians and nurses.

Almost all licensed physicians are paid by their respective provincial government for all relevant services according to a schedule of benefits bargained collectively between each provincial government (or its delegate) and the relevant provincial medical association. Their economic structure as bilateral monopolies is an essential feature of these labour markets. As is understood from the basic Rubinstein (1982) bargaining model, the party in a bilateral monopoly that has greater success in negotiation is the one with the higher outside option and/or lower discount rate. The contest is, therefore, between the relative strengths of factors such as opportunities for physicians in other jurisdictions, and on the other side, pressure on governments to lower taxes and/or reduce deficits.

Most physicians are self-employed, with the right to bill the relevant provincial government for all services the physicians deem, within professional norms, to be medically necessary. One way for the provinces to control costs is to manage the supply of practising physicians. With consultation, the provinces set the number of domestic applicants admitted to medical schools, as well as the number of international medical graduates admitted to practice. In determining the number of open slots

Figure 6.1 Real per capita total and public health human resource expenditures, 1975–2011

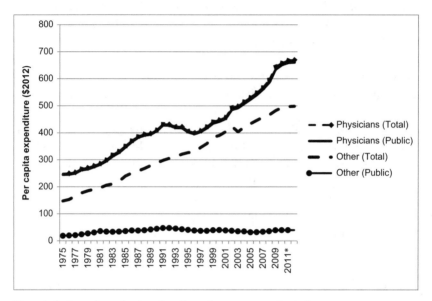

Note: Inflation adjusted using the all-goods consumer price index.
* The year 2011 is a forecasted number.
Sources: CIHI 2012a; Statistics Canada.

for new physicians, provinces balance the health-care requirements of their populations against the need to generate tax revenue or public debt to fund those positions. Political considerations often play a role also, and public-sector collective bargaining frequently has a substantial media component accompanied by public debate. Moreover, even though it directly affects only physicians and hospitals (and thereby most nurses and others employed in hospitals), Canada's single-payer system's influence is substantial. As a result, the affected labour markets are not competitive and what economists conceptualize as the market forces of supply and demand do not operate. Addressing health human resources requires a political economy model quite different from the standard economic models employed for most other sectors. In addition, there is a certain degree of centralized planning within each province but little coordination across provinces.

Turning to the health human resource cost trends that have evolved in this context, as seen in Figure 6.1, the headline observation is the substantial growth rate in real per capita public expenditures for physician billings, but not "Other" professions, and the simultaneous growth in private-sector remuneration for "Other" providers. The dip in public-sector physician expenditures in the 1990s is particularly noteworthy and discussed in the third section. Unfortunately, the accounting system generating these numbers captures only the initial recipient of funds; so, for example, nurses' earnings are not identified but are subsumed in the funding to their employers (mostly hospitals and physicians). Also, total and public expenditures on physicians are almost identical, since non-public expenditures are extremely small. Overall, average inflation-adjusted spending per Canadian for both physician and "Other" private health provider services has increased about two and two-thirds times since 1975. However, *public-sector* spending on "Other" health professions has been much flatter. Although the scale of the plot makes it difficult to see, the public "Other" category increased substantially before the early 1990s, at which point it declined and then flattened out, while the growth in costs for both private-sector "other" and physicians was astounding.[3]

Three possible paths to cost reduction

Sustainability in health-care financing can be achieved by decreasing costs and/or increasing revenue. Although the focus here is on cost reduction, increasing revenue cannot be dismissed. We posit three cost-reduction paths: providing less, paying less, and higher productivity.

Publicly funded health-care service reductions

In the early to mid-1990s, a key approach by which provincial governments contained costs was to appreciably reduce public health-service provision. This included both limiting resources for services in the public sphere and switching some services from the public to the private sector. Reducing enrolment in medical school is an example of the first, which ultimately led to an unacceptable reduction in service provision (e.g., CAPER 2012; Chan 2002; Duckett 2012; Tuohy 2002). Although nominally motivated by an effort to alleviate supplier-induced demand in the context of a perceived physician surplus, as discussed by Barer and Stoddart (1991), actual events seem to have been mostly unrelated to

---

3 The value of health-care spending is notoriously difficult to judge, but it is worth noting that the CIHI (2009) reports that Canadian life expectancy increased from 78 to 81 years between 1996 and 2006. Interestingly, as observed by Eggleston and Fuchs (2012), in this period— and in contrast to a century earlier—most such gains accrued in the post-age 65 years of life. Inasmuch as the growth in health-care costs is buying this increase in longevity, to say nothing of increases in quality, the value for money may be judged by most patients to be substantial.

their set of proposals, motivated instead by fiscal pressures—especially in terms of the duration of the reductions. Also, the appreciable reduction in transfers to hospitals in the early to mid 1990s affected nurses and other staff paid from hospital budgets (see, for example, Figures 18 and 19 in CIHI 2012b).

Given current public perceptions of "doctor shortages," emergency department crowding, and the substantial aversion to increased wait times for various medical/hospital services, it seems unlikely that any policy that reduces the supply of physicians or hospital services will be pursued with vigour in the near future. Moreover, it is unclear that this route delivers long-run cost containment, as evidenced in Figure 6.1 by the return to high expenditure growth rates immediately following the cutbacks and the extremely high rates of growth starting around 2008, near the peak of the business cycle.[4] Even if substantial expenditure reductions in the near future are not feasible through service reductions, nonetheless, avoiding future cost escalation implies managing the number of physicians and other providers, which is starting to trend upward at a rapid rate. Alternatively, tax revenue needs to be increased to fund higher levels of service.

A second policy option pursued by some provinces in the 1990s involved full or partial delisting of several health-care services not covered by the *Canada Health Act*, such as optometry, chiropractic, and physiotherapy (Stabile and Ward 2006). This appears to have had a permanent effect on public-sector expenditures in this area that is reflected in the "Other (Public)" curve in Figure 6.1. However, the magnitude is small. Sweetman and Yang (2012) find that the savings accrued from a mixture of reduced service delivery and increased private-sector payments. Some practitioners, such as chiropractors, saw appreciable earnings reductions.

Overall there is a need for ongoing public policy decisions regarding the apportionment of particular services to the public and private sectors, as discussed by Flood, Stabile, and Tuohy (2006). Managing the public-sector basket of coverage/subsidized services is one way to manage public-sector costs. However, akin to management of the number of physicians, there are relatively few savings that can be had on this front, since the relatively easy cuts have been enacted already. In stark contrast, there are calls from many quarters—see, for example, Duckett (2012) and Grignon and Bernier (2012)—to extend the universal basket of public services to long-term care facilities and other health human resource–intensive operations that could

---

4 Of course, the expenditures in Figure 6.1 combine rates of pay per service and number of services per capita, or total remuneration per provider with the number of providers. Distinctions among these issues will be addressed below.

raise public sector spending appreciably.[5] Undertaking such publicly funded expansions may be in the public interest, but any such move towards universality or increased coverage must simultaneously consider sources of revenue to fund these benefits.

Redistribution among providers and taxpayers

Lowering the hourly (or per service) remuneration of the health workforce is one way to redistribute funds from providers to taxpayers and reduce costs. This occurs on a regular basis in wage negotiations; reductions can take the form of salary caps, as occurred in the mid to late 1990s (see, for example, Kantarevic, Kralj, and Weinkauf 2008). While most citizens do not want to underpay the health workforce, taxpayers also want to obtain value for money and not overpay. Defining an "appropriate" wage in health care is extremely difficult, given that the industry is a highly regulated bilateral monopoly. International comparisons do not help, since other developed countries also have highly distorted health labour markets.

Remuneration in the health sector is also tied partly to moral or ethical issues stemming from society's aversion to (or taste for) income inequality. The recent Occupy Movement, with its focus on the top 1% of wage earners, highlighted this on an international scale. Veall (2012) and Fortin and colleagues (2012) show that the share of national income accruing to the uppermost echelons of the earnings distribution has increased dramatically in the past three decades. Since, as will be seen below, health-care workers form a substantial portion of the top 1%, discussions regarding income inequality necessarily affect them. Of course, wage reductions have ramifications for the international mobility of health professionals, but even in relatively low-wage periods Canada has always been a net recipient of health professionals in global labour markets.

Improved efficiency of health-care delivery

Probably the most important, though also the most challenging, approach to cost containment involves improving the efficiency of health-care delivery. Proposals for productivity-enhancing reforms are numerous, with the extensive literature summarized by Duckett (2012); recent primary-care reforms are surveyed by Hutchison and colleagues (2011), although the expected productivity enhancements remain a promise yet to be verified.

---

5 We recognize that there is already appreciable public funding for the sectors under discussion, but the issue is the fiscal sustainability of any expansions.

Many observers believe that these types of changes represent the best and most enduring approach to cost containment (and quality improvements). However, in practice, while these types of reforms may achieve some of their intended objectives, they often do not produce the expected cost savings. In some cases costs are not a primary concern; for example, Henry and colleagues (2012) illustrate that the primary-care reforms in Ontario did not target cost containment and were associated with very substantial increases in physician remuneration.

Many productivity-enhancing proposals have been advocated over many years, yet few have been broadly implemented. As valuable as some of the proposals may be, the hurdles to undertaking these reforms are non-trivial. On the health human resource side, examples range from changes in practitioner scopes of practice for pharmacists to the introduction of nurse practitioners and physician assistants. A central idea is that practitioners should be operating near the top of their scope of practice; that is, no profession should normally provide what a lower-paid profession can safely and effectively deliver. These changes permit tasks previously restricted to the purview of (especially) physicians to be shifted to others. In some cases it moves the tasks beyond the scope of the *Canada Health Act* and (perhaps) into the private sector. It also frees up physicians to operate nearer the top of their scope of practice and has merit for public-sector cost containment if it can reduce physician services and public billings. However, it is not yet clear to what degree these types of measures are indeed cost-reducing, although they may enhance quality. In the presence of a physician shortage or supplier-induced demand and an excess supply of physicians, such policies may simply increase the total number of services provided across the various health professionals. The behavioural responses of practitioners and patients need to be actively measured at various intervals following a policy change to understand its impacts. It is also useful to recall that, from an economic perspective, if services are appropriately priced, then whichever particular practitioner provides them is not economically relevant; the move to alter scopes of practice suggests that the schedule of benefits may not correctly price high- versus low-skill tasks. However, it may also be that allowing a range of practitioners to perform the same tasks provides leverage in negotiations over the price schedule.

Closely related to this type of approach is the move to team-based care. While this approach holds much promise for quality as well as cost savings, it is not clear that we have gained sufficient experience and institutional knowledge to understand the most efficient manner with which to implement such care. For example, there are coordination costs involved in team-based care, and we do not understand the relative value of the savings compared to the cost of coordination. Also, in the short run, transaction costs are involved in moving from one institutional form to another. This is an area in which ongoing monitoring and evaluation are required to ensure that outcomes evolve as expected. These activities also point to the payer's responsibility regarding system-wide efficiency.

A more broad-ranging approach involves developing an "efficiency culture" in the health-care workplace. This has substantial implications for human resource management since in the continuous-improvement model, efficiency-improving suggestions frequently emanate from the general workforce. Saskatchewan's introduction of LEAN management techniques, which involve staff in reducing waste and increasing productivity, is an example; it represents more active management (or proactive governance) by the province than has been the tradition in Canadian health care.

Increased preventive care and the diligent management of chronic diseases to reduce future health-care costs are important elements of this approach that are just beginning to be explored. Provincial governments are coming to realize that responsibility for patients' long-term health-care costs rests primarily with the province—the payer—and that under Canadian medicare, patients, their families, and physicians do not have sufficient incentives to pursue preventive care in a medically and economically optimal manner. As with continuous-improvement models, this implies the need for more active governance and/or management of the health-care system by the payer/province. Or, taking a stronger view, it requires the development of Canadian provincial health-care *systems,* as opposed to payment mechanisms. Sinclair (2003) argues that productivity gains in health care should be comparable to those in the rest of the economy as advances in knowledge and technology are implemented, and this seems quite sensible even if productivity is difficult to measure in health care. The move to regional and province-wide wait lists for cardiac and cancer care are specific examples of this type of coordinated activity to promote system-wide efficiency. While these efforts are broad, with many clinical aspects, they also have substantial implications for human resource management.

Actions by some provinces, especially Ontario and Manitoba, to alter provider payment mechanisms so as to encourage clinically optimal preventive care are important initiatives on this front. Although Hurley and Li (see Chapter 2) and Van Herck et al. (2010) suggest that the pay-for-performance schemes commonly employed in support of preventive care activities—and within health care more generally—have at best mixed results, this does not take away from the provinces' increasing recognition that as the health-care payers they also have a substantial stake in supporting preventive care, and that there is therefore a need to understand how to design pay-for-performance systems.

Overall, much work remains to ensure that any proposed efficiency-enhancing activities are indeed cost-reducing, or at least lead to cost-effective quality improvements, and this needs to be a high priority for human resource planning.[6] The track record to date, as clearly evidenced in Hurley and Li's chapter in this volume (Chapter 2), is that pay-for-performance in health care all too frequently fails to achieve its goals.

Canada in international perspective

Akin to but slightly more extreme than most Anglo-American countries, Canada has historically had a low physician-to-population ratio, as depicted in Figure 6.2, where substantial cross-national gaps are evident. Of

Figure 6.2 Physicians per 1,000 population, selected OECD countries, 1995–2010

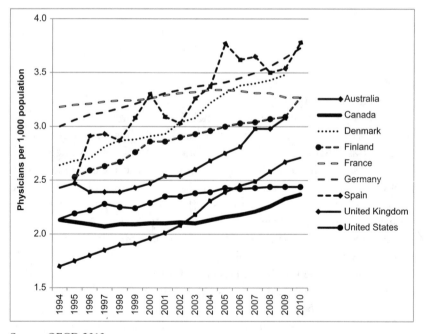

Source: OECD 2012.

---

6 And, of course, there is still much clinical work to be done in establishing best-practice guidelines for preventive care in many contexts.

Figure 6.3 Nurses per 1,000 population, selected OECD countries, 1995–2010

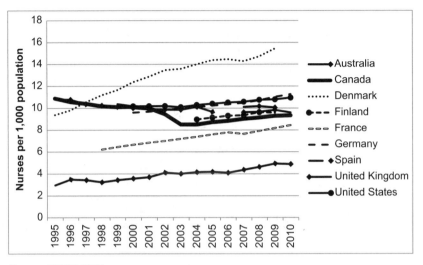

Source: OECD 2012.

course, these gaps do not necessarily imply fewer services per capita, since a simple head count of physicians does not take account of hours of work and norms regarding the allocation of activities within the broader health-care sector. Nevertheless, comparing trends over time among countries can provide evidence on where Canada sits (and where it is going) relative to other countries. Almost all nations in this set are seen to have experienced substantial increases in their physician-to-population ratio, with Canada being a notable outlier, especially in the early years. Starting around 2005, however, Canada begins to trend upward, so that by the end of this time period it has almost caught up with the United States. Canada's constraint has been easing.

In contrast, with respect to nurses per capita, Canada is on the high end of the distribution for the nations presented in Figure 6.3, although Canada trends down over the years under study, with a decline just after the turn of the millennium. For some services, physicians and nurses are substitutes; countries with high physician-to-population ratios tend to have low nurse-to-population ones (and vice versa). However, with the exception of Denmark, the nations in Figure 6.3 did not seem to experience the same dramatic increase in nursing labour supply as was observed for physicians. Overall therefore, the physician-to-nurse ratio is shifting upward in most of these nations.

Provincial trends in physician supply and expenditures

Physician billings are a key element of health human resource costs. To this end, figures for eastern and western Canada (see Figures 6.4 and 6.5) depict physicians per 1,000 population across provinces and over time. Overall,

Figure 6.4 Physicians per 1,000 population, eastern Canada, 1971–2005

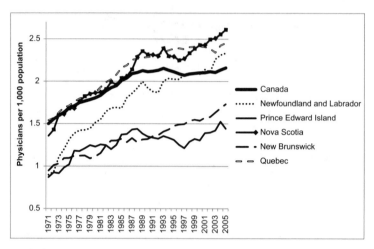

Note: Includes interns and residents.
Source: CIHI 2006.

Figure 6.5 Physicians per 1,000 population, western Canada, 1971–2005

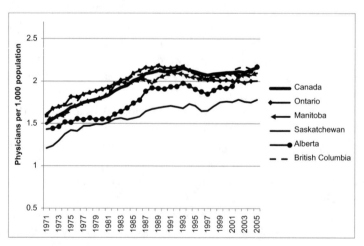

Note: Includes interns and residents.
Source: CIHI 2006.

Figure 6.6 Real per capita provincial public-sector spending on physicians, 1975–2012

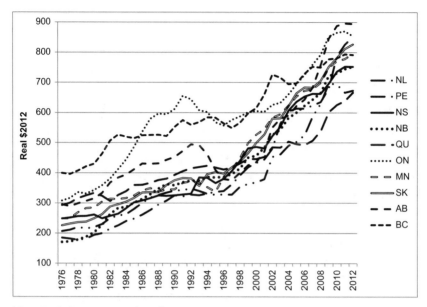

Note: Includes interns and residents.
Source: CIHI 2012.

while there are notable differences across the provinces, they are substantially smaller than those seen across nations in Figure 6.2. Over time, a clear move to increased physician density is obvious from the early 1970s until around 1990 in almost all jurisdictions. Subsequent to this period there is divergence, with some provinces continuing to increase, albeit at a lower rate, while others flatten out and some contract. In particular, British Columbia, Alberta, Manitoba, and Ontario all experience a contraction in their physician per 1,000 population ratio. However, the contractions are never to ratios below those observed in the late 1970s and early 1980s.

Real per capita provincial public expenditures on physicians are presented in Figure 6.6. The contrast with Figures 6.4 and 6.5 is remarkable. Although declines in the early to mid 1990s can be observed for a few provinces, there is a short-lived decline in the rate of growth of physician expenditures in most provinces, rather than a contraction. Moreover, in all provinces except British Columbia and to a lesser extent Ontario, expenditures increase appreciably between around 2000 and 2005, in contrast to the relatively flat profile for physicians per 1,000 population. Moreover, Figure 6.6 extends several years beyond 2005, which is the final year in

Figure 6.7 Real per physician provincial public-sector spending on physicians, 1975–2005

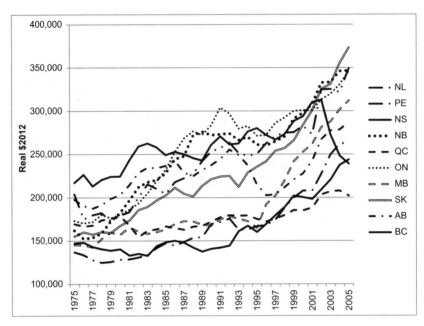

Note: Includes interns and residents.
Source: CIHI 2012.

Figure 6.5. In these final five years, real per capita expenditures increase quite dramatically in all provinces except British Columbia.

Figure 6.7 explores these issues from a different angle by looking at real provincial public-sector spending per physician to 2005. Again there is an appreciable spread across provinces, and that spread appears to increase as the years go by. While there are a few short periods of contraction, overall provincial trends suggest that expenditures per physician are accelerating at a rate greater than inflation, particularly near the end of the decade (see also CIHI 2012a). Overall, these data suggest substantial increases in both real per capita and real per physician public expenditures on physicians over most of the period under study. This points to the redistribution of funds from taxpayers to health practitioners (discussed above in the second section) as a potentially important source of Canada's increasing health-care costs. It also suggests that, much of the time over the past few decades, the bilateral negotiations between governments and physicians have been "won" by physicians, despite contractions associated with the fiscal restraint following the recession of the early 1990s and the public-sector fiscal pressures of that period.

Figure 6.8 Canadian and international medical graduates entering first-year post-MD positions, 2002–2012

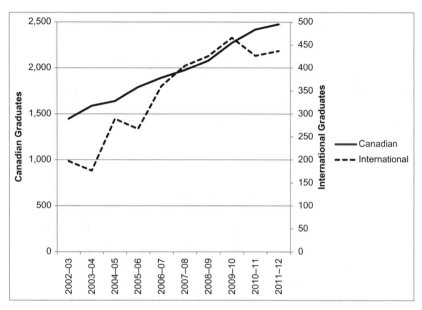

Source: Canadian Post-MD Education Registry (CAPER) 2012.

Looking forward, Figure 6.8 depicts graduates from Canadian medical schools and internationally trained MDs in funded positions in residency programs who would normally be employed in Canada. Both have trended up so substantially in the past decade that it is entirely plausible that Canada may be shifting from the current period of physician shortages to a forthcoming one of surpluses. If this is the case, then physician billings to provincial medicare programs (and other payers such as Workers' Compensation Boards) will increase as in the 1980s. This has implications for other aspects of the health-care system and other provincially funded programs, since hiring new physicians is effectively a commitment to future health-care billings that may crowd out other expenditures. For more on internationally trained physicians, see Grignon, Owusu, and Sweetman (2013). Note however, that a large portion of the growth in physician billings has been growth in billings by specialists, as documented by CIHI (2013), rather than by family physicians. Overall, two of the most important issues in terms of public-sector health-care costs are managing workforce growth and its composition. Given the structure of the Canadian medicare system, outlined above, this is one of the most important areas where policy decisions taken now will have long-term health-care cost implications.

Trends in income for physicians and registered nurses

To better understand the growth in expenditures on health practitioners, in this section we examine the income levels of health workers. We first show the growth and distribution of physician and nurse salaries using density plots and then make comparisons of where health-care workers sit in the distribution of earnings of the entire population.

Density plots of annual earnings

To examine the incomes of physicians and nurses relative to the rest of society—that is, the non-health sector workforce—we undertake a series of simple exercises using annual earnings data from the 1991, 1996, 2001, and 2006 censuses (which are for the previous calendar year), adjusted using the all-goods CPI to 2012 dollars. For each of physicians, registered nurses, and the entire non-health workforce, we examine (the logarithm of) annual labour market earnings, defined as employment plus positive self-employment earnings. Unlike most measures of physician expenditures (including those in the fifth section, which omit non-medicare income and comprise total billings that contain not only take-home pay but also overhead that supports non-physician activities in the practice), the census captures total employment income before taxes. Of course, if some individuals (physicians and others) are self-employed and elect to incorporate their business activities and receive some of their income in the form of dividends as opposed to employment income, then measuring their taxable income becomes more difficult and is not fully captured in the measure employed here. Owners of incorporated businesses may elect to spread the receipt of remuneration across time and potentially distribute some of the corporation's profits to other owners. However, inasmuch as such practices are constant over time, shifts in the distribution of earnings will still be informative.

Trends across census years for the entire distribution of earnings can be observed by comparing Figure 6.9 for the non-health workforce, Figure 6.10 for physicians, and Figure 6.11 for registered nurses, which present density plots of the logarithm of annual earnings. For those not in the health sector, the four density plots in Figure 6.9 have substantial overlap, indicating little change from one census year to the next, although that for 2006 has less mass in the centre of the distribution, more in the left (lower earnings)

Figure 6.9 Gross real annual (ln)earnings for non-health earners, census years 1990–2005

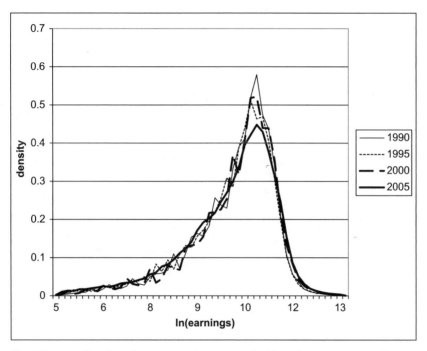

Note: Density plot of total pre-tax employment and self-employment earnings for Canada for all earners not in the health industry.
Source: Census master files.

tail, and slightly more in the right tail. This is frequently referred to as income polarization or, popularly, as a hollowing out or decline of the middle class, with more people at either extreme of the earnings distribution.[7]

In contrast, the density curves for physicians (Figure 6.10) show appreciable shifts of the entire distribution, indicating widespread increases or decreases in earnings. Interestingly, there is a shift to the left (lower earnings) between 1991 and 1996, consistent with the contraction in expenditures observed earlier in the CIHI data; this seems to have hit the entire distribution more or less evenly and is not highly concentrated among the high or low earners. Clearly the contraction reduced not only

---

7 Of course, there are a variety of popular opinions regarding income inequality. See, for example the *Globe and Mail*'s editorial "Hug the 1 Per Cent" (2013). Also, income reflects in part a return on investment, and as provincial governments have increased tuition at medical schools, a greater income is required to offset the increased investment.

Figure 6.10 Gross annual real (ln)earnings for physicians, census years 1990–2005

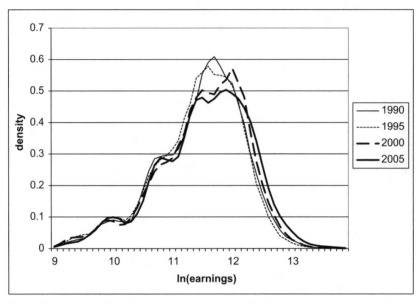

Note: Density plot of total pre-tax employment and self-employment earnings of physicians in Canada.
Source: Census master files.

the number of physicians but also take-home earnings per physician. However, by 2001 this had more than reversed and the inflation-adjusted curve shifted to the right (higher earnings); by 2006 it had shifted even further to the right. In both cases mass appears to be removed primarily from the middle of the distribution, although some is also removed from the left-hand tail. Thus the shifts in the distribution of earnings among physicians and those of the entire workforce outside the health-care sector are moving in quite different directions. Overall, unlike the non–health care population, in inflation-adjusted terms the annual earnings of physicians increased across this 15-year period. Moreover, as seen in Figure 6.6, the largest expansions in physician expenditures started only in the early to mid 2000s, so the shift towards higher physician earnings reported in the 2001 and 2006 censuses may well continue, and be extended, in the years following.

For registered nurses, Figure 6.11 shows annual earnings increases without any reductions between 1991 and 1996. Rather, the entire distribution shifts to the right each year and no mass is lost from the centre of the

Figure 6.11 Gross annual real (ln)earnings for registered nurses, census years 1990–2005

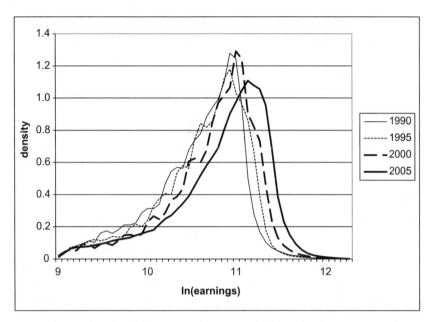

Note: Density plot of total pre-tax employment and self-employment earnings of nurses in Canada.
Source: Census master files.

distribution. Although the CIHI does not capture this type of information regarding nurses, it appears that the incomes of practising nurses—or at least registered nurses—have increased substantially across these years, which is remarkable given that 1990 represents the peak of the business cycle before the cutbacks in health care.

Of course, these plots are of annual earnings and they could be affected by changes in hours or weeks of work or compositional issues within each profession (e.g., an increasing share of physicians might be specialists). The hours issue is explored in some detail in the appendix tables. While there is evidence of a small increase in work intensity for nurses, so that some of the increase observed in Figure 6.11 is attributable to increases in hours per year as opposed to dollars per hour, the work intensity for physicians appears to decrease slightly across this interval. Overall, the plots suggest strongly that the earnings of individual workers in these health professions have increased at a substantially higher rate than experienced by the workforce outside of the health sector.

Distributions and relative distributions of earnings for physicians and nurses

Descriptive statistics of the distribution of earnings for physicians are presented in Table 6.1 in constant 2012 dollars. For each province and census year, the mean and the 20th, 50th, and 80th percentiles of the earnings distribution are tabulated; the results make it evident that the distribution is highly skewed. Overall, the contraction from 1991 to 1996 is apparent, as is the subsequent expansion. Moreover, substantial differences can be observed across provinces. For example, in 2005 the median physician is most highly remunerated in Ontario, Québec, and Newfoundland but mean earnings are much higher in Ontario and Saskatchewan, as a result of the long right tail of the distribution witnessed by the earnings at the 80th percentile in those provinces. Also, in most provinces and particularly since 2000, the 80th percentile is increasing faster than the median, implying increasing inequality in the profession. In contrast, the median-earning physicians in Québec and in Ontario are quite similar, whereas the mean and the 80th percentile are substantially higher in Ontario.

Clearly, characterizing the "middle" of the earnings distribution with the mean, as opposed to the median, makes an appreciable difference to the interpretation and appearance of pay differences across provinces. In total, the observations are consistent with those seen earlier: physicians have seen appreciable real wage increases over the 15-year period, and there is considerable diversity in the distributions across the provinces. However, unlike the earlier plots, this table also makes it clear that the shapes of the distributions also vary markedly across provinces.

A different tack is employed in Table 6.2, where various points of the physician distribution of earnings (e.g., the physician at the 20th percentile) are mapped onto the earnings distribution of the non-health workforce. For example, the 91.0 in the upper left-hand corner of the table, in the 20th percentile row, indicates that in 1991 the Newfoundland and Labrador physician at the 20th percentile of the physician distribution of earnings in that province had the same earnings as the person at the 91st percentile of the distribution of earnings of workers in the non-health sector in the province. In Newfoundland and Labrador in 1991, all physicians above the median (i.e., at least half of the physicians) had earnings in the top 1% of the non-health earners—in other words, well above most income-earners in the province. In interpreting these statistics it is worth recalling the substantial gap in earnings associated with small changes in the percentiles of earnings distribution in the right tail. Within the top one percentile of the earnings distribution, a shift of half a percentage point is associated with an extremely large absolute change in annual earnings; continuing to focus on

Table 6.1 Real pre-tax physician annual earnings, by province and census year (2012 dollars)

Year		NL	PE	NS	NB	QC	ON	MB	SK	AB	BC	Canada
1990	Mean	165,293	179,761	145,843	189,155	150,518	175,086	141,249	152,224	143,277	145,317	159,344
	20th %ile	65,917	75,756	51,792	109,769	67,098	61,842	51,019	55,335	57,204	61,842	61,842
	50th %ile	150,575	142,235	123,683	160,787	139,144	154,603	123,683	131,413	115,953	123,683	139,144
	80th %ile	230,434	278,286	231,906	272,102	216,445	262,826	216,445	231,906	210,162	219,537	231,906
1995	Mean	156,422	169,504	142,557	158,604	150,054	164,125	136,239	176,593	131,527	137,376	152,290
	20th %ile	57,528	107,682	49,309	82,183	68,485	61,637	44,538	68,485	51,879	63,048	61,637
	50th %ile	136,971	144,861	120,818	143,819	136,971	139,094	121,903	145,530	109,577	109,577	134,700
	80th %ile	222,851	250,348	219,153	207,740	219,153	246,548	211,275	246,548	197,237	205,456	226,002
2000	Mean	171,771	155,694	152,543	171,367	166,236	179,903	166,443	175,584	146,954	147,660	166,968
	20th %ile	69,355	56,746	54,224	71,500	70,326	63,446	50,441	75,660	63,051	63,051	63,051
	50th %ile	151,322	158,452	126,102	143,756	151,322	151,322	142,889	157,627	126,102	113,491	141,625
	80th %ile	252,203	252,203	239,594	252,203	252,203	264,813	252,203	252,960	221,343	226,984	252,203
2005	Mean	189,107	136,115	134,975	160,010	178,931	205,977	174,354	204,238	167,052	146,747	182,532
	20th %ile	58,691	48,938	57,062	87,758	69,135	64,552	63,209	70,435	62,644	65,481	64,758
	50th %ile	170,002	125,077	113,335	132,331	163,985	166,325	136,924	147,843	120,611	115,231	146,939
	80th %ile	297,569	213,329	197,427	235,361	263,366	310,551	270,534	304,667	260,670	205,142	274,281

Note: Real annual employment and self-employment earnings.
Source: Census master files.

Newfoundland and Labrador in 1991, the shift from the 99.5th to the 99.9th percentile in Table 6.2 can be seen as the difference between $150,000 per year and $230,000 per year, in the upper left-hand corner of Table 6.1. In total, in most provinces and in most years, the median physician is well within the top 2%—and frequently within the top 1%—of the distribution of earnings for what can be considered the "general population."

Interestingly, physicians residing in equalization-receiving provinces on the east coast of the country (and in Saskatchewan) tend to rank much more highly in the earnings distribution of their provinces than do physicians in the centre and west of the country. Also, compared to the right tail of the earnings distribution, the median physician has fallen slightly, from the 98.6th percentile to the 98.0th percentile, between the start and end of this period. Although more research is required on this point, physician earnings (and public-sector earnings more generally) may be partly responsible for driving the increase in inequality popularized by the Occupy movement and discussed by Veall (2012). Fortin and colleagues (2012, Table 6.1) identify professionals in health as comprising 11.6% of the top 1%, in contrast to professionals in business and finance, who represent only 7.1% in 2006. In fact, the contrast between the substantial increase in purchasing power evidenced in Table 6.1 and the relative stability of physicians within the earnings distribution seen in Table 6.2 raises interesting ethical questions about the public sector's (and the health-care sector's) role in driving and responding to increasing earnings inequality within Canadian society.

For registered nurses, in Table 6.3, inflation-adjusted annual earnings are seen to increase very substantially across the census years. Of course, as mentioned and as seen in the appendix, some of this reflects a small increase in hours/weeks of work. Looking across provinces, some of the differences are remarkable, with, for example, in 2006 the median nurses in Newfoundland and Labrador and Ontario having extremely similar earnings, at $62,300, whereas the median nurse in Quebec made only $51,200. However, in the context of the earnings distribution of their respective provinces (Table 6.4), the earnings of median nurses in Quebec and Ontario look extremely similar, at approximately the 77th percentile of the non-health earnings distribution, whereas the median registered nurse in Newfoundland is located at the 86th percentile of that province's non-health earnings distribution. Clearly, equalizing earning capacity relative to one's provincial counterparts is not equivalent to equalizing the dollar value of earnings! Another interesting observation is that, in general, equalization-receiving provinces appear to pay their nursing staff at higher rates relative to their provincial populations than do provinces where taxpayers make net contributions to equalization.

Table 6.2 Physician income percentiles relative to annual earnings distribution of non-health workforce (per cent), by province and census year

Year		NL	PE	NS	NB	QC	ON	MB	SK	AB	BC	Canada
1990	20th %ile doctor	91.0	95.5	78.3	98.6	87.1	77.5	78.1	82.1	77.7	79.1	80.5
	Median-earning doctor	99.5	99.4	99.0	99.6	99.0	98.6	98.9	99.1	97.4	98.1	98.6
	80th %ile doctor	99.9	99.9	99.9	99.9	99.7	99.7	99.8	99.9	99.6	99.6	99.7
1995	20th %ile doctor	85.5	98.9	78.8	95.7	87.9	79.5	73.0	90.3	74.7	81.5	82.6
	Median-earning doctor	99.3	99.5	99.0	99.5	99.0	98.4	98.8	99.4	96.7	97.0	98.6
	80th %ile doctor	99.9	99.9	99.8	99.8	99.8	99.6	99.7	99.8	99.4	99.5	99.6
2000	20th %ile doctor	90.7	88.4	80.1	91.7	87.9	77.9	75.7	91.3	80.0	81.4	81.4
	Median-earning doctor	99.4	99.6	98.7	99.3	99.0	97.9	99.0	99.4	97.0	96.9	98.2
	80th %ile doctor	99.8	99.9	99.7	99.9	99.7	99.4	99.8	99.8	99.3	99.5	99.6
2005	20th %ile doctor	83.8	82.2	82.3	95.4	87.5	78.4	85.0	87.5	75.5	82.4	81.3
	Median-earning doctor	99.6	99.6	97.3	99.0	99.1	98.2	98.8	99.1	94.5	96.5	98.0
	80th %ile doctor	99.9	99.9	99.5	99.8	99.7	99.5	99.7	99.8	99.0	99.2	99.5

Note: This table shows where a physician from a given jurisdiction falls in the annual earnings distribution of all workers (excluding those in the health sector) in that jurisdiction. For example, the first value shows that a 20th percentile–earning physician in Newfoundland and Labrador (who earns $65,917) earns more than 91.0% of that province's non-health workforce.
Source: Census master files.

Table 6.3 Real pre-tax registered nurse annual earnings, by province and census year (2012 dollars)

Year		NL	PE	NS	NB	QC	ON	MB	SK	AB	BC	Canada
1990	Mean	41,211	31,552	40,059	38,881	44,630	43,188	40,572	41,174	41,979	42,188	42,712
	20th %ile	26,282	18,552	22,861	23,191	27,933	24,575	23,191	24,153	23,191	23,191	24,736
	50th %ile	44,114	30,920	40,914	40,197	46,381	44,835	41,743	40,996	41,743	43,289	43,823
	80th %ile	56,611	46,406	57,351	54,111	60,295	61,230	57,489	58,749	61,225	60,295	59,935
1995	Mean	40,844	34,513	38,618	40,031	45,051	47,610	42,032	43,094	41,000	47,340	45,139
	20th %ile	27,640	20,875	22,340	25,335	28,763	27,395	26,929	26,857	21,916	28,468	27,395
	50th %ile	45,201	34,243	40,399	41,091	46,569	47,939	43,333	44,073	41,091	47,939	46,553
	80th %ile	54,311	51,849	54,788	56,158	60,267	68,485	58,580	58,408	60,479	67,115	62,370
2000	Mean	47,839	41,602	45,242	43,624	49,886	52,900	46,451	49,177	47,673	52,527	50,512
	20th %ile	33,897	29,004	29,004	29,004	32,787	31,526	28,954	33,359	27,743	34,048	31,526
	50th %ile	51,702	42,875	49,124	47,919	51,297	52,963	48,446	51,702	49,683	55,485	51,170
	80th %ile	60,529	56,746	59,320	56,746	65,411	75,660	63,051	64,312	65,573	68,915	68,095
2005	Mean	54,464	46,655	52,708	54,785	49,135	60,303	55,936	56,588	57,037	57,524	56,127
	20th %ile	36,783	29,756	32,039	34,343	30,334	36,071	34,001	36,268	29,200	33,255	33,246
	50th %ile	62,334	50,172	56,104	60,782	51,177	62,328	58,080	61,110	59,067	60,038	57,726
	80th %ile	68,475	65,124	71,544	71,834	65,645	83,364	74,801	73,668	82,530	78,695	77,927

Note: Real annual employment and self-employment earnings.
Source: Census master files.

Table 6.4 Registered nurse earning percentiles relative to annual earnings distribution of non-health workforce (per cent), by province and census year

Year		NL	PE	NS	NB	QC	ON	MB	SK	AB	BC	Canada
1990	20th %ile nurse	59.3	47.1	43.8	48.4	44.3	34.4	43.6	48.9	39.5	38.8	39.8
	Median-earning nurse	77.5	66.4	67.5	69.3	68.1	60.5	67.6	69.3	62.5	62.5	63.8
	80th %ile nurse	86.0	82.9	82.9	82.6	81.9	77.3	83.2	84.2	80.1	78.2	79.6
1995	20th %ile nurse	60.5	52.3	47.6	53.7	49.0	42.6	49.8	53.3	40.2	46.7	46.9
	Median-earning nurse	77.4	71.6	69.9	73.6	71.5	67.3	71.5	74.6	65.5	68.8	68.7
	80th %ile nurse	83.0	86.9	83.1	85.3	83.6	82.7	85.1	85.2	81.6	83.7	82.8
2000	20th %ile nurse	65.0	60.7	52.7	54.6	51.2	43.5	49.2	58.2	42.2	51.3	48.3
	Median-earning nurse	81.8	78.1	74.9	76.9	75.3	69.1	74.4	78.2	67.6	74.3	71.5
	80th %ile nurse	86.8	88.4	83.4	83.7	85.2	83.6	86.5	86.3	81.2	84.1	83.8
2005	20th %ile nurse	68.3	60.4	62.8	64.0	52.7	53.5	58.1	61.1	44.8	54.9	53.4
	Median-earning nurse	86.0	83.3	81.6	86.3	76.2	77.0	81.9	82.3	73.1	79.2	77.0
	80th %ile nurse	89.1	92.2	89.0	91.4	85.7	87.5	90.5	89.1	85.4	88.9	87.7

Note: This table shows where a nurse from a given jurisdiction falls in the annual earnings distribution of all workers (excluding those in the health sector) of that jurisdiction. For example, the first value shows that a 20th percentile–earning nurse in Newfoundland and Labrador (who earns $26,282) earns more than 59.3% of that province's non-health workforce.
Source: Census master files.

Discussion

What actions can provincial governments, which have particular responsibilities as "single payers," undertake to constrain costs and, more important, to ensure value for money on the health human resource side? At the outset it is worth recognizing that there are no easy solutions to rising health-care costs in general and increasing health human resource remuneration specifically. They are both pervasive and difficult to manage. As visualized in Figure 6.1, it is not at all clear that the private sector in Canada is any better—and in fact it might be worse—at managing the rate of growth of real per capita health-care expenditures compared to Canadian governments. Moreover, as discussed in the fourth section, dramatically rising health-care human resource costs appear to be virtually ubiquitous across developed countries.

Three broad approaches to cost containment are discussed in the third section, with the evidence to evaluate the plausibility of each presented elsewhere in the paper. The first involves a reduction in public-sector service provision through reducing services received by patients, and/or by transferring services to the private sector. However, given that this route was an important element of the fiscal restraint of the 1990s, and that the cutbacks and the ensuing restrictions on access to health care of the mid 1990s are still fresh in the minds—and the experiences—of Canadians, there is little room to manoeuvre on this front. Nevertheless, there may be some scope for shifting publicly funded services to, or cost-sharing with, the private sector if taxpayers are unwilling to bear the fiscal burden. However, it is not clear that the private sector would provide better value for money in health care, and there are associated equity implications. Personal cost-benefit ratios might be quite heterogeneous, and the gap between the winners and losers could be large.

Looking forward and focusing not so much on reducing current costs as on preventing future cost escalation, the increases in entry into residency programs (see Figure 6.8) are perhaps one of the most important issues requiring attention. While it seems unlikely that there is any scope to reduce current levels of service provision (in fact there are arguably ongoing shortages), there is a need to guard against future physician and other health professional surpluses and the associated costs, given Canada's single-payer system, where prices need not adjust in the face of surpluses.

The second approach to reducing health human resource costs involves reducing rates of pay for health-care practitioners. The analysis in the fifth and sixth sections of this paper suggests that earnings in the health-care sector have risen substantially in inflation-adjusted terms, and have also risen quite appreciably relative to increases seen in the non-health workforce. For provincial governments this raises not only issues of escalating costs but also ethical issues about income inequality and the public and health sectors' role in exacerbating income inequality in Canada. If the bilateral monopoly model correctly depicts the economic structure of labour markets in the health-care sector in Canada, then the current extreme fiscal situation raises the opportunity cost for provinces and makes it likely that near-term bargaining outcomes will favour the provinces in negotiations with health practitioners. It also suggests that the federal government's 2012 decision to tie the rate of growth of health-care transfers to the provinces to the economy's rate of growth will provide greater discipline for provinces in future contract negotiations.

More generally, if provincial fiscal situations improve, one can expect future provincial governments to acquiesce in negotiations to rates of wage growth in the short run that exceed what is fiscally sustainable in the long run. There is no obvious mechanism to ensure that voters will elect governments that have learned from previous fiscal crises so as to prevent future crises. Moreover, in accord with predictions from the bilateral monopoly model, the short duration of political terms in office does not support long-term planning as part of provincial negotiations. Overall, therefore, reductions in rates of pay for health-care practitioners seem likely to occur in the short run but not necessarily to be sustained if the fiscal situation improves appreciably.

The third approach to cost containment is probably the most difficult but simultaneously the most fruitful. It involves improving the efficiency and productivity of health care—making it more of a "system." Many voices are calling for health human resource changes that fall into this broad category. However, implementation is relatively slow and the challenges are substantial. All too frequently, as outlined by Hurley and Li's chapter in this volume with respect to pay-for-performance schemes, the results of policy changes are mixed and the intended goals not always achieved. It is clearly worthwhile to push forward with initiatives in this class, but it is at least as important to ensure that adequate monitoring and evaluation are undertaken to make sure that the cost-containment and/or quality-improvement goals of each project are actually met. Hard decisions will be necessary for cost savings to be realized. In the end, however, this approach is very worthwhile, since experiments of this type that are successful have the potential to improve efficiency and provide savings and quality improvements that endure.

References

Barer, M., and G. Stoddart. 1991. *Toward Integrated Medical Resource Policies for Canada: Background Document.* HPRU 91:06D. Vancouver: Center for Health Services and Policy Research, University of British Columbia.

Canadian Post-MD Education Registry (CAPER). 2012. *Annual Census of Post-MD Trainees, 2011–2012.* Ottawa: Association of Faculties of Medicine of Canada.

Chan, B. T. B. 2002. *From Perceived Surplus to Perceived Shortage: What Happened to Canada's Physician Workforce in the 1990s?* Ottawa: Canadian Institute for Health Information.

CIHI (Canadian Institute for Health Information). 2006. "Supply, Distribution, and Migration of Canadian Physicians 2005." Ottawa: CIHI.

———. 2009. "Health Care in Canada 2009: A Decade in Review." Ottawa: CIHI.

———. 2012a. "Healthcare Cost Drivers: Physician Expenditure – Technical Report." Ottawa: CIHI.

———. 2012b. National Health Expenditure Trends, 1975 to 2012. Ottawa: CIHI.

———. 2013. National Physician Database, 2010–2011. Ottawa: CIHI.

Deber, R. 2009. "Canada." In *Cost Containment and Efficiency in National Health Systems: A Global Comparison,* edited by J. Rapoport, J. Philip, and E. Jonsson, 15–39. Weinheim, Germany: Wiley-Blackwell.

Di Matteo, L., and R. Di Matteo. 2012. *The Fiscal Sustainability of Canadian Publicly Funded Healthcare Systems and the Policy Response to the Fiscal Gap.* Ottawa: Canadian Health Research Foundation.

Dodge, D. A., and R. Dion. 2011. "Chronic Healthcare Spending Disease: A Macro Diagnosis and Prognosis." Commentary no. 327. Toronto: C. D. Howe Institute.

Duckett, S. 2012. *Where to from Here? Keeping Medicare Sustainable.* Montreal: McGill-Queen's University Press.

Eggleston, K. N., and V. R. Fuchs. 2012. "The New Demographic Transition: Most Gains in Life Expectancy Now Realized Late in Life." *Journal of Economic Perspectives* 26, no. 3: 137–56. http://dx.doi.org/10.1257/jep.26.3.137.

Flood, C., M. Stabile, and C. Tuohy. 2006. "What's In and Out of Medicare? Who Decides?" In *Just Medicare: What's in, What's out, How We Decide,* edited by C. M. Flood, 15–41. Toronto: University of Toronto Press.

Fortin, N., D. A. Green, T. Lemieux, K. Milligan, and W. C. Riddell. 2012. "Canadian Inequality: Recent Developments and Policy Options." *Canadian Public Policy* 38, no. 2: 121–45. http://dx.doi.org/10.3138/cpp.38.2.121.

Globe and Mail . 2013. "Hug the 1 Per Cent." Editorial, 30 January, A12.

Grignon, M., and N. F. Bernier. 2012. *Financing Long-Term Care in Canada.* IRPP Study no. 33. Montreal: Institute for Research in Public Policy.

Grignon, M., Y. Owusu, and A. Sweetman. 2013. "The International Migration of Health Professionals." In *The International Handbook on the Economics of Migration,* edited by A. F. Constant and K. F. Zimmermann, 75–97. Cheltenham, UK: Edward Elgar.

Henry, D. A., S. E. Schultz, R. H. Glazier, R. S. Bhatia, I. A. Dhalla, and A. Laupacis. 2012. *Payments to Ontario Physicians from Ministry of Health and Long-Term Care Sources, 1992/93 to 2009/10.* ICES Investigative Report. Toronto: Institute for Clinical Evaluative Sciences.

Hutchison, B., J.-F. Levesque, E. Strumpf, and N. Coyle. 2011. "Primary Healthcare in Canada: Systems in Motion." *Milbank Quarterly* 89, no. 2: 256–88. http://dx.doi.org/10.1111/j.1468-0009.2011.00628.x.

Kantarevic, J., B. Kralj, and D. Weinkauf. 2008. "Income Effects and Physician Labour Supply: Evidence from the Threshold System in Ontario." *Canadian Journal of Economics/Revue canadienne d'économique* 41, no. 4: 1262–84. http://dx.doi.org/10.1111/j.1540-5982.2008.00503.x.

Marchildon, G. P. 2013. "Canada: Health System Review." *Health Systems in Transition* 15, no. 1: 1–179.

OECD (Organisation for Economic Co-operation and Development). 2012. "Health Policies and Data." Accessed 17 August 2012. http://www.oecd.org/health/health policiesanddata/oecdhealthdata2012-frequentlyrequesteddata.htm.

Parliamentary Budget Officer. 2012. *Fiscal Sustainability Report 2012*. www.pbo-dpb.gc.ca

Rapoport, J., J. Philip, and E. Jonsson, eds. 2009. *Cost Containment and Efficiency in National Health Systems: A Global Comparison*. Weinheim, Germany: Wiley-Blackwell.

Rubinstein, A. 1982. "Perfect Equilibrium in a Bargaining Model." *Econometrica* 50, no. 1: 97–109. http://dx.doi.org/10.2307/1912531.

Sinclair, D. G. 2003. "Notes from the Editor." *Healthcare Papers* 3, no. 4: 4–9.

Stabile, M., and C. Ward. 2006. "The Effect of De-listing Publicly Funded Healthcare Services." In *Health Services Restructuring in Canada: New Evidence and New Directions*, edited by C. Beach, R. Chaykowski, S. Shortt, F. St-Hilaire, and A. Sweetman, 83–110. Kingston: McGill-Queen's University Press.

Sweetman, A. 2002. "Working Smarter: Productivity and Education." In *The Review of Economic and Social Progress: Productivity*, edited by K. Banting, A. Sharpe, and F. St-Hilaire, 157–80. Montreal/Ottawa: CSLS and IRPP.

Sweetman, A., and W. Yang. 2012. "On the Margins of Medicare: Delisting Services from Canadian Public Health Insurance." Department of Economics, McMaster University.

Tuohy, C. H. 2002. "The Costs of Constraint and Prospects for Health Care Reform in Canada." *Health Affairs* 21, no. 3: 32–46. http://dx.doi.org/10.1377/hlthaff.21.3.32.

Van Herck, P., D. De Smedt, L. Annemans, R. Remmen, M. B. Rosenthal, and W. Sermeus. 2010. "Systematic Review: Effects, Design Choices, and Context of Pay-for-Performance in Health Care." *BMC Health Services Research* 10, no. 1: 247. http://dx.doi.org/10.1186/1472-6963-10-247.

Veall, M. R. 2012. "Top Income Shares in Canada: Recent Trends and Policy Implications." *Canadian Journal of Economics/Revue canadienne d'économique* 45, no. 4: 1247–72. http://dx.doi.org/10.1111/j.1540-5982.2012.01744.x.

Appendix

Table 6.5 Nurse and physician working times, by province and census year

Year		NL	PE	NS	NB	QC	ON	MB	SK	AB	BC	Canada
Physicians												
1990	Mean weeks/year	48.4	50.0	48.2	48.4	47.5	48.2	48.2	47.6	47.8	47.3	47.9
2005	Mean weeks/year	47.3	47.4	47.0	46.8	46.2	47.2	48.1	47.4	46.7	46.4	46.8
1990	Mean hours/week	53.7	55.1	52.2	53.1	45.0	49.6	49.0	54.6	50.7	48.3	48.7
2005	Mean hours/week	52.0	43.0	49.0	49.1	44.8	47.7	51.3	49.5	50.9	45.6	47.3
Nurses												
1990	Mean weeks/year	44.3	43.9	44.7	45.4	46.7	45.4	44.6	44.5	43.6	43.8	45.2
2005	Mean weeks/year	47.0	45.0	46.5	47.2	46.0	46.5	45.5	46.2	44.4	44.8	45.9
1990	Mean hours/week	29.9	29.4	30.4	30.9	28.5	30.1	29.5	29.6	28.3	28.2	29.3
2005	Mean hours/week	32.4	30.5	32.9	32.0	29.6	32.9	30.6	32.4	29.7	30.7	31.4

Source: Census master files.

seven

Three Federal Approaches to Cost Containment in Health Care

KATHERINE FIERLBECK

> We decided, as provinces, we don't need the federal government ...
> We run the health care system. This is a process, not an event.
> — Saskatchewan Premier Brad Wall
> (*Globe and Mail*, 26 July 2012)

Introduction

The dynamics of health-care federalism in Canada have changed dramatically. What will this mean for attempts to bend the cost curve? Two quite distinct theories addressing the relationship between federalism and cost containment are prevalent in Canadian policy debates. In Canada, perhaps the most common perspective on federalism is that it is highly cost-inefficient because of the existence of multiple veto points (e.g., Jordan 2009; Pierson 1994; Schaltegger and Feld 2009) and jurisdictional overlap (Banzhaf and Chupp 2012; Rodden 2003; although cf. Brown 1994; Hollander 2010). According to this account, a strong central presence is useful, if not essential, in controlling expenditure (e.g., Crivelli, Filippini, and Mosca 2006; Pedersen, Christiansen, and Bech 2005; Haardt 2013). The contrary argument is that federalism, at least where jurisdiction is sharply defined, can be quite effective in constraining expenditure because of competitive behaviour between substate actors (e.g., Leachman et al. 2007; Neyapti 2010; Qian and Weingast 1997; Weingast 1995).

The larger discussion over what to do about cost escalation in Canadian health care seems to oscillate between these two arguments. Unsurprisingly, each approach is informed by a particular ideological outlook: the left tends to see the merits of greater central control, while the right favours competition between discrete jurisdictions. Of course, the question of whether federal health-care systems in general have a more difficult time containing health-care costs than unitary ones has been with us for some time. And the best answer to this question, quite sensibly, is that it depends upon the peculiarities of the federal or unitary structures themselves: disparate federal systems may have quite different reasons for poor cost containment, while the institutional structure of some unitary states, such as France, may make it more difficult for them to bend the cost curve compared to other unitary states, such as the United Kingdom.

Certainly federal systems have two obvious disadvantages. The first is that 21st-century health care is a complex and interdependent system that works best when communication and coordination are facilitated, qualities not easily attained within an inherently decentralized federal system. The second disadvantage is simply that regional quarrels can distract from other kinds of policy debates, crowding key issues off the political agenda.

The discussion of the relationship between health care, the structure of federalism, and cost containment has become so politicized that it is well worth asking whether there are any gains to be made from such discourse at all. Admittedly, many of the most useful solutions to bending the cost curve will likely be found at a micro level, where the perception of ideological neutrality is greater and political constraints are highly localized. Yet if we remain complacent in thinking that a larger discussion can be avoided completely, we seriously risk remaining "a country of perpetual pilot projects" (Bégin, Eggerton, and Macdonald 2009). Others have described numerous successes with implementing less expensive optimal standardized procedures but note that "unless such programs are ramped up on a nationwide scale, they aren't going to do much to improve health care for most people or reduce the explosive growth of health-care costs" (Gawande 2012, 58). Sound micro-policies and programs are essential, but the capacity to implement them is important too, and that is directly affected both by the larger federal structures and by political gaming, where health care is often as much about the consolidation of power as it is about good policymaking. Thus, despite the frustrating intractability of the discussion about the relationship between health-care cost containment and federal structures or processes, we cannot afford to lose sight altogether of the larger picture.

This chapter examines three broadly different approaches to cost containment within federal systems. As the following section explains, the theoretical perspective that links all three approaches is the insight that institutions and structures matter for provincial behaviour. What is at issue, of course, is precisely how these causal relationships are to be interpreted. The chapter then discusses each of these approaches in turn (federal conditionality, decentralized competition, and decentralized coordination), focusing upon both the logic and the externalities presented by each.

Bending the cost curve: an instrumental analysis of political behaviour in a federal context

In what follows, three distinct approaches to provincial behaviour in health-care cost containment are presented; all have specific approaches to the issue of bending the cost curve, but the mechanisms (and the consequences) of each are quite distinct. Again, while these are presented here as ideal approaches, the way in which they actually manifest themselves in Canadian politics is much more poorly defined. Nonetheless, it is possible to identify a "critical juncture" of change away from the model of federal conditionality that has been in play for decades, and it is important to be able to identify why this shift has occurred, as well as what the consequences of the change may be.

In the first approach, constraints are imposed hierarchically by an overarching political entity. Within Canada, the federal government has in the past directly structured the institutional and political context to influence the behaviour of the provinces. The provinces, in other words, have been accountable to the federal government for the way in which they structure their health-care systems. Historically the emphasis upon conditionality has not focused on cost containment directly (indeed, one might even argue that the emphasis on national standards has been very inflationary). However, exponents of this approach point out that federal leadership is essential for implementing programs (such as pharmacare) and policies (based upon benchmarks or best practices) that effectively have the capacity to bend the cost curve over time. Others might object that it is not correct to say that the provinces are "inferior" to the federal government—they are equal constitutional partners—especially as they have clear jurisdiction over the provision and funding of health care and are legally not answerable to Ottawa in this area. Technically this is absolutely true. However, by committing specific revenues to the provinces (i.e., transfer payments) and by using a legislative framework as the basis for determining the rules of this distribution (the *Canada Health Act*), Ottawa became the de facto principal to whom the provinces adapted their behaviour. This implies a clear hierarchical relationship, and it became the norm in health-care federalism for such a considerable time that Ottawa was generally expected to continue to play this role on expiration of the 2003 and 2004 interprovincial health-care agreements. If any change was anticipated, it was that the federal government would impose even more stringent conditionality upon funding arrangements.

Not only did Ottawa refuse to impose more stringent conditionality, by the end of 2011 it was insisting that the provinces take full responsibility

for the administration of health care, attempts at health policy innovation, and any failure to contain health costs. At this point the federal
Conservatives renounced their supervisory role and attempted to restructure the institutional dynamics indirectly, so that the provinces would face
harder constraints and thus put more political effort into bending the cost
curve individually. This model of hard constraints in a competitive environment is the second approach. And while one might object that "provincial
responsibility" is a misnomer, given that provincial governments are in
essence still directly answerable to their taxpayers, the fact remains that
under this model they are required to keep a much sharper eye on their fiscal
capacity. Within academic literature, much of the theoretical discussion of
ways to restructure federalism to enhance cost containment has occurred
within the school of market-preserving federalism.

The third approach is that of decentralized coordination (or "polycentric governance"). In this instance, governments of relatively equal
formal stature agree among themselves to set objectives and benchmarks
and to account for any divergence from those goals. Communication is
a major aspect of this approach, so as to articulate best practices and to
identify ways in which collaborative action might be useful in restraining
costs. Hard sanctions are rare; the force of this account rests more upon
a pervasive transparency, not only to horizontal units but more widely
to the citizenry itself. Adherence depends upon participants' perceptions
that collaborative behaviour produces greater economic efficiencies without
unduly restricting provincial autonomy. Like market-preserving federalism,
this theory of federalism has become much more refined in the past decade.
References to intergovernmental accountability are not new to the discussion
of Canadian health care; there was limited discussion of the concept in the
development of the Social Union Framework Agreement (SUFA) and in
studies presented to the Romanow Commission, as well as in the Romanow
Report itself, and in the debate over establishment of the Health Council of
Canada. However, the past decade has seen more determined attempts (especially outside Canada) to think about the kinds of structures and mechanisms
that might facilitate collaborative activity in federal systems more effectively.

Conditional federal funding

Health policy analysts view good health care as an end in itself, yet historically it has often been part of a much larger enterprise of nation-building.
Regardless of any particular constellation of constitutional boundaries, a
national government that wishes to construct a policy to strengthen the
national presence will use all the tools at its disposal to do so. It is thus

unsurprising to find the development of a "Canadian" health-care system coming to fruition in the 1960s, when Canada was attempting to define itself more broadly as a coherent political entity. And in the 1980s, during heightened constitutional crises, the federal Liberal administration became attentive to measures that would strengthen the relevance of the federal government in the minds of the voting public. As former federal health minister Monique Bégin recounts (2002), realization of the considerable popular support for public health care in Canada led the federal Liberals to embrace public health care as a means of reinforcing a national sensibility (at the same time neutralizing the more nationalist New Democratic Party). Thus was the *Canada Health Act* (CHA) born.

The two previous pieces of legislation upon which the CHA was based—the 1957 *Hospital Insurance and Diagnostic Services Act* and the 1966 *Medical Care Act*—did of course impose sets of conditions upon participating provinces, but the 1984 CHA (along with the 1995 Marleau letter) effectively codified these conditions. The political battles over these conditions (most pointedly the *Chaoulli* case and subsequent challenges) have been heated, but the conditions themselves have nonetheless remained the formal status quo. Underlying the principle of conditionality, however, is a top-down logic that became unfashionable during the 1990s, when the theory of "new public management" emphasized the need for responsiveness provided by a more bottom-up system. Interestingly, the past two decades of experimentation with regionalization and decentralization have illustrated that decentralizing decision-making often leads to a surfeit of "responsiveness," sometimes manifested as a form of clientelism and sometimes as simple incapacity that resulted in poor policy performance. This has resulted in a concerted move towards greater provincial centralization, driven very specifically by the need of provincial governments to better control health expenditures (see Marchildon 2012, 38–39; Saltman 2008).

The logic underlying a relationship based upon federal conditionality is that it allows Ottawa to coordinate policy design across the country in a way that could maximize efficiencies and thus reduce cost pressures over time. The identification, development, and communication of best practices; assistance in establishing IT systems in diagnosis, treatment, and record-keeping; coordination of purchasing power; and the potential to centralize comparative effectiveness research have all been suggested as ways in which federal leadership is essential to bend the cost curve. On this account, the carrot of federal funding, which allows provinces (especially those with little fiscal capacity) to undertake investment in effective reforms, works in tandem with the stick of conditional funding, ensuring that provinces execute these programs as stipulated.

But there are several problems with such an approach. The first is political: there are few strategic gains to be made by a federal neoliberal administration in buying in to such an arrangement. Taking responsibility for achieving change in such a complex and unwieldy area is a daunting prospect; where costs are potentially high and the likelihood of significant change is low, the idea of a leadership role for the federal government is, politically, not a sound strategic choice. Moreover, any attempt to present a coherent and viable conditional funding strategy requires establishing sophisticated benchmarks and performance criteria that could be viewed suspiciously as excessive state micromanagement by any pro-market governing party.

Such political realities are underscored by the perception of negative externalities underlying a policy of federal conditionality. The first, often cited by provinces in the past, is the distortion of regional priorities implicit in the practice of conditional funding at a national level. If conditions are determined unilaterally by a central body, the nuances and variability of regional needs can easily be overlooked and exacerbated by such a strategy. This does not, of course, diminish the principle of conditional funding per se, but it does emphasize that the practice is a great deal more complicated and uncertain than most proponents of conditionality often recognize. The second problem is overlap, as higher costs can result when measures provided by one level of government partially cover the same area as measures provided by another (Savail 1992). However, others have pointedly argued that the explicit separation of powers has been unable to eliminate overlap in several instances, and that jurisdictional overlap can in fact be quite useful in providing opportunities for debate, increasing government responsiveness, and promoting a wide variety of problem-solving approaches (Hollander 2010). Brown (1994) reinforces this view, pointing out that no Canadian study has successfully proven that overlap actually causes inefficiency, and suggests that it promotes greater efficiency by providing greater responsiveness.

The third issue is that of moral hazard: by committing to any level of funding, some argue, Ottawa may be changing the behaviour of provinces by obscuring the true costs of health care. Kneebone (2012), for example, argues that taxpayers experience "fiscal illusion" because there is a gap between the government expenditure covered by taxes paid by voters, on the one hand, and expenditure supported by intergovernmental transfers, on the other hand. This in turn leads provincial voters to pressure their governments to supply health-care services beyond what provincial taxpayers would otherwise be likely to bear. The theory of federal funding as moral hazard, of course, is highly speculative; provincial health-care spending is the cumulative result of several different factors, and demands by residents for certain services (e.g., keeping rural hospitals open) may not necessarily be tied to consideration of the tax burden. There are also competing comparative accounts (e.g., Switzerland) arguing that fewer deficits occur when a sub-national region is more dependent upon intergovernmental transfers (Freitag and Vatter 2008). Moreover, there is the not insignificant normative argument that provinces that receive interprovincial transfers have a right to make demands that are beyond their capacity to support, simply because this underscores the principle of intergovernmental equalization articulated in section 36(2) of the Canadian Constitution.

Regardless of the academic debate over the utility of federal conditionality, the idea that the federal relationship can be used effectively to control costs through the mechanism of conditional funding has little support in a neoliberal administration. Continued exhortations that Ottawa return to this role may be useful in a constructivist sense, but there is little possibility that it will have much impact upon the key policymakers themselves. On the contrary, the theoretical logic underlying the federal Conservatives' approach to health care is based on the assumption that the market is a much more formidable disciplinarian than any government could be. In this account the objective is to rework the structures of federalism so that provincial governments become more answerable to their electorates for how effectively health-care resources are used.

Hard(er) constraints: Decentralized competition

If you assume that "government spending responds more strongly to an extra dollar of income received by way of intergovernmental transfers than it does to an extra dollar of income received from voters" (Kneebone 2012, 22), then you are likely to see shared-cost programs as a significant liability for cost containment. From this perspective, the solution for cost escalation involves modifying the behaviour of provincial governments by isolating their fiscal responsibilities and imposing harder economic constraints on them. This reduces moral hazard and puts the pressure for cost containment directly on the provinces.

An offshoot of the Virginia School of economics (perhaps best known to political scientists for its espousal of constitutional limits on government spending), the theory of market-preserving federalism posits that federalism be used to achieve and maintain a propitious economic environment. As Weingast (1995) suggests, the strategy is to use the structure of federalism to impose competition between sub-national units and to force them to compete by imposing "hard budget constraints" upon them (e.g., no bailouts from the federal government to compensate for overspending). The theory was originally designed to promote economic growth in developing economies such as China and India. Weingast and his colleagues have distilled the principles of market-preserving federalism down to the following five ideal conditions, the first two of which are based on Riker's definition of federalism (1964, 11):

1. A hierarchy of governments with a delineated scope of authority (for example, between the national and subnational governments) exists so that each government is autonomous within its own sphere of authority.
2. The subnational governments have primary authority over the economy within their jurisdictions.
3. The national government has the authority to police the common market and to ensure the mobility of goods and factors across subgovernment jurisdictions.
4. Revenue sharing among governments is limited and borrowing by governments is constrained so that all governments face hard budget constraints.
5. The allocation of authority and responsibility has an institutionalized degree of durability so that it cannot be altered by the national government either unilaterally or under the pressures from subnational governments. (Montinola, Qian, and Weingast 1995, 55; see also Weingast 1995, 4)

To what extent do these conditions obtain in Canada? Proponents have argued that, while there is some overlapping of jurisdiction between Ottawa and the provinces, the country's constitution has often been said to be based upon the principle of "watertight compartments." And while the federal government has specific jurisdiction over certain aspects of the economy, provincial governments do have clear authority to tax their citizens and to make decisions governing the economic management of their polities. The need for a clear division of authority also explains the current federal government's position that health care is under provincial jurisdiction and that provinces must therefore take full responsibility for the implementation of health care within their borders

The third point is somewhat more contentious. While Ottawa does have constitutional authority over the regulation of trade and commerce, currency, and banking, the provinces maintain authority over regional regulation of various industries and professions. This has resulted in substantial barriers to a Canadian "common market." Although some of the barriers have been reduced (especially in the 1995 Agreement on Internal Trade), there remain significant obstacles to interprovincial trade. After winning a majority government in 2011, Prime Minister Harper outlined a new approach to intergovernmental relations. A key point was having Ottawa play "a more active role in promoting the economic union," particularly by "tearing down the walls of provincial interest" that hampered the growth of the economy (Curry, Scoffield, and Perkins 2012, A1, A4). More recently these measures include renewed efforts to establish a national securities regulator and a proposal to allow federally incorporated credit unions that can operate more efficiently across provincial boundaries.

The fourth point—the imposition of "hard budget constraints"—is reflected in unilateral changes made not only to the total amount of health-care transfers but also, more importantly, to the way in which those transfers are calculated (i.e., on an equal per capita basis). Arguably the current funding structure hardly meets the requirement for "hard" budget constraints, which is simply not a political option in Canada. Moreover, provinces can raise additional revenues to change their budget constraints, although the point of inducing competition between units is that there are both economic and political limits to doing so. Nonetheless, the new pure per capita funding structure for the Canada Health Transfer (CHT), which will be implemented in 2014–15, does impose greater fiscal pressures on all the provinces (except Alberta, which will be the only province to see an increase in its cash CHT transfer as a result of this change). As the Office of the Parliamentary Budget Officer (2012) outlines, the projected average growth in CHT cash transfers to provinces (with the exception of Alberta) is less than the projected growth in health spending. Moreover, Ottawa has increasingly been offloading health-care costs to the provinces in several areas, such as immigrants' health-care benefits. When asked how the provinces could cope with cuts in federal funding just as they were entering a period of deep austerity, the prime minister replied that provincial affairs were not his concern (Curry, Scoffield, and Perkins 2012, A1, A4).

The dynamic underlying the theory of market-preserving federalism is that, because sub-national units can no longer depend on intergovernmental transfers, they must rely more heavily on direct taxation within their own jurisdictions. Such an approach in a common market leads, *ceteris paribus*, to capital flight, thus restricting economic growth even further. Thus, as Qian and Weingast (1997) argue, the jurisdictional competition between federal units itself imposes a kind of hard constraint upon public spending. Given that health care constitutes such a large proportion of provincial expenditure, the impact of such structural constraints on health care cannot be avoided. As a consequence, most provinces face some stark choices: they can continue to provide the same level of health services despite reduced capacity to do so, by engaging in greater deficit spending (leading to even less long-term capacity); they can restrict public services while continuing to limit access to private payment systems for health care and health insurance (likely leading to greater public dissatisfaction); or they can restrict public services while allowing easier access to private payment systems. Given that these decisions are made by provincial governments individually, there is little reason to hold Ottawa responsible for any movement towards greater privatization of health care.

To what extent has federal behaviour been a deliberate attempt to impose market-preserving federalism, or is it simply an extension of the federal Conservatives' stated commitment to "open federalism"? The fundamental premise of open federalism is clarity of (and respect for) the constitutional jurisdiction of each province in specific policy areas, regardless of outcome. Market-preserving federalism, on the other hand, is the application of open federalism only in specific areas—Ottawa willingly encroaches on provincial jurisdiction when the goal is enhancing the economic union—and with a particular purpose in mind, such as achieving and maintaining a market-friendly environment. Overall, the intellectual basis of the Conservatives' current economic strategies seems to fit better with the school of market-preserving federalism than with that of open federalism.

The principal objection to market-preserving federalism vis-à-vis health policy is that it seems to be a poor fit for cost containment in health care, which is (and has been for decades) accepted by most health economists as something rather distinct and *sui generis* relative to other goods and services. Again, the logic of competitive federalism holds that strengthening a national common market and constraining access to fiscal resources require provinces to compete for limited skills and capital. It is fairly easy to understand how this logic contributes to a reduction in public spending per se, but how effective is it in achieving cost containment in health care? The obvious problem is that the most politically palatable means of reducing public spending on health care may be to offload it to the private sector, which in the absence of effective regulation leads to higher overall spending. Yet another way in which a more competitive federal structure increases costs rather than decreasing them is by encouraging rent-seeking behaviour on the part of professionals whose skills are highly in demand. Discrete jurisdictions competing for scarce medical personnel will simply attempt to outbid each other; those with greater resources will have more success in obtaining those personnel but less success in bending the cost curve.

The effectiveness of such disengaged federalism depends largely on estimation of dependence on transfers as a major driver of health-care expenditure. But if this cost driver is only one among many—to the extent that it exists in any significant form at all—then "open" or "market-preserving" federalism merely eliminates moral hazard without addressing any other underlying cost drivers. It also produces greater disparities between provinces and can lead to escalation in the cost of limited health-care resources. There is also the objection that the emphasis on discrete jurisdictions is increasingly an ill fit with the very nature of contemporary health care. To the extent that both open and market-preserving federalism must assume the existence of clearly delineated spheres of authority ("watertight compartments") to work effectively, they are a poor fit with the sprawling and interconnected nature of modern health-care provision. From determination of best practices and increasing dependence on IT systems to coordination of projected health human resource needs, very few cost drivers can be effectively contained at an isolated level, especially for less populous and less wealthy Canadian provinces.

Looking sideways: Decentralized coordination

The idea of horizontal accountability as a mode of cost containment is counterintuitive. Unlike hierarchical ("command and control") or competitive versions, which depend on firm conditionality and hard fiscal constraints, this approach holds that a softer and more diffuse manifestation of accountability can in fact produce more significant results. Approaches based on the principle of "polycentric" (Ostrom 2009; Tollefson, Zito, and Gale 2012) or "plurilateral" (Zielonka 2007) governance begin with a different set of premises. Provocatively, these accounts loosen—and even sever—the link between behaviour and consequence. The key here is that the immediate objectives are in this approach somewhat different from simply enforcing behaviour. Rather, the emphasis is more upon securing participation per se when a more stringent approach would simply reinforce isolation. This approach can be useful, for example, in conditions of stalemate or radical uncertainty (Sabel and Zeitlin 2008, 208). Importantly, it attempts to minimize the opportunity costs of participation. The focus in the first place tends to be on knowledge sharing, voluntary performance standards, accommodation of diversity (e.g., accepting different objectives or strategies for different actors), flexibility and revisability, and experimentation. There are no strict demands to which participants must adhere, but they are required to articulate their positions and their justifications: at the very least, they are obliged to acknowledge the "potential externalities of their political preferences" and to explain why these costs to others are nonetheless justifiable (Ebenstein and Kerwen 2004, 129). The direct consequences to themselves are minimal to negligible, but there is nonetheless a relatively strong requirement of accountability insofar as actors are "held to account" and must articulate an explicit defence of their behaviour—a feature that is notably lacking in the other approaches discussed. Whether and to what extent this approach can actually facilitate political change is the subject of a lively debate in political science between institutional realists and institutional constructivists (see, e.g., Bell 2011; Blyth 2002; Hay 2004; Schmidt 2008, 2010). But there are arguably areas in which more traditional approaches to accountability do not work particularly well. As Scott and Trubek describe, these are areas of increasing complexity and uncertainty, often coupled with rapid and unpredictable change; "irreducible diversity" between participants or jurisdictions; and often "competence creep," where those bodies best equipped to deal with an issue simply do not enjoy the legal jurisdiction to do so (2002, 6–7) .

The specific forms of this decentralized coordination are quite varied. As the organizational and jurisdictional issues mirror those of Canada in many ways, the discussions over social policy within the European Union may be relevant to discussions of the Canadian social union. The focus on polycentric governance in the European Union has exploded in the past two decades. It has been driven by, first, the need to coordinate policy areas in a federal system in which much jurisdiction remains with member states (precluding federal policymaking), and second, the neoliberal structure of the European Union itself, the raison d'être of which is primarily achievement of an effective common market. For political reasons—including the fears of member states that they were losing the ability to maintain stable control over public services such as health care—many attempts were made to think about coordinating non-economic policymaking (especially social policy) to deal with legislative uncertainty in these areas, and to forestall competition between member states that could lead to serious negative spillover effects. Even the formal units of the European Community began to recognize the utility of these approaches; in 2001, for example, the European Commission published a white paper on governance that noted the way in which "softer" forms of governance could achieve policy goals (2001, 428).

The past few years have seen a wave of publications focusing on evaluation of these various methods (e.g., de Búrca 2010; Carrigan and Coglianese 2011; Greer 2011; Mendez 2011; Tollefson, Zito, and Gale 2012). No meta-survey of these articles has yet been published, but certain observations can be discerned. One conclusion is that the wider the policy area, the less success there is in achieving policy change. The formal Open Method of Coordination (OMC) in health policy was in 2006 amalgamated into a "social inclusion" OMC that incorporated planning on pensions and long-term care. While the rationale for this move was to take advantage of synergies among the three areas, there is little evidence that considerable achievements have been made (see, e.g., Kröger 2011). At the same time, however, there is evidence that the development of policy networks was instrumental in the development of very specific policy goals across the European Union, including cooperation on rare diseases (Greer 2011), HIV/AIDS policy (Steffen 2012), and cancer-care policy. The more specific the policy field and the more widespread the support, the more likely coherent policy development will occur. As Greer notes, "[b]y drawing on smaller networks with clearer preferences, more specific data concerns, greater lobby support, and professional engagement, [this kind of specific sectoral initiative] can create coordination and rule-making where there were only informal shared ideas" (Greer 2011, 198). This underscores earlier evidence that moving decision-making into the realm of functional specialties, where possible, constrains the capacity of "high politics" to hinder decision-making (Peters 1997).

Despite the economic turmoil present in Europe over the past few years, which has overshadowed most discussions of social policy development, these experiments with new forms of government have provided modest but real results in some areas under specific conditions. The basic rules of politics still apply: when parties are clearly and firmly opposed to policy development, the possibility of success is negligible. But when parties stand to gain from cooperation, and when experts and policy navigators with experience in the field are willing to guide discussions, the likelihood of policy collaboration is much more positive. This is not necessarily reduced to simple rational calculations of individual gain.

There is very little theoretical discussion of these new approaches in Canadian health policy, even though there is some precedent for the use of "soft" governance in health policy in Canada. The unexpected decision by Ottawa to offload cost containment to the provinces in the mid 1990s was the critical juncture that led to several different horizontal proposals for health-care governance. As many have argued, when shifting policy formation to softer forms of governance, crisis appears to be a "necessary factor" (e.g., Steffen 2012, 19). In 1995 the perception of crisis was quite apparent. "That the provinces would shoulder two-thirds of the increase in the deficit arising from a major recession," notes Courchene, was "unprecedented in modern Canadian fiscal history, and probably in the fiscal history of any federation" (2006, 16).

The first clear articulation of a provincial response to Ottawa's 1995 budget proposal was the Report to the Premiers, published by the Ministerial Council on Social Policy and Renewal (1995), which called for greater clarity in the roles and responsibilities of federal and provincial governments, especially in the area of social policy. Following soon after, Thomas Courchene, at the request of the Ontario government, produced two models of federalism (the ACCESS models) that reconsidered the economic and social relationship between federal and provincial governments. What is remarkable is how inconceivable those models were seen to be at the time, especially in comparison to the much more extensive de facto provincial autonomy over health care that now exists. Courchene's most radical option, for example, contained an enforceable pan-provincial accord (excluding Ottawa) that set out overarching principles and national standards, as well as an equalization program that guaranteed sufficient redistribution between provinces to allow reasonably comparable services across the country (Courchene 1997). Intriguingly, one of the biggest obstacles to possible implementation of such a plan was seen to be the intransigence of the federal government in surrendering its role (Maioni 1999). Another was the observation that some provinces would be unwilling to limit their autonomy to the extent that would be required by an enforceable accord or equalization plan (Maioni 1999; Richards 1999).

Three years later, a second negotiation attempted to accommodate federal participation. The Social Union Framework Agreement (SUFA), ratified (with the exception of Québec) in 1999, established a normative and a procedural armature for an intergovernmental approach to social policy. The procedural aspect (including the exercise of federal spending power and development of an intergovernmental dispute avoidance and resolution mechanism) received a great deal of initial attention. But the normative aspect of the agreement is also quite remarkable, as it clearly articulates a different kind of accountability than that implied by models such as ACCESS. In addition to setting out a reconfirmation of CHA values, the document outlined an approach to accountability that looked beyond the more traditional approach—each level of government being responsible to its citizenry within well-defined spheres of jurisdiction—and instead discussed it as involving the willingness of both levels of government to commit to greater transparency and accountability towards each other and to Canadians of all regions.

The design of SUFA led some commentators to note the possibilities of reform contained in the plan. The minister of human resources, Pierre Pettigrew, saw SUFA as an opportunity to "reinvent the country" (Canadian Council on Social Development 2002, 6), while Lazar observed that SUFA had "the potential to be the most far reaching reform in the workings of the federation since the changes associated with the Constitution Act, 1982" (2002, 1). But SUFA fell victim to a common paradox of potential transformation: the provinces held that it would have no transformational power unless it was tied to significant federal spending (Lazar 2002, 3), while it was the infusions of federal cash negotiated in 2000, 2003, and 2004 that effectively neutralized any political will for radical change.

What we have at present seems to be negation of the only viable options available for bending the cost curve. On the one hand, there are no enforceable sanctions (as ACCESS outlined); on the other hand, there is no leadership role for Ottawa. Is the resulting state of disarray and discontinuity destined to failure? Not necessarily. There are several advantages to a pluri-lateral strategy: First, it is more likely to secure provincial participation, for the very reason that it does not require a formal co-decision process; the ability to compel behaviour is consequently low, but at least there remains a forum for discussion. Second, the lack of direct federal participation shifts provinces' strategizing away from merely securing more funding to a much more substantive discussion of how existing funding can be made to work better. Third, it avoids the tired mantra that all that is required is clear delineation of matters into either federal or provincial jurisdiction. The problem is that effective health care is no longer a policy area that can be addressed by individual jurisdictions—especially the smaller ones—in isolation. What is needed are processes that accommodate this reality, not ones that attempt to assume it away. A complex and slightly messy model of accountability, in other words, could be a more accurate representation of how health care actually works.

Can Canadian health-care federalism exist without enforceable accountabilities?

Two phenomena marked the end of the regime of federal conditionality. The first was the announcement by the federal minister of finance in December 2011 that federal transfers would be linked to the country's rate of economic growth; that funds would be calculated on a strict per capita basis; and that beyond that, Ottawa would leave policy development to the provinces themselves. This seemed to augur a shift from strict federal conditionality to a regime of no accountability. Yet by placing clear limits on transfers (which did not address the trend of cost escalation in health care), by underlining provinces' jurisdictional responsibility for health care, and by reinforcing a more efficient economic union, the regime change was in fact a move from one form of hard constraints (federal conditionality) to another (the market).

The second notable occurrence was the decision by the provinces to fill the "policy leadership gap" left by Ottawa with a pan-provincial approach. In January 2012, through the mechanism of the Council of the Federation (COF), the provinces established the Health Care Working Group "to identify innovations in health delivery that could be shared across Canada." Six months later the group published a report that focused on specific recommendations for clinical practice (chronic-care guidelines for cardiovascular disease and foot ulcers caused by diabetes); team-based health-care provision; health human resource initiatives; and the purchasing of generic drugs. Commentators' reactions were mixed, ranging from congratulatory to dismissive. The position of the latter—that the strategy fell well short of what was needed to overhaul the fundamental structural problems of health care in Canada—focused not only on the limited measures that were being taken but also on the fact that they were not happening quickly or forcefully enough.

There are many who agree with Gibbins (1996,10) that "[i]nterprovincial agreements as an effective substitute for Parliamentary action are a mirage." Bolleyer, for example, holds that "intergovernmental agreements set up within the weakly institutionalized Canadian arrangements usually do not transcend position taking against federal plans or the demand for more funds" (2006, 473), while Brock goes even further and declares that the "philosophy embraced by the COF" would lead inexorably to a self-interested regime of intergovernmental relations that would destroy any sense of national unity (2008, 140). The assumption common to these positions is that the only states that will succeed in formulating satisfactory social policy regimes are those that can control and enforce substate behaviour, or those that have strongly integrated co-determination processes. This criticism, however, ignores the numerous bodies recently established in the field of health care—such as CADTH, CIHI, the Health Council of Canada, Canadian Blood Services, and the Canadian Partnership Against Cancer—that perform limited but productive roles in coordinating health services. It also sees the function of coordinating bodies to be overarching, that is, providing extensive policy development across many health-care fields, and compulsory.

But one must ask whether hierarchical control and strong co-determination processes are the best means of achieving cost containment. If bending the cost curve depends on innovative practices—doing things differently—then this may be precisely the wrong strategy. A regime of hard constraint does not seem well designed for a policy field that is by nature diffuse, overlapping, and built to accommodate and even encourage rapid change in treatment options. Hard constraints can be simply counterproductive when imposed under the wrong conditions. Competitive pressures between provinces to lower overall costs, for example, can lead to short-sighted and mutually defeating short-term strategies. Moreover, stringent directives from Ottawa can impede policy development and coordination by distorting priorities, facilitating moral hazard, and allowing provinces to focus on securing funding rather than redesigning policy.

Proponents of hard constraints in the form of conditional federal funding are not incorrect in arguing that they can play an important role in preserving the geographical equity of health care across Canada. A larger question, of course, is the degree to which transnational equity in health care—the concept of a social union—is still important to Canadians, and especially to those in the more populous and wealthier provinces. A separate and distinct issue is the extent to which these hard constraints can ensure equitable health care for Canadians *within* each discrete province. To the extent that one defends the decommodification of health care, hard constraints of this kind are very important indeed, and a key responsibility for any federal government. But what needs to be stressed here is that this federal activity is, at least for the present, simply not forthcoming. The issue, then, is whether coordinated activity, however limited, is better than disjointed policymaking.

Skepticism towards any attempt at pan-Canadian policymaking that does not involve hard constraints has been a common theme in discussions about Canadian federalism, and it has generally been well supported. But the contours of both policy and politics change over time. Within the field of health policy, the movement away from hierarchical structures in government has been developing for years. For example, the provision of health services is increasingly focusing on inter-professional collaborative health teams. Organizational and management theory has for decades grappled with the problem of how to operationalize the ideas presented first by proponents of general systems theory (Bertalanffy 1968), and later by more refined versions such as complex adaptive systems (Ford 2008), for the provision of complex health-care provider teams. Another notable shift in health policy has been greater utilization of policy networks in the field of health care. Network governance is not a new trend, but the principles underlying it—structured relationships that transcend the formal institutions of representative government, the absence of clear hierarchy, and the use of bargaining over the exercise of centralized authority (Farrelly, Jeffares, and Skelcher 2010, 89)—have proven to be productive frameworks for effective policy development and execution.

Scholars of federalism, especially health-care federalism, must carefully consider not only the ways in which the traditional institutional structures and processes of federalism influence health care but also the ways in which 21st-century health care is changing how we think about those institutions and processes. As P.-G. Forest notes in Chapter 8, the complexity and interdependency of contemporary health care require a different kind of organizational structure than the traditional linear Weberian model of bureaucratic government, and certainly a different kind of federalism than the myth of watertight compartments supports. Much more policy development in health care is accomplished through voluntary and informal processes than ever before. This includes both the relationships between provinces and the use of commercial and private not-for-profit organizations to provide specialized policy capacity (see Atkinson et al. 2013, especially 49–52). In health care, the use of nongovernmental bodies is especially useful when those organizations have transnational structures that can provide integrative regulatory functions (e.g., codifying practices or positions, formulating guidelines, accrediting services). It is perhaps more promising than attempts by provinces to establish policy at the interprovincial level. Any common front formed by the provinces will be sorely tested by the new federal funding formula for the CHT, by renegotiation of the equalization formulas, and by other non-health-related issues (such as energy policies) in which provincial interests are quite divided and therefore have the potential to damage cordial interprovincial relationships. As Courchene (2010) has noted, while the vertical fiscal imbalance was integral to the establishment of provincial solidarity upon which the Council of the Federation was established, the development of an acute horizontal fiscal imbalance may destroy it.

The final paradox here is that the political actor best placed to facilitate an effective form of polycentric governance—the federal government—is the very body whose absence created the conditions that made these alternative forms of governance a real possibility in the first place. Ottawa arguably has both the resources and the expertise to facilitate precisely what the Council is already doing—providing infrastructure and impetus to a process that requires the provinces to be active participants and to tap into a series of policy networks. That Ottawa currently refuses to do so may, in the end, prove to be an advantage. The model of federal conditionality that existed up to 2011, as its critics point out, tended to encourage provinces to focus their energies on getting more funding from Ottawa. It was Ottawa's withdrawal from the policy sphere that impelled provincial governments to direct their health ministries to collaborate in policy development in a way that had never been attempted. Nonetheless, there is a hope that several years of groping towards a model of polycentric governance may in time solidify a modus operandi that will permit a future federal government, after several years in the wilderness, to become engaged in health policy formulation within a new intergovernmental dynamic. Provinces are already discussing the possibility of constructive federal engagement should the political landscape change in 2015.

Health-care federalism is no longer characterized by federal conditionality. That this shift may be able to bend the cost curve is quite possible, but not because of innovative efficiencies to be gained from unrestrained competition between jurisdictions. The promise of this critical juncture is largely political rather than economic. What the shift away from federal conditionality has accomplished in the first place is simply to goad provinces to focus on executing many small and unremarkable policy reforms that, systematically deployed, may potentially have real financial consequences. Importantly, it has also obliged provinces to devote scarce resources to thinking through longer-term policy strategies that have languished at the bottom of their priority lists because of lack of political will. It may solidify a way of communicating and designing policies—for example, though better utilization of policy networks—that may be better able to weather the usual ups and downs of interprovincial rivalry.

For better or for worse, we are entering a new way of thinking about health-care federalism. Ottawa is not interested in policy development. The federal minister of health has categorically declared that "decision-making about health care is best left to the provincial, territorial and local levels. As federal minister of health, I will not dictate to the provinces and territories how they will deliver services or set their priorities" (Picard 2012, A5). A pessimistic reading of this situation predicts a race to the bottom, with wary provinces unwilling to trust or to believe that more coordinated activity is either possible or beneficial. A more optimistic view acknowledges that there is good reason to believe that enough enabling conditions exist to stave off a descent into policy anarchy or hasty privatization. It is even possible to foresee a future in which the federal government once again becomes actively engaged in health-care policy—not driving the bus, of course, but certainly willing to keep the windshield clean.

References

Atkinson, M. M., D. Béland, G. P. Marchildon, K. McNutt, P. W. B. Phillips, and K. Rasmussen. 2013. *Governance and Public Policy in Canada: A View from the Provinces*. Toronto: University of Toronto Press.

Banzhaf, H. S., and B. A. Chupp. 2012. "Fiscal Federalism and Interjurisdictional Externalities: New Results and an Application to US Air Pollution." *Journal of Public Economics* 96, no. 5/6: 449–64. http://dx.doi.org/10.1016/j.jpubeco.2012.01.001.

Bégin, M. 2002. "Revisiting the Canada Health Act 1984: What Are the Impediments for Change?" Speech given to Institute for Research on Public Policy, Ottawa, 20 February.

Bégin, M., L. Eggerton, and N. Macdonald. 2009. "A Country of Perpetual Pilot Projects." *Canadian Medical Association Journal* 180, no. 12: 1185. http://dx.doi.org/10.1503/cmaj.090808.

Bertalanffy, L. v. 1968. *General System Theory: Foundations, Development, Applications.* New York: George Braziller.

Bell, S. 2011. "Do We Really Need a New "Constructivist Institutionalism" to Explain Institutional Change?" *British Journal of Political Science* 41, no. 4: 883–906. http://dx.doi.org/10.1017/S0007123411000147.

Blyth, M. 2002. *Great Transformations: Economic Ideas and Institutional Change in the Twentieth Century.* Cambridge: Cambridge University Press. http://dx.doi.org/10.1017/CBO9781139087230.

Bolleyer, Nicole. 2006. "Federal Dynamics in Canada, the United States, and Switzerland: How Substates' Internal Organization Affects Intergovernmental Relations." *Publius* 36, no. 4: 471–502. http://dx.doi.org/10.1093/publius/pjl003.

Brock, K. 2008. "The Politics of Asymmetrical Federalism: Reconsidering the Role and Responsibilities of Ottawa." *Canadian Public Policy* 34, no. 2: 143–61. http://dx.doi.org/10.3138/cpp.34.2.143.

Brown, G. R. 1994. "'Canadian Federal-Provincial Overlap and Presumed Government Inefficiency." *Publius* 24, no. 1: 21–37.

Canadian Council on Social Development. 2002. CCSD "Submission: Social Union Framework Agreement (SUFA) Third Year Review." Accessed July 2012. http://www.ccsd.ca/index.php/component/content/article?id=101.

Carrigan, C., and C. Coglianese. 2011. "The Politics of Regulation: From New Institutionalism to New Governance." *Annual Review of Political Science* 14: 107–29. http://dx.doi.org/10.1146/annurev.polisci.032408.171344.

Courchene, T. 1997. "ACCESS: A Convention on the Canadian Economic and Social Systems." In *Assessing ACCESS: Towards a New Social Union.* Proceedings of the Symposium on the Courchene Proposal, Queen's University, 1996. Kingston: Institute of Intergovernment Relations, Queen's University. Accessed 7 July 2011. http://www.queensu.ca/iigr/pub/archive/books/AssessingAccess-TowardsaNewSocialUnion.pdf.

———. 2006. "Accountability and Federalism in the Era of Federal Surpluses: The Paul Martin Legacy, Part II." IRPP Working Paper Series no. 2006–01. Montreal: Institute for Research on Public Policy.

———. 2010. "Intergovernmental Transfers and Canadian Values: Retrospect and Prospect." *Policy Options* 31, no. 5: 32–40

Crivelli, L., M. Filippini, and I. Mosca. 2006. "Federalism and Regional Health Care Expenditures: An Empirical Analysis for the Swiss Cantons." *Health Economics* 15, no. 5: 535–41. http://dx.doi.org/10.1002/hec.1072.

Curry, B., H. Scoffield, and T. Perkins. 2012. "Feds Warn Provinces: Get in Line." *Globe and Mail*, 24 February, A1, A4.

de Búrca, G. 2010. "New Governance and Experimentalism: An Introduction." *Wisconsin Law Review* 2010, no. 2: 227–38.

Eberlein, B., and D. Kerwen. 2004. "New Governance in the European Union: A The-oretical Perspective." *Journal of Common Market Studies* 42, no. 1: 121–42. http://dx.doi.org/10.1111/j.0021-9886.2004.00479.x.

European Commission. 2001. "European Governance: A White Paper." COM (2001) 428. Brussels: European Commission.

Farrelly, M., S. Jeffares, and C. Skelcher. 2010. "Rethinking Network Governance: New Forms of Analysis and the Implications for IGR/MLG." In *Governance and Intergovernmental Relations in the European Union and the United States*, edited by E. Ongaro, A. Massey, M. Holzer, and E. Wayenberg, 87–107. Cheltenham, UK: Edward Elgar. http://dx.doi.org/10.4337/9781849807067.00010.

Ford, R. 2008. "Complex Adaptive Systems and Improvisation Theory: Toward Fram-ing a Model to Enable Continuous Change." *Journal of Change Management* 8, no. 3/4: 173–98. http://dx.doi.org/10.1080/14697010802567543.

Freitag, M., and A. Vatter. 2008. "Decentralization and Fiscal Discipline in Sub-national Governments: Evidence from the Swiss Federal System." *Publius* 38, no. 2: 272–94. http://dx.doi.org/10.1093/publius/pjm038.

Gawande, A. 2012. "Big Med." *New Yorker*, August. http://www.newyorker.com/reporting/2012/08/13/120813fa_fact_gawande?currentPage=all.

Gibbins, R. 1996. "Decentralization and National Standards: 'This Dog Won't Hunt.'" *Policy Options* 17: 7–10.

Greer, S. 2011. "The Weakness of Strong Policies and the Strength of Weak Poli-cies: Law, Experimentalist Governance, and Supporting Coalitions in European Union Health Policy." *Regulation and Governance* 5, no. 2: 187–203. http://dx.doi.org/10.1111/j.1748-5991.2011.01107.x.

Haardt, D. 2013. "The Economics of Health Care Federalism: What Do We Know?" In *Health Care Federalism in Canada*, edited by K. Fierlbeck and W. Lahey, 27–44. Montreal: McGill-Queen's University Press.

Hay, C. 2004. "Ideas, Interests, and Institutions in the Comparative Political Economy of Great Transformations." *Review of International Political Economy* 11, no. 1: 204–26. http://dx.doi.org/10.1080/0969229042000179811.

Hollander, R. 2010. "Rethinking Overlap and Duplication: Federalism and Envi-ronmental Assessment in Australia." *Publius* 40, no. 1: 136–70. http://dx.doi.org/10.1093/publius/pjp028.

Jordan, J. 2009. "Federalism and Health Care Cost Containment in Comparative Perspective." *Publius* 39, no. 1: 164–86. http://dx.doi.org/10.1093/publius/pjn022.

Kneebone, R. 2012. "How You Pay Determines What You Get: Alternative Financing Options as a Determinant of Publicly Funded Health Care in Canada." School of Public Policy Research Papers 5, no. 20. Calgary: University of Calgary. http://dx.doi.org/10.2139/ssrn.2099844.

Kröger, S. 2011. "Five Years Down the Road: An Evaluation of the Streamlining of the Open Method of Coordination in Social Policy Fields." Brussels: OSE Briefing Papers no. 8. Brussels: OSE Europe.

Lazar, H. 2002. "The Social Union Framework Agreement: Lost Opportunity or New Beginning?" School of Policy Studies Working Papers no. 3. Kingston: Queen's University.

Leachman, L. L., G. Rosas, P. Lange, and A. Bester. 2007. "The Political Economy of Budget Deficits." *Economics and Politics* 19, no. 3: 369–420. http://dx.doi.org/10.1111/j.1468-0343.2007.00320.x.

Maioni, A. 1999. "Decentralization in Health Policy: Comments on the ACCESS Proposal." In *Stretching the Federation: The State of the Art in Canada*, edited by R. Young, 97–121. Kingston, ON: IIGR.

Marchildon, G. P. 2012. "Canada: Health System Review." *Health Systems in Transition* 14, no. 7: 1–179.

Mendez, C. 2011. "The Lisbonization of EU Cohesion Policy: A Successful Case of Experimentalism Governance?" *European Planning Studies* 19, no. 3: 519–37. http://dx.doi.org/10.1080/09654313.2011.548368.

Montinola, G., Y. Qian, and B. Weingast. 1995. "Federalism, Chinese Style: The Political Basis for Economic Success in China." *World Politics* 48, no. 1: 50–81. http://dx.doi.org/10.1353/wp.1995.0003.

Natali, D., and B. Vanhercke, eds. 2012. *Social Developments in the European Union 2011*. Brussels: European Social Observatory and European Trade Union Institute.

Neyapti, B. 2010. "Fiscal Decentralization and Deficits: International Evidence." *European Journal of Political Economy* 26, no. 2: 155–66. http://dx.doi.org/10.1016/j.ejpoleco.2010.01.001.

Office of the Parliamentary Budget Officer. 2012. Projected Growth in Provincial and Territorial Government Health Spending. Accessed July 2012. http://www.parl.gc.ca/PBO-DPB/documents/Health_spending_growth.pdf.

Ostrom, E. 2009. "A 'Polycentric' Approach for Coping with Climate Change." Policy Research Working Papers no. 5095. Washington, DC: World Bank.

Pedersen, K. M., T. Christiansen, and M. Bech. 2005. "The Danish Health Care System: Evolution—Not Revolution—in a Decentralized System." *Health Economics* 14 (Suppl. 1): S41–57. http://dx.doi.org/10.1002/hec.1028.

Peters, B. G. 1997. "Escaping the Joint-Decision Trap: Repetition and Sectoral Politics in the European Union." *West European Politics* 20, no. 2: 22–36. http://dx.doi.org/10.1080/01402389708425189.

Picard, A. 2012. "Aglukkag Defends Ottawa's Hands-off Role in Health-Care Funding." *Globe and Mail*, 14 August, A5.

Pierson, P. 1994. *Dismantling the Welfare State? Reagan, Thatcher and the Politics of Retrenchment*. Cambridge: Cambridge University Press. http://dx.doi.org/10.1017/CBO9780511805288.

Qian, Y., and B. Weingast. 1997. "Federalism as a Commitment to Preserving Market Incentives." *Journal of Economic Perspectives* 11, no. 4: 83–92. http://dx.doi.org/10.1257/jep.11.4.83.

Richards, J. 1999. "Comment." In ed. *Stretching the Federation: The State of the Art in Canada*, edited by R. Young, 122–28. Kingston, ON: IIGR.

Riker, W. 1964. *Federalism: Origin, Operation, and Significance*. Boston: Little, Brown.

Rodden, J. 2003. "Reviving Leviathan: Fiscal Federalism and the Growth of Government." *International Organization* 57, no. 4: 695–729. http://dx.doi.org/10.1017/S0020818303574021.

Sabel, C., and J. Zeitlin. 2008. "Learning from Difference: The New Architecture of Experimentalist Governance in the EU." *European Law Review* 14, no. 3: 271–327. http://dx.doi.org/10.1111/j.1468-0386.2008.00415.x.

Saltman, R. 2008. "Decentralization, Re-centralization and Future European Health Policy." *European Journal of Public Health* 18, no. 2: 104–6. http://dx.doi.org/10.1093/eurpub/ckn013.

Savail, M. 1992. "Federal-Provincial Program Overlap." Ottawa: Government of Canada. http://publications.gc.ca/collections/Collection-R/LoPBdP/BP/bp321-e.htm.

Schaltegger, C. A., and L. Feld. 2009. "Are Fiscal Adjustments Less Successful in Decentralized Governments?" *European Journal of Political Economy* 25, no. 1: 115–23. http://dx.doi.org/10.1016/j.ejpoleco.2008.08.002.

Schmidt, V. 2008. "Discursive Institutionalism: The Explanatory Power of Ideas and Discourse." *Annual Review of Political Science* 11, no. 1: 303–26. http://dx.doi.org/10.1146/annurev.polisci.11.060606.135342.

———. 2010. "Taking Ideas and Discourse Seriously: Explaining Change through Discursive Institutionalism as the Fourth 'New Institutionalism.'" *European Political Science Review* 2, no. 1: 1–25. http://dx.doi.org/10.1017/S175577390999021X.

Scott, J., and D. Trubek. 2002. "Mind the Gap: Law and New Approaches to Governance in the European Union." *European Law Journal* 8, no. 1: 1–18. http://dx.doi.org/10.1111/1468-0386.00139.

Steffen, M. 2012. "The Europeanization of Public Health: How Does It Work?" Paper presented at International Political Science Association, Madrid, July 2012. Forthcoming in *Journal of Health Policy, Politics, and Law*, 2013. http://dx.doi.org/10.1215/03616878-1813845.

Tollefson, C., A. R. Zito, and F. Gale. 2012. "Symposium Overview: Conceptualizing New Governance Arrangements." *Public Administration* 90, no. 1: 3–18. http://dx.doi.org/10.1111/j.1467-9299.2011.02003.x.

Weingast, B. R. 1995. "The Economic Role of Political Institutions: Market-Preserving Federalism and Economic Development." *Journal of Law Economics and Organization* 11, no. 1: 1–31.

Zielonka, J. 2007. "Plurilateral Governance in the Enlarged European Union." *Journal of Common Market Studies* 45, no. 1: 187–209. http://dx.doi.org/10.1111/j.1468-5965.2007.00708.x.

eight

The Federal Role in Health Care

PIERRE-GERLIER FOREST

Introduction

Health was given short shrift by the founding fathers of the Canadian federation. Their vision of the common good, as famously stated in the *Constitution Act* of 1867, was "peace, order and good government." Those are all determinants of health in good standing, of course, and good government may even be a necessary condition to the institution of any sort of health-care system. But the truth is, health did not merit much attention in Canada's founding documents, where it appears in the most limited or indirect language in just two brief sections of the constitution.

Section 92.7 gave the provinces power over hospitals and other care-giving institutions. Section 91.11 granted the federal parliament authority over public health, defined as it was at the end of the 19th century as the control of infectious disease. The provincial role in health-care delivery was strengthened by the provinces' power to regulate professions and insurance markets. The federal role in public health was reinforced by Ottawa's criminal law powers, which were used in the early 20th century to expand its responsibilities in food and drug safety as well as environmental health.

Health did not fare much better at the time of the great constitutional revision of 1982. Its architects should have known better, given the popularity of the national health program established in previous decades and the wealth of knowledge about health and health care displayed by some of the protagonists—including some of the prime minister's most senior advisors. In the end, however, the new Charter of Rights ignored the issue while making room for public values such as "life, liberty, and security of the person."

The national health program established over the past 50 years is, in fact, the product of a succession of complex political arrangements distinct from, if respectful of, the constitutional order. The story has been told many times (Maioni 1998; Taylor 1978; Tuohy 1999). Provinces and the federal government found a common interest in providing health services to the Canadian population and agreed to share the cost under certain conditions. Responsibility for the organization and the management of health-care services rested with the provinces, while the federal government used its superior fiscal capacity to sustain comparable levels and types of services across the country.

Despite its highly decentralized structure, the resulting system is surprisingly homogeneous. A large number of hospitals were built at the same time, reflecting a similar understanding of the requirements of medical care, while the training and norms of practice of professionals such as physicians and nurses are nearly identical in every province. It is true that the overarching governance structure is prone to delays and timid solutions because it requires the participation and consent of many partners with divergent interests. However, at least until recently, it was perceived as a successful example of executive federalism, characterized by "a continuous process of federal-provincial consultation and negotiation" (Banting and Boadway 2004; Watts 1989).

The Canadian health-care compact

Historians suggest that the common dimensions of our public health system date back to the 1930s, when the Canadian Medical Association and a few provinces, notably Alberta and British Columbia, started considering the idea. Whatever its genesis, it would be almost 30 years later before a national health-care system took shape through the different pieces of federal legislation that would come to define it, from the *Hospital Insurance and Diagnostic Services Act* of 1957 to the *Medical Care Act* of 1966 and the *Canada Health Act* of 1984 (Marchildon 2012).

The five principles currently enshrined in the *Canada Health Act* emerged progressively as well. There were initially just three in 1957: universality, portability, and public administration. In 1966 that increased to four when we added comprehensiveness to the package. They expanded to five in 1984, when we distinguished more clearly between universality and accessibility.

Our history might have been much different. In 1940 the provinces consented to a constitutional amendment granting the federal government responsibility for unemployment insurance. It is doubtful that the provinces would have willingly relinquished authority over such an important and diverse area of social policy, but in theory there is no reason why Canada could not have developed a national health service along the same lines (MacDougall 2012). Yet another possibility would have been to use federal spending power to impose a mandate on the provinces, much like what happened in the United States after the establishment of Medicaid and Medicare in the 1960s (Blumenthal and Morone 2009; Funigiello 2005;

Sparer, France, and Clinton 2011). However, this has not traditionally been the Canadian way. Major decisions and most program initiatives were invariably achieved once the federal government and the provinces agreed on the objectives and the funding mechanism. The process was cumbersome and trying but in line with the Canadian political culture of accommodation and compromise.

Given the size of the country and the nature of the union, the original division of roles and responsibilities between the provinces and the federal government made a lot of sense. Each province was able to develop a health system reflecting the needs and values of its population, while the federal government took care of risks and threats that could affect the country as a whole. This legal structure reflected an underlying social compact that engaged many partners, including provincial governments, physicians' associations, hospitals, and all sorts of other stakeholders (Lavis 2004). Canadian citizens overwhelmingly supported the compact, which was framed for public purposes as a simple but solemn promise: in Canada, anyone could see a doctor when sick, independently of his or her capacity to pay, and when very sick, anyone could go to a hospital, once again without worrying about what it might cost.

In the eyes of many, the federal government would be the guarantor of this engagement and was expected to enforce its terms on any group or government tempted to stray. Although the provinces never consented to what would amount to federal supervision, in practice it happened. On a few occasions, with the assent of the public, Ottawa had to remind a particular government of its obligations.

The compact was respectful of the logic and the letter of the Canadian constitution. The provinces were in charge of organizing and delivering health-care services, except for the few domains where the federal government was legally required to step in directly—for instance, correctional institutions and the military. Ottawa's influence was felt, however, not only because of the fiscal capacity of the central government but also because of its persistence in seeking harmonization of policies and practices through a variety of roundtables, networks, and working groups, all supported by federal funding. Beginning in the 1990s, financial support has also been extended to a few intergovernmental bodies, agencies, and "foundations" tasked with providing data and evaluation results to participating governments.

National norms and standards, when they existed, were usually issued and enforced by professional organizations, licensing bodies, or trade associations outside federal or provincial control; they were all too happy to exert influence on a system they had often intensely opposed at the time of its creation. Too often the legal or academic discussions of constitutional design and allocation of power among the federal government and the provinces ignore the role and contribution of this dense web of organizations. From teaching hospitals to nurses' associations and from primary care to mental health, the Canadian health system benefits from this dynamic. It makes good use of the knowledge and leadership of competent and highly motivated practitioners instead of resorting to bureaucrats who are too remote from the front lines. In fact, in many domains the asymmetry resulting from the federal and (therefore) decentralized structure of the health system is well balanced by the centralizing action of nongovernmental organizations.

The end of executive federalism

As with every other large, complex system, a national health program requires constant adjustments. Some of these adjustments originate within the system itself, from the bottom up, and the need for national authorities to act is, in point of fact, quite limited. By necessity, however, important structural policy decisions must result from new political arrangements. Moreover, in a democracy like Canada there exists an expectation that decisions will be preceded by public discussion.

Until recently, most policies with a decisive impact on the structure, cost, or functioning of the national health system were the subject of intense public debate before adoption. This was true for the major pieces of legislation that created the system in 1957 and 1966, it was true of the *Canada Health Act* in 1984, and it was certainly the case again with the first ministers' health accords of 2003–04. Recognizing Canadians' deep attachment to medicare and meeting the public's wish to have a say in the accords' content was the inspiration behind the national consultation orchestrated by the so-called Romanow Commission: the Royal Commission on the Future of Health Care in Canada (McIntosh and Forest 2010).

This level of transparency and public deliberation is not always expected in a culture of executive federalism, but in the case of health care, the stakes were too high for politicians and bureaucrats to ignore public sentiment. In her book on the fight for the *Canada Health Act* in the early 1980s, former Liberal health minister Monique Bégin recalls how citizen mobilization in defence of the public provision of health-care services countered the influence of provincial governments and other elite interest groups (Bégin 1987). Many other examples abound, including massive opinion campaigns at the federal and provincial levels.

After decades of conferring with (if not always deferring to) Canadians and ensuring inclusion of the public's perspective before launching health initiatives, the current federal Conservative government has ended this approach. Executive federalism may not be totally dead, given that Canada is still a federation and that some issues still require common solutions, but multilateral negotiations in health are now reserved for a limited number of technical decisions related to matters such as vaccines or labour market issues.

Prime Minister Harper has resisted all pressures to renew the tradition of intergovernmental meetings and joint governance, not just in health care but also in all other sectors. He has repeatedly demonstrated that he is ready to make decisions that are not popular with most citizens, from criminal justice to the environment, and does not seem to be interested in public debate outside of electoral periods. In a dramatic breach with past practice, the federal government now tends to operate exclusively in its own sphere and not to seek alliances or coalitions with the provinces. Even when responsibilities are shared for constitutional reasons or otherwise, such as health and health care, the government defines its own policy in splendid isolation, according to its own priorities and its own principles.

Putting this philosophy into practice, Canada's minister of finance, Jim Flaherty, announced on 19 December 2011 a new federal funding framework for health care, without prior consultation with the provinces and without any attempt to mobilize interest groups or any concession to public opinion. For many observers and health policy leaders, this announcement came as a shock—not so much because of the dollar amounts involved (which were not unreasonable) but because the underlying message was one of disentanglement. The co-funding of health-care services by the central government will continue into the future, as Ottawa will pay its share, but its active participation in co-management of the national system is clearly over. In the blunt words of the federal minister of health, Leona Aglukkaq, "Decision-making about health care is best left to the provincial, territorial and local levels" (Aglukkaq 2012).

This new approach will clearly not satisfy those who have called for an "empowered" federal government imposing conditions on the provinces to foster bold reforms (Marchildon 2013). It was a real blow to those who dreamed of expansion of the system, notably into fields such as pharmaceuticals and home care. In Ottawa, interest groups and coalitions that were preparing themselves for federal-provincial discussions on renewal of the 2003 and 2004 health accords found themselves adrift and directionless.

The provinces and territories also expressed reservations. Certainty of funding has always been part of their long-term objectives in past negotiations with Ottawa, but in the absence of any discussion, there would be no opportunity to examine the benefits and hazards of the new federal formula. Even provinces such as Québec and Alberta, which are constantly pleading for freedom of action, looked rather uncomfortable, if only because the new framework was ambiguous about the limits that provinces should respect when "experimenting" with reforms. In effect, while the federal government did not insist on the conditionality of its future financial contribution, the prime minister nonetheless reaffirmed his government's support for the *Canada Health Act* and, supposedly, for the restrictions it imposes on privately funded health care and other market-oriented solutions.

It is much too early to say if this new approach will achieve the results expected by the Conservative government. It is highly improbable that the national health system will change radically in just a few years, and just as unlikely that it will suddenly collapse. Like other large social systems, public health care is both resilient and resistant to change, and often for the same reasons. It is more important to determine whether the differences in governance structure—as they evolve from a tradition of executive federalism tempered by citizen engagement to a vision of limited federal-provincial exchanges regarding fiscal transfers and technical cooperation—will actually deliver the decisions needed to preserve the adaptive capacity of the health system and bend the cost curve in the right direction. Ottawa's position seems to be that the national dimension of the governance structure has become an obstacle to problem solving, especially in the face of new and difficult circumstances, such as population aging and cost increases, that require innovative solutions.

Experiences in other sectors and in other federations do not necessarily support this point of view. The changes instituted could be questioned for three different reasons. First, it is obvious that the federal government underestimates—or chooses to dismiss—the interdependencies among its own policies and what happens at the "provincial, territorial, and local level," to use the language of Minister Aglukkaq. Beyond jurisdictional debates, the modern concept of health encompasses more than just health care, including all sorts of health-enhancing and health-damaging factors. Some of these "determinants of health" are rooted in the policy domains of federal jurisdiction and cannot be ignored without consequences.

Second, it would be useful to know if the provinces can actually cooperate in a meaningful way in the absence of federal leadership. Although Ottawa has never been a major source of innovation in health care, it has played the dual role of relay and sponsor of other health actors' initiatives. The most famous example is of course the decision to establish a national health system based on Saskatchewan's experiment with hospital and medical-care insurance. It is not clear how the provinces might assume this role as they simultaneously spur much-needed innovation, especially when confronted with unprecedented growth in health expenditures since 1997.

Finally, the new regime encourages nongovernmental actors to play an active role in fostering collaboration and positive change. It is tempting to see the multiplication of partnerships and private undertakings as a sign of vitality and progress. However, in the end, the outcomes of all these initiatives ought to be judged according to the same criteria used to evaluate public health care in general, from quality to appropriateness and from transparency to affordability. The jury is still out.

Health as a shared responsibility

The current federal administration's insistence on a role in health policy limited to providing funds to the provinces is a departure from the cautious course favoured by previous governments, which were aware of the many intertwined factors in play and, therefore, eager to keep their options open. Even a hurried reader of the reports tabled by a succession of committees of inquiry and other commissions, from the first Hall Report of 1964 to the National Forum of Health in 1997, would know that building a national health system is forever an unfinished business.

It is possible that no policy document ever expressed the interdependencies in Canada's health system better than the federal Lalonde Report of 1974, *A New Perspective on the Health of Canadians*. This green paper was issued just four years after Québec joined the federal-provincial agreement over medical care, thereby making medicare a reality (Lalonde 1974; McKay 2000). The report is known for its audacious vision of health and its pioneering use of the concept of "determinants of health." Its core message—that health is more than health care—has had a lasting impact on the way health policy is conceived in Canada and around the world. Its most immediate goal, however, was more practical: it was to define the new limits of the federal health sphere, given Ottawa's self-assigned role of building and funding the national health system. Hence policy domains that were within federal purview, such as environment and science policy, were recognized as essential to the achievement of health goals at both population and individual levels. Other domains such as education and social policy, over which the provinces had uncontested jurisdiction, were also targeted, given their impacts on health outcomes.

At the time of the report, admittedly, the evidence about determinants of health was not what it is today. The Lalonde Report never became legal or constitutional doctrine and barely influenced federal policy outside of the health sector (Lavis 2002). But it was a convincing rebuttal to those who wanted to limit the federal role in health, and its vision survived, notably in the ranks of the bureaucracy and its closer allies. Moreover, many of its conjectures have been vindicated by decades of research. Given the proper financial incentives, even physicians who operate in the wasteful culture of "defensive medicine" now recognize the importance of looking at the social determinants of health. In policy circles, efforts to narrow health inequalities are now commonplace, from fiscal measures intended to encourage people to adopt healthier lifestyles to bold initiatives aiming at improving living standards of deprived populations (Oliver 2010).

The Supreme Court of Canada has also unambiguously and repeatedly affirmed the interdependence of the federal and provincial roles in health. In a recent decision, for example, the Chief Justice insisted that the need to safeguard the public's health—a legitimate federal responsibility well established in the constitution—interferes by necessity with the provincial authority over health care: "The federal role in the domain of health makes it impossible to precisely define what falls in or out of the proposed provincial 'core.' Overlapping federal jurisdiction and the sheer size and diversity of provincial health power render daunting the task of drawing a bright line around a protected provincial core of health where federal legislation may not tread" (2011 SCC 44, 68). This is a bold statement that runs against the thesis that the two orders of government can operate in isolation. It is well grounded in the current scientific understanding of how health is determined, or "produced," at the population and individual levels.

Whoever is responsible for promoting and protecting good health cannot ignore the signals sent by the health-care system, whether in the form of high utilization rates or poorer health indicators (Stuckler, Basu, and McKee 2010). Whoever is in charge of the medical treatment of diseases must be aware that the root determinants of death and disability cannot be addressed without collaboration from all policy sectors, at all levels of government. In the strong and direct words of a previous Supreme Court decision, "Health is a jurisdiction shared by both the provinces and the federal government" (2010 SCC 61, 52).

It is possible to see the federal-provincial dyad as a vast supply-and-demand system. The provinces are the main agents on the supply side. They decide how many health professionals are required and where they will work. In many cases—nurses, for example—they provide the pay and determine the working conditions through collective agreements with the provincial nurses' unions. Provinces also fund hospitals. In the last instance, they choose what is included in the basket of publicly insured services and what is not. The federal government does not have much to say about any of these issues. In cases where Ottawa provides health insurance or health services to a few specific groups or populations, the federal government never seems to be particularly innovative and could rarely claim that it possesses any unique knowledge or experience of benefit to provincial governments.

In sharp contrast, however, the federal government has a major role on the demand side. Economic policy, immigration policy, and agricultural policy have immediate consequences on the population's health and well-being. Science policy influences both the type and intensity of research that is performed in health organizations and the demand for new technology. Federal power impinges on social and behavioural factors such as smoking, drug use, toxic agents, and firearms, among other things. Ottawa regulates the sale of pharmaceuticals in Canada and decides their market price. It plays an essential role in the surveillance and control of epidemics and contagious diseases.

And that is not all. The federal government also contributes to the general solvency of the health-care system. The cash portion of health-care costs covered by direct federal transfers may not be what it was when the system was first established, but it is still significant. Even a rich province such as Alberta seems to believe that participation in the national program and receiving its share of federal money is a better deal than devising a system on its own. It is also worth mentioning that in the past decade, when the federal government increased its funding, a corresponding increase in expenditures and costs was observed, notably for health professionals—an almost textbook example of the impact on demand of fiscal stimulus.

On a symbolic level, finally, the mere fact that Ottawa keeps alive the fundamental promise that all Canadian citizens have a right to necessary health care, wherever they live and without financial barriers, is doubtless a key driver of the demand for medical services. It is well known that Canadians' attachment to the *Canada Health Act* is not related to the Act's actual content (of which most are probably ignorant) but has much to do with the message of empowerment it conveys (Forest 2012). In poll after national poll, to receive care when needed is seen by most Canadians as a guaranteed right of citizenship, a right that trumps the authority of a provincial government engaged in rationing or a health professional tempted to dismiss his or her patient's wants.

Four visions of system governance

It should be no wonder that the two levels of government have no option but to cooperate; in such an interdependent system one cannot achieve much without the assistance of the other. Of course, some factors may contribute to make collaboration less than automatic, from party politics to individual leaders' personalities, and from fiscal capacity to policy understanding. But on the whole, when required by circumstances, Ottawa and the provinces know that they need to find common ground.

In fact, conflicts and quarrels are a perfectly normal feature of federalism, and Canada is no exception to this general rule. Knowing when to compromise is the key, and it involves a commitment to the values of national welfare. Other health actors are well accustomed to this situation. They have learned to maintain working relationships with provincial governments while pleading for Ottawa to take over more responsibilities, and vice versa. They also understand how to play one level against the other, if necessary, to gain political or financial advantage.

The professed indifference of the current federal government to health-care issues is creating a new state of affairs. As Katherine Fierlbeck puts it in her contribution to this book (Chapter 7), "Not only did Ottawa refuse to impose more stringent conditionality but, by the end of 2011, it was insisting that provinces had to take full responsibility for the administration of health care, attempts at health policy innovation, and any failure to contain health costs." From a financial management point of view, to use Fierlbeck's language, the government is promoting an unprecedented option, inspired by a very narrow understanding of the country's constitution and a surprising indifference to tradition.

Because of the Canadian system's design, it is expected that health and health-sector challenges will initially be perceived and defined through the prism of each province's specific economic, demographic, or cultural reality. For a productive national conversation to take place, it is usual and necessary for someone to step in and suggest that a given issue has broader dimensions and implications. Common solutions that respect the interests and political sensitivities of all can then be devised that advance the greater public good. This is supposedly where the influence of the federal government is most needed. But instead of arguing for the provinces to pay more attention to national issues, it now becomes essential to remind Ottawa that no other government can speak for the country as a whole.

What make the current federal-provincial environment particularly unsatisfactory are the lack of a debate on the motives behind Ottawa's recent decision and a clear sense of where it intends to go next. The Conservative government seems to have abandoned the traditional definition of the federal role in health care, but it is also sending signals that it won't be satisfied for very long with the position it has just taken and that it may attempt to define yet another position in the future. Where that will leave Canadians, who are profoundly attached to the health-care system as they have traditionally known it, is open to debate.

There are four different ways of thinking about governance of the Canadian health system, depending on role the central government is expected to perform. To simplify,

1. A national health service that would have the federal government making all the essential decisions and enacting federal laws to pre-empt or supersede provincial and local actions anytime they conflict. Although this vision is hardly compatible with the constitution, it never lacked supporters in the health policy community, who lament the existence of "fourteen distinct health systems" and suggest that "a fragmented and province-centred approach" is responsible for unacceptable variations in performance and quality (Lewis et al. 2001).

2. A governance structure in which the federal government is *primus inter pares*: a senior government leading a group of equals. This vision arose naturally from the arrangements that established the health system, reflecting a long tradition of intergovernmental relations. Until very recently it was the default position of the Government of Canada and was used to justify federal contributions to a multitude of agencies and other collective endeavours, as well as the tradition of Ottawa's co-chairing all meetings, roundtables, and other management processes.

3. An approach in which the federal government is only one among many by virtue of its specific responsibilities in the health sector and its limited but tangible financial contribution to the operation of the health system. In the past, for example, when provincial premiers were unhappy with Ottawa's support for health care, they would argue that the central government should not exert more influence than what it actually paid for (Kneebone 2012). In the past few years, however, especially after the minister of finance announced the new funding formula in December 2012, the federal government appears to be basing its own position on this vision. The wording of a letter sent to her colleagues by the federal minister of health in January 2012 is particularly telling, notably when she intimated she wanted a seat among the provincial ministers studying health innovation (Wells 2012).

4. A fully decentralized governance structure with very limited coordination but with what its proponents would call "real accountability," because of exact apportionment (at the provincial

level) of health expenditures and taxation. This approach is close
to the "provincialist" vision traditionally championed by Québec
and Alberta, which states that health is an exclusive provincial
jurisdiction. But it adds two new dimensions. First, it supposes
that the federal government would abandon all its health-related
activities, starting with health care but eventually including most
of its health protection and promotion portfolios. Second, as
explained in a much circulated policy piece written by a former
advisor to the prime minister (Boessenkool 2010), it postulates that
decentralization requires full fiscal autonomy and suggests phasing
out direct federal cash contributions.

Recent initiatives on the part of the federal government indicate that it
is very much tempted by the last and most radical of these four positions,
a position that may be closest to the ideological sensitivities and constitutional vision of the Conservative Party. The decision to relinquish the federal government's role as health insurer for the Royal Canadian Mounted
Police, announced in the 2012 federal budget, is a good indication of
a new policy course. It is the same with the decision to transfer federal
responsibility for Aboriginal health in British Columbia to the province.
Program cuts at Health Canada and other central agencies seem to obey a
similar logic. While it is true that the funding engagement is not supposed
to change soon, it has been taken out of the realm of provincial-federal
(electoral) politics, a necessary first step in any serious fiscal conversation.

Let's acknowledge that all this does not amount to an attack against
public health care. At the moment it is a change with only a few consequences, limited to the implicit governance structure of the national health
system. Yet it is a radical departure from a federal-provincial governance
model that has been in place for close to 50 years and to which all health-
sector actors, not to mention Canada's citizens, are perfectly accustomed.
For those who were expecting more from Ottawa, and in particular new
national programs or important program expansion, it is a resounding
defeat. In essence, the new structure is intended to limit the capacity of
the central government to pursue policy initiatives in the health sector or,
framed differently, to encourage provinces to innovate—the widely hailed
solution to all that currently ails the health system. For the majority of
interested parties, though, it raises a series of empirical questions on the
ability of the system to adjust to the new rules of engagement. How probable it is that the provinces will be able to take on this new policy leadership role? How much innovation can the system generate? How much
variability can it tolerate?

The system at risk

Scholars of federalism are well aware that federated entities such as states or provinces do not cooperate spontaneously (Imbeau et al. 2000). Left to themselves, they would rather compete—for investments, for jobs, for immigrants, for qualified workers, for access to markets, and so forth. Taxation rates, both individual and corporate, are essential factors in this competition. The type and quality of public services count as well, including infrastructure and public safety, of course, but also education, social services, and health care.

Market-oriented analysts will submit that competition entices states or provinces to be more efficient, offering better services for a smaller tax burden. Others worry about a "race to the bottom," as it is popularly known, as each jurisdiction tries to get away with the lowest possible taxes, with dire effects on public services. The federalist solution to this dilemma is to make use of a central authority to level the playing field (Forest and Bergeron 2005).

If every state or province is forced to offer a health insurance program, for example, it will still compete with others in quality and efficiency but it will not be tempted to deprive its population of an essential service. In Canada, where section 36.2 of the *Constitution Act* (1982) guarantees all citizens "reasonably comparable levels of public services at reasonably comparable levels of taxation," federal transfer payments are supposed to help all provincial governments to provide a level of service close to the national average. In fact the expectation is really to "universalise the best," to borrow from Aneurin Bevan's famous quote on Britain's nascent National Health Service. Small provinces with a narrow tax base and large provinces with a diverse and demanding population should cover the same medically necessary services, regardless of their individual circumstances.

The risk associated with the new federal approach may be less on the funding side than in terms of the historic tendency of the provinces to level up their health services to a relatively common basket of universally available services. As long as the services that are publicly insured stay the same in all provinces, the federal financial contribution could be effective in restricting interprovincial fluctuations in quality and coverage, even when the health transfer's yearly growth will be reduced to its "floor value" of approximately 3% after 2016. The problem is rather that the composition of the basket of insured services may itself begin to fluctuate as provinces look for ways to cost-contain in the short run and bend the cost curve in the longer run.

In health care, after all, limiting access is the easy way out in case of financial difficulties. It is the path of least resistance, especially compared to painstaking reforms of delivery systems. During the HMO (health maintenance organization) debacle in the United States in the 1990s, for example, organizations that were supposed to compete on efficiency quickly ended up competing on access (Rochefort 2001). It could be argued that, if allowed to do so, the Canadian provinces would have acted identically at the end of the same decade, in response to both their own fiscal crises and massive federal cuts in transfer payments. They resisted the temptation because they were still subject to a federal mandate that forced them to provide services at a certain level. The cuts and restrictions imposed at the same time on the services provinces covered, over and above the "CHA basket" of hospital and medical services, are a case in point (Marchildon 2006).

In the past, a province could always decide to upgrade its basket of services if it was ready to tax more or if it was in a fiscal position to do so, and most provinces did opt for an expanded basket that could include anything from physical therapy to pharmaceuticals. In times of hardship it was also possible for a province to downgrade its basket of services, such as when provinces started to "delist" some of those same services in the 1990s to lessen financial pressures. But the constraints of the *Canada Health Act* meant that it was nearly impossible to play with the core medical and hospital services. In the current environment it is highly possible that provinces could be given more flexibility—in the name of innovation, of course, but also because Ottawa will probably not veto initiatives that respect the letter of the *Canada Health Act* if not its spirit. By contrast, a decade ago it insisted that calling a hospital by some other name would mean that it would not be allowed to charge user fees to patients.

Towards a narrower health system

One other dimension of the Canadian system, from a fiscal point of view, is its redistributive character. In insurance terms, federal funding ensures that the pooling of health risks takes place at the national level. Until 2007, the complex formula used to determine the cash portion of the Canada Health Transfer, the federal funding vehicle for hospital and medical care, even included an "equalization amount" to reflect and partially compensate for the unequal distribution of wealth among provinces.

In recent years the federal government has pursued a direction that entails more interprovincial equity but less redistribution, notably because of a decision to calculate all transfers on a strict per capita basis, including the Canada Health Transfer (Gauthier 2011). Provinces are being given time to adapt, but in the long term it is clear that this approach changes the actuarial logic that underlies the current health system. Inevitably it will evolve towards a series of nearly independent provincial risk pools. For provinces favoured by demographics and wealth, this means enhanced capacity to expand or improve their health-care programs. For the others, particularly provinces challenged by an aging population or a declining industrial base, this may mean shrinking the basket of services through delisting or providing the same services but with poorer access and deteriorating quality.

As long as federal funding ensures that cost sharing is taking place at the national level, and if all the provinces continue to abide by common principles, is there much to fret about? The answer is twofold. First, as mentioned before, the system is not at risk of imminent collapse. It will, though, become more rigid because of its declining capacity for common problem-solving. Provincial programs will grow apart, with gradually fewer opportunities for sharing good ideas and best practices.

Second, a narrowing of the official perspective on health issues is to be expected. During the dark hours of the 1990s program cuts, public health suffered throughout the country, with a few dramatic crises as a consequence. This could happen again. Population health, which can develop only in an intellectual climate in which it is possible to question policy choices in any sector, from public safety to the environment, could suffer as well from Ottawa's new definition of its role (Brown 2010). It is said that the federal minister of health is personally sensitive to the impact of social conditions on people's health, and the Canadian Medical Association has discovered that physicians can be inspired to pay more attention to the economic realities of their patients. But these statements are not a substitute for a government actively engaged, through policy programs, in reduction of inequalities and the resulting distribution of better health.

Silver linings

In the past few years there has been intense criticism of governments across the country for their management of innovation (or lack thereof) in the health system. Despite massive reinvestment by Ottawa and some significant efforts from the provinces, none of the expected transformations—primary-care reform, electronic health records, a common pharmaceutical policy, and so on—seem to have materialized. Echoing the opinion of many other observers, a departing president of the Canadian Medical Association, Dr. Jeff Turnbull, spoke in his valedictory address of the "mediocrity" of the health system: "Illnesses prolonged because of unaffordable medications. Operations cancelled because of hospital overcapacity. Debilitating pain because of delayed knee joint replacements. Millions of Canadians without family doctors. This is Canada's health care system. And it's a system Canadians can no longer take pride in" (Collier 2011).

The government may not be open to the kind of solutions Dr. Turnbull would like to pursue, but this does not mean that it is not taking the diagnosis seriously. Its solution—one of "strategic restraint," so to speak—is a drastic remedy; it has the merit of being simple and, most interestingly in this case, it has never been tried. This interpretation of the minister's announcement of December 2011 has not gained much traction in the public discourse. Indeed, the first reaction to the federal government's announcement of its change in approach was almost unanimously negative. Expert after expert decried what was seen as abandonment of federal responsibility. Provincial policymakers gave interviews in which they envisioned the worst-case scenarios that they had been working for years to avoid: delisting of services, imposition of user fees, abandonment of the principle of portability as provinces refused to reimburse residents treated out of province.

But what if leaving the door open to provinces for experimentation is, in reality, an opportunity for innovative solutions? What if the end of a regime in which it was only possible to reach the lowest common denominator is, in fact, a blessing? What if some degree of healthy rivalry between jurisdictions entices health actors to lead change rather than to test the water indefinitely? The easy answer is that only the future will tell. Most of the dire predictions that immediately followed Jim Flaherty's announcement were aimed at a situation that will unfold incrementally, with plenty of time for everybody to adapt. The message is that the federal government wants its health-related transfers to the provinces to be more sustainable. However, for the time being, it is as generous as were its most profligate predecessors. A cynic would say there is no better time to experiment—risk is still limited (given the level of funding) and there is a sense that success will be rewarded.

Another way of looking at the problem is to think about the capacity of this large and complex system to adapt and evolve. It is well known that complexity brings costliness and declining returns (Tainter 1988); in that sense, the government's scheme could be seen as an honest attempt to return to a level of "lower complexity." In effect it could be that provincial units are better placed to satisfy demand according to the circumstances of their populations, with limited waste and shorter response rates. The health regionalization movement in the 1990s was inspired by quite similar considerations (Forest and Palley 2008). This is not far either from the decentralized vision associated with the 1867 constitution, and should, therefore, not be cast as a total departure from the Canadian tradition.

Breaking up is hard to do

The real problem with an exclusive provincial focus is that some issues require solutions at another level. This is not only true for contagious diseases and other public health threats; it applies as well to certain medical specialties that require a combination of expertise and volume that cannot be found in a single province, such as pediatric surgery. It applies to the procurement of costly pharmaceuticals, which would work better if negotiations with manufacturers involved more players with a bigger budget. It applies to human resources planning, which cannot be done in isolation without a good knowledge of the demographics and working conditions in other jurisdictions.

For the time being, the bundle of intergovernmental bodies charged with health information gathering or with knowledge development and dissemination is still quite active, from the Canadian Institute of Health Information to the Health Council. Their dependency on federal funding, however, leaves these organizations quite exposed in case of further policy changes and budget cuts. All have proved their utility, but if difficult decisions had to be made, given the resources available at the provincial level for such endeavours, few would survive Ottawa's pullback.

Back in 2003 the provinces established a permanent structure to foster and support their collaborative efforts independently from Ottawa. The Council of the Federation, as it is known, behaved at first more like a lobby group pleading for unconditional federal funding of provincial programs than a service organization or a common policy unit. Furthermore, on many topics it is clear that, past the expression of a few banalities, competing provincial interests hinder policy formulation. In recent years, however, the Council has taken it upon itself to develop policy platforms in several different areas related to health care. These include a "purchasing alliance" for drugs, medical supplies, and equipment; an "innovation working group" preoccupied with clinical practice guidelines, human resources management, and scope-of-practice issues; and a more traditional study of fiscal arrangements. The products of these efforts are not particularly original or especially profound (Council of the Federation 2012a; 2012b); nonetheless, they fulfill an essential purpose: to establish that a constructive conversation on health care is still possible at the national level, even if Ottawa has deserted the table.

The Council of the Federation's process also demonstrates that cooperation among the provinces will take place if it is profitable. This is less trivial than it may look at first glance. The Canadian federation is extremely decentralized, and many factors are contributing to movement towards an even more dispersed political community. Provinces are separated by distance, culture, and politics. Their resources differ in nature and in importance, especially in the energy sector. The demographics of a large province like Ontario places it a world apart from Prince Edward Island or Nunavut. Competition, not cooperation, is the iron law of federalism. Frankly, if pursuit of their economic interests were to counterbalance just for a while the powerful centrifugal forces at play in the federation, it would be for the better.

Another encouraging reality is the fact that voluntary organizations and professional groups that have taken charge of the development and enforcement of national norms and standards in the Canadian health system have not been eliminated or emasculated as a result of recent changes. On the contrary, a host of new initiatives has seen the light of day, all of them contributing to keeping the national system together. Well-established private groups with a historical national presence, such as the Canadian Medical Association and the Canada Nurses Association, remain determined to play a role in the new interprovincial process and have worked hand-in-hand with the Council of the Federation on issues relevant to their areas of interest and expertise.

New partnerships are also forming. An interesting development has seen health actors from very different institutional backgrounds coming together to share ideas and to develop policy options in areas such as cancer care, mental health, and patient safety. The list of participants in these undertakings can include voluntary organizations, patient groups, health organizations, research institutions, and—most interesting—governments from the local, the provincial, and even the federal level. Although it is too early to say if these initiatives will all be successful, it is encouraging that common policy approaches are being adopted nationally, such as in cancer care. The Canadian Partnership against Cancer, for example, already goes far beyond anything achieved through traditional intergovernmental processes, in which every jurisdiction vigorously affirmed its status and jealously guarded its independence; best practices are shared, standards of care are defined and implemented, and costs are scrupulously examined.

Be careful what you wish for

Some might argue that the current federal approach simply complies with the provinces' long-standing demand for greater autonomy. For decades

Canadian provinces told Ottawa that they wanted the federal government out of "their" health-care systems. They wished for sustained, substantial, predictable, and unconditional funding from the central government, but they protested and resisted every time Ottawa tried to carve out a role for itself that involved more than just being rich and benevolent.

In the provinces' defence, it must be said that the Government of Canada has not been very consistent about establishing its health priorities. In the recent past, Ottawa has successively identified its definitive "first priority" as patient safety (in 2001), public health (after the SARS crisis in 2003), waiting times (after the 2006 election), and performance measurement (in 2011). This might be normal practice for a government that does not deliver care on a daily basis, but it can be irritating for governments and organizations that have a day-to-day responsibility to administer and deliver health services.

There even exists a small possibility that Ottawa might change its mind about the current policy, without mentioning the scenario of an election, probable public outcry if the CHA's perceived "sacred trust" is breached, or a potential change in the governing party. The federal government was tempted to do so once before, when it revisited its transfer payments policy at the very end of the 1970s to put an end to cost sharing. It is doubtful that it will happen this time, however, given that the current orientation is rooted in a constitutional doctrine prescribing that each order of government must operate in its own separate sphere, and in a philosophy that calls for a smaller bureaucracy.

Without prejudging the chances that the government's strategy to achieve some essential results, and especially to foster experimentation and innovation in Canada's health system, will be accomplished, a sobering conclusion is inescapable: in the long term, health will remain a shared responsibility in need of the full attention of all interested parties, including Ottawa. The development of essential policies will not happen if the initiative is left to the provinces, not because they are obtuse or incapable but because they have neither the mandate nor the instruments.

To give just one example, to declare success in primary care, it will be essential to address socioeconomic inequalities in health. Our society cannot redeem itself simply by offering free access to health care to those it has made sick in the first place, like those employers of the early 20th century who would agree to subscribe to a workers' safety insurance plan but would not change anything in the work environment. This issue is obviously related to the distribution of health services, but also to the production and redistribution of wealth—a domain over which Ottawa very much has control. Social choices and their impact on economic and fiscal policies would need to be exposed and debated in a "vigorous democratic discussion" at the national level, something which cannot take place if the federal government is not involved (Gostin 2000).

Canadians are invariably willing to tackle such questions, as consultations under the Romanow Commission underscored (Maxwell, Rosell, and Forest 2003)—members of the public were among the first to say that the system could be better organized. People know when doctors, nurses, and hospitals are doing a lousy job, and they are ready to fight for something they have traditionally had that has been taken away. Regardless of what governments may have in mind, based on health's consistently high ranking in public opinion polls, it seems highly unlikely that Canadians will "go gently into that good night."

The outcomes of any policy process are always uncertain. The recent decision on the part of the federal government to distance itself from the health sector is no exception. The fairest appraisal at this time is that it puts the national system at risk, given the inherent dynamics of the federation, but it also creates unusual opportunities for reform. The provinces got what they had been seeking for decades, and with the right mix of courage, intelligence, and good fortune, they may well be able to move forward this most important of our national programs.

References

Aglukkaq, L. (2012). Speaking notes by the Honourable Leona Aglukkaq, Minister of Health and the Canadian Northern Economic Development Agency, opening remarks, Canadian Medical Association 145th annual meeting, Yellowknife, NT. http://www.hc-sc.gc.ca/ahc-asc/minist/speeches-discours/_2012/2012_08_13-eng.php.

Banting, K., and R. Boadway. (2004). "Defining the Sharing Community: The Federal Role in Health Care." In Money, Politics and Health Care: Reconstructing the Federal-Provincial Partnership, edited by H. Lazar and F. St-Hilaire, 1–77. Montreal: Institute for Research on Public Policy.

Bégin, M. 1987. L'Assurance santé: Plaidoyer pour le modèle canadien. Montreal: Boreal.

Blumenthal, D., and J. A. Morone. 2009. The Heart of Power: Health and Politics in the Oval Office. Berkeley: University of California Press.

Boessenkool, K. J. 2010. "Fixing the Fiscal Imbalance: Turning GST Revenues over to the Provinces in Exchange for Lower Transfers." School of Public Policy Research Papers 3, no. 10. Calgary: University of Calgary.

Brown, L. D. 2010. "The Political Face of Public Health." Public Health Reviews 32, no. 1: 155–73.

Collier, Roger. 2011. "Mediocrity Has Become the Norm, Turnbull Asserts in Valedictory Address." Canadian Medical Association Journal 183, no. 1: E995–96. http://dx.doi.org/10.1503/cmaj.109-3982.

Council of the Federation. 2012a. From Innovation to Action: The First Report of the Health Care Innovation Working Group. Ottawa: Council of the Federation.

————. 2012b. *Report of the Council of the Federation Working Group on Fiscal Arrangements: Assessment of the Fiscal Impact of the Current Federal Fiscal Proposals*. Ottawa: Council of the Federation.

Forest, P.-G. 2012. "Is Our Healthcare System's Future Tied to the Canada Health Act? Part 2" *Health Innovation Report* 4: 12–16. Accessed 15 April 2014. http://www .healthinnovationforum.org/en/article/is-our-healthcare-systems-future-tied-to -the-canada-health-act/#.

Forest, P.-G., and K. M. Bergeron. 2005. "Les politiques de réforme du système de santé dans cinq fédérations : une analyse de travaux scientifiques récents." In *Politiques publiques comparées dans les états fédérés*, edited by L. Imbeau, 59–90. Quebec: Presses de l'Université Laval.

Forest, P.-G., and H. A. Palley. 2008. "Examining Fiscal Federalism, Regionalization, and Community-Based Initiatives in Canada's Health Care Delivery System." *Social Work in Public Health* 23, no. 4: 69–88. http://dx.doi.org/10.1080/ 19371910802162280.

Funigiello, P. J. 2005. *Chronic Politics: Health Care Security from FDR to George W. Bush*. Lawrence: University of Kansas Press.

Gauthier, J. 2011. "The Canada Health Transfer: Changes to Provinces Allocation." Library of Parliament Background Papers no. 2011-02-E. Ottawa: Library of Parliament.

Gostin, L. O. 2000. "Public Health Law in a New Century. Part 1: Law as a Tool to Advance the Community's Health." *Journal of the American Medical Association* 283, no. 21: 2837–41. http://dx.doi.org/10.1001/jama.283.21.2837.

Imbeau, L. M., R. Landry, H. Milner, F. Pétry, J. Crête, P.-G. Forest, Gerlier, and V. Lemieux. 2000. "Comparative Provincial Policy Analysis: A Research Agenda." *Canadian Journal of Political Science* 33, no. 4: 779–804.

Kneebone, R. 2012. "How You Pay Determines What You Get: Alternative Financing Options as a Determinant of Publicly Funded Health Care in Canada." School of Public Policy Research Papers 5, no. 20. Calgary: University of Calgary.

Lalonde, M. 1974. *A New Perspective on the Health of Canadians: A Working Document*. Ottawa: Department of Health and Welfare.

Lavis, J. N. 2002. "Ideas at the Margin or Marginalized Ideas? Non-medical Determinants of Health in Canada." *Health Affairs* 21, no. 2: 107–12. http://dx.doi .org/10.1377/hlthaff.21.2.107.

————. 2004. "Political Elites and Their Influence on Health Care Reforms in Canada." In *The Governance of Health Care in Canada*, edited by T. McIntosh, P.-G. Forest, and G. P. Marchildon, 257–79. Toronto: University of Toronto Press.

Lewis, S., C. Donaldson, C. Mitton, and G. Currie. 2001. "The Future of Health Care in Canada." *British Medical Journal* 323, no. 7318: 926–29. http://dx.doi .org/10.1136/bmj.323.7318.926.

MacDougall, H. 2012. "Into Thin Air: Making National Health Policy, 1939–1945." In *Making Medicare: New Perspectives on the History of Medicare in Canada*, edited by G. P. Marchildon, 41–70. Toronto: University of Toronto Press.

Maioni, A. 1998. *Parting at the Crossroads: The Emergence of Health Insurance in the United States and Canada*. Princeton, NJ: Princeton University Press.

Marchildon, G. P. 2006. *Health Systems in Transition: Canada*. Toronto: University of Toronto Press.

————. 2012. "Canadian Medicare: Why History Matters." In *Making Medicare: New Perspectives in the History of Medicare in Canada*, edited by G. P. Marchildon, 3–18. Toronto: University of Toronto Press.

———. 2013. "The Future of the Federal Role in Canadian Health Care." In *Health Care Federalism in Canada: Critical Junctures and Critical Perspectives*, edited by K. Fierlbeck and W. Lahey, 177–91. Montreal: McGill-Queen's University Press.

Maxwell, J., S. Rosell, and P.-G. Forest. 2003. "Giving Citizens a Voice in Healthcare Policy in Canada." *British Medical Journal* 326, no. 7397: 1031–33. http://dx.doi.org/10.1136/bmj.326.7397.1031.

McIntosh, T., and P.-G. Forest. 2010. "Talking to and with Canadians: Citizen Engagement and the Politics of the Romanow Commission." *Southern Journal of Canadian Studies* 3, no. 1: 28–50.

McKay, L. 2000. "Making the Lalonde Report." Background paper. Ottawa: Canadian Policy Research Networks. http://cprn.org/documents/ACFQQqr3M.PDF

Oliver, A. 2010. "Reflections on the Development of Health Inequities Policy in England." *Health Care Analysis* 18, no. 4: 402–20. http://dx.doi.org/10.1007/s10728-010-0144-x.

Rochefort, D. 2001. "The Backlash against Managed Care." In *The New Politics of State Health Policy* edited by R. B. Hackey and D. A. Rochefort, 113–41. Lawrence: University of Kansas Press.

SCC (Supreme Court of Canada). 2010. Reference re: *Assisted Reproduction Act*, 2010 SCC 61.

———. 2011. *Canada (Attorney General) v. PHS Community Services Society*, 2011 SCC 44.

Sparer, M. S., G. B. France, and C. Clinton. 2011. "Inching toward Incrementalism: Federalism, Devolution, and Health Policy in the United States and the United Kingdom." *Journal of Health Politics, Policy and Law* 36, no. 1: 33–57. http://dx.doi.org/10.1215/03616878-1191099.

Stuckler, D., S. Basu, and M. McKee. 2010. "Budget Crises, Health, and Social Welfare Programs." *British Medical Journal* 340: c3311. http://dx.doi.org/10.1136/bmj.c3311.

Tainter, J. A. 1988. *The Collapse of Complex Societies*. Cambridge: Cambridge University Press.

Taylor, M. G. 1978. *Health Insurance and Canadian Public Policy: The Seven Decisions that Created the Canadian Health Insurance System*. Montreal: McGill-Queen's University Press.

Tuohy, C. H. 1999. *Accidental Logics: The Dynamics of Change in the Health Care Arena in the United States, Britain, and Canada*. New York: Oxford University Press.

Watts, R. L. 1989. *Executive Federalism: A Comparative Analysis*. Institute of Intergovernmental Relations Research Papers no. 26. Kingston, ON: Queen's University.

Wells, P. 2012. "Aglukkaq's Letter to Provincial Health Ministers: Slip-Slidin' Away." *Maclean's*, 19 January. http://www.macleans.ca/2012/01/19/aglukkaqs-letter-to-provincial-health-ministers-slip-slidin-away/.

PART III

Provincial Experiences
in Canada

nine

Ontario: Changing Policies, Changing Categories

RAISA DEBER AND SARA ALLIN

Health spending in Ontario

Internationally, increases in health expenditures have led to concern that these costs are not sustainable. Rhetoric has evoked the need for "system transformation," although it often carefully does not specify what needs to be transformed. However, the extent to which these concerns are supported by the data is far from clear.

For this paper we have focused heavily on data provided by the Canadian Institute for Health Information (CIHI). Most published comparisons are between Ontario and Canada as a whole. Spending patterns in Ontario often resemble the Canadian average because Ontario makes up almost 40% of the Canadian population, so where possible we have also added information about what we will call the "rest of Canada"—an average of the remaining nine provinces, excluding the territories, weighted by population size.

Figure 9.1 illustrates that health spending in Ontario has tracked the trends in the other Canadian provinces. These patterns apply both over time and for the most recent data available.

Figure 9.1 Total health spending per capita in Ontario, rest of Canada, and Canada, 1975–2011 (current dollars)

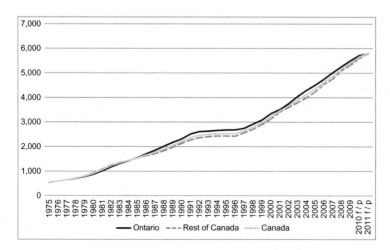

However, closer analysis of the data does reveal some slight differences. For example, examining the shares of spending across sub-sectors shows that Ontario spends relatively more on physicians and relatively less on hospitals than the rest of the country. Table 9.1 provides data on per capita spending as forecast by CIHI for 2011, which we have collapsed into three sources of funds (provincial governments; other public sources, including federal direct spending and social security funds; and private), with more detailed information for selected uses of fund categories that together account for the bulk of provincial spending.

In CIHI's 2011 forecasts for total health expenditures per capita, Ontario resembles the rest of Canada in that the growth of provincial spending per capita has been similar to that in other provinces. In addition, the effect of population growth and aging in Ontario is quite similar to patterns in Canada as a whole, although there is clearly variation across provinces.

Examining these patterns by use of funds, we see that Ontario spent less on hospitals than the rest of Canada. Ontario's per capita hospital

Table 9.1 Spending per capita (dollars), selected use of funds, Ontario, Canada, and rest of Canada, 2011

Category	Provincial	Other Public	Private	Total
Ontario				
Hospitals	1,317	18	243	1,579
Other institutions	317	3	183	502
Physicians	897	14	8	920
Drugs (Rx)	335	19	432	785
Public health	370	67	0	437
All other	409	147	1,014	1,569
Total	**3,645**	**267**	**1,880**	**5,792**
Canada				
Hospitals	1,510	21	162	1,693
Other institutions	409	4	173	586
Physicians	785	17	13	814
Drugs (Rx)	301	48	438	788
Public health	286	76	0	362
All other	487	142	939	1,568
Total	**3,778**	**308**	**1,725**	**5,811**

Table 9.1 (Continued)

Category	Provincial	Other Public	Private	Total
Rest of Canada				
Hospitals	1,620	23	108	1,755
Other institutions	467	4	171	638
Physicians	710	18	16	746
Drugs (Rx)	281	67	454	801
Public health	235	79	0	310
All other	532	136	880	1,549
Total	**3,843**	**327**	**1,628**	**5,799**

Source: CIHI 2011b.

Notes

Rest of Canada = population-weighted average across the nine other provinces.

All other = remainder of health expenditures, including over-the-counter drugs, capital, administration, and "other" categories from CIHI data (items such as home care, medical transportation/ambulances, hearing aids, other appliances, training of health workers, voluntary health associations, and occupational health to promote and enhance health and safety at the workplace).

Other institutions = primarily LTC facilities licensed and/or funded by provincial governments.

Total per capita spending on average in Canada is slightly higher than for Ontario and the rest of Canada because it includes the three territories, where spending ranges from $8,996 (Northwest Territories) to $11,929 (Nunavut), and because the only two provinces spending less than Ontario—British Columbia ($5,450) and Québec ($5,261)—account for more than half of the rest of Canada.

spending also rose more slowly: a 1.1% increase between 2010 and 2011 versus 2.6% for Canada and 3.5% for the rest of Canada. However, it is important to recognize that comparing short-term trends in hospital spending is difficult because the Ontario government occasionally steps in to cover hospital deficits; this means that a few years of lower spending may be followed by a few years of higher spending. Nonetheless, the average annual growth rate on hospital spending for the period 2004–11 was 4.3% in Ontario, compared to 5.4% for the rest of Canada. In terms of expenditures by provincial governments, Ontario also spent less for hospitals than did other provinces: its $1,317 per capita accounted for 36% of provincial health spending as compared to 42% for the rest of Canada. Indeed, the proportion of provincial spending allocated to hospitals has been lower in Ontario than in the rest of Canada since the early 1980s, and since then the proportion spent on hospitals has been declining at a faster rate than in the rest of Canada.

Provincial spending on other institutions, the majority of which are long-term care homes, was also considerably lower in Ontario ($317 per capita in 2011) than in the other nine provinces ($467 per capita). This was not balanced by private spending; Ontario private spending on other institutions ($183 per capita) only slightly exceeded the average of $171 in the rest of Canada. The relatively low spending on both hospitals and other institutions reflects long-standing efforts in Ontario to shift care to the community, as discussed below.

The second largest component of provincial spending is physicians. Since 1975, provincial spending on physicians has been consistently higher in Ontario than in the rest of Canada, although the growth rates were comparable. Ontario spent considerably more in the physicians category ($920 per capita versus $814 for Canada and $746 for the rest of Canada). The share was also higher: 15.9% of total spending (24.6% of provincial spending) in Ontario versus 14% of total spending (21% of provincial spending) in Canada and 12.9% of total spending (18.5% of provincial spending) for the rest of Canada. However, it is difficult to compare spending across jurisdictions, as there are some differences in classification (see below).

Until 2011, spending on drugs had been the third largest provincial expense in health care in Ontario. CIHI data show that the province's drug spending was roughly comparable to the national average, at $939 per capita in Ontario versus $929 in Canada and $924 in the rest of Canada. As well, 16.2% of total spending in Ontario was for drugs, versus 16% for both Canada and the rest of Canada. However, because non-prescription drugs are paid entirely through private-sector sources, Table 9.1 places them in the "other" category and looks separately at spending for prescription drugs; Ontario's total spending for that sub-category was $785 per capita, as compared to $801 as the average for the rest of Canada. More of these prescription drug costs were paid by the Ontario government, in part a reflection of more generous provincial coverage. Another factor is that some of this spending reflects a shifting of drug expenditures out of hospitals and into the outpatient drug category. The annual increase in total drug spending per capita in Ontario was less than the national figure (1.5% versus 2.8%, and 3.7% in the rest of Canada), partially because of policy initiatives that included cuts to generic pricing (Law, Ystma, and Morgan 2011).

Another striking observation is that public health has become the third largest component of Ontario's provincial health spending (10.2%, compared to 7.6% in Canada as a whole). The growth in public health spending has been significant: from 2% of the provincial health budget in 1975 ($7 per capita) to 10.2% ($370 per capita) in 2011. If one considers total public spending on public health rather than spending only by provincial governments, one notes that the total was $437 per capita in Ontario compared to $310 in the rest of Canada ($362 in Canada). However, although some of this increase reflects traditional public health (catalyzed by such events as the SARS outbreak), much reflects how spending is classified (see the next section).

The CIHI cost-driver analysis noted several factors affecting the growth in health spending over the period 1998–2008 (CIHI 2011a, 2011b). A portion of the increase resulted from high economic growth during that period, which allowed governments to spend more and at the same time to reduce tax rates. Some of these factors related to the general economy, some to demography (population growth and population aging), and some to policy decisions. In summary, CIHI divided the 7.4% annual increase in health spending for the 1998–2008 growth period as follows: 2.8% arising from general inflation; 2.8% from health-specific inflation, including new technology and increased use of services; 1% from population growth; and 0.8% from population aging (CIHI 2011a). Hospital cost drivers were similar, with a slightly greater impact from population aging at 1% per year (CIHI 2012b).

CIHI argued that the main cost drivers were "rents"—higher wages/fees paid for similar care (although some of this reflected catch-up). However, there was also an increase in the number of physician services used per Canadian, and in the supply of physicians; between 2000 and 2010 there was an 8.4% increase in the number of physicians per capita in Canada and a 4.8% increase in Ontario (CIHI 2011c). CIHI analyses of cost drivers of Ontario physician spending for the period 1998–2008 suggest that per capita age-adjusted utilization was relatively more important and prices relatively less important than for the rest of Canada. One policy implication is that a focus on cutting fee schedules, as Ontario is trying to do, may or may not "bend the cost curve," depending in part on how these policies affect utilization. Note that it is very difficult to predict what effect these fee cuts could have on utilization, as there are numerous factors other than physician fees that may affect use patterns.

Cost pressures: Is the devil in the details?

As noted, at first glance, Ontario has good control over hospital costs. Physician costs seem higher, as do (to a lesser degree) drugs and "public health." However, scrutiny of the CIHI data clarifies several caveats about interpreting these findings. Some of the differences found by analyzing expenditure patterns represent substantive interprovincial differences, while others represent differences in how provinces have chosen to organize and fund particular activities, rather than real differences in overall costs.

How are things classified?

Although CIHI has standardized how health spending is reported, different ways of delivering care may make things fall into a different category. Accordingly, changing how particular services are delivered may shift their costs into a different category. For example, as care moves out of hospitals, pharmaceutical costs shift from the Hospitals to the Drugs category. In Ontario, the decision to move many mental health services from provincial psychiatric hospitals into "community mental health" also meant that the same services, often delivered by the same people, were coded as Public Health rather than Hospitals. Similarly, CIHI classifies what Ontario calls "independent health facilities" under physician services; to the extent that the province has sought to move some specialized services (including diagnostic imaging and laser eye surgery) into such clinics, they appear as increases in the costs of physician services. Given Ontario's continuing efforts to provide care as cost-efficiently as possible, it is likely that this trend to deliver services in non-hospital settings will accelerate over time.

What costs are being captured?

Some costs may not be captured by the system of health statistics reported to CIHI. For example, in the Other Institutions category, unregulated residential care facilities (whose costs are private) are often not captured by the system of health statistics. Home care, a growing sub-sector, is also problematic. Most provinces do not report data about home care, including Ontario, which has not reported home-care spending data to CIHI since 2004–05. CIHI's national health expenditure (NHEX) framework also excludes some home-care services not provided by health professionals. Some of this spending is captured in the Other residual category, but some is not in the data at all. Particularly given decisions by the Ontario government to encourage home-care services, this omission from the national data complicates comparative analysis in this growing health sector.

Who is paying for what?

Are we talking about total spending or public spending? Within public spending, are we focusing only on what provincial governments pay? For example, because of the way Ontario has organized public health, some of those costs are classified as being municipal rather than provincial expenditures, which is not the case in other provinces. Municipal governments in Ontario also have some responsibility for funding long-term care, including owning and operating about one-sixth of long-term care homes in the province. Partly for these reasons, Ontario municipalities spent $44 per capita on health in 2011 compared to the average of $12 per capita in the remaining nine provinces.

Who is generating which costs?

Although information is usually presented as expenditures per capita, it is important to recognize that health-care spending is heavily skewed, with a small proportion of the population accounting for the bulk of spending. This pattern exists across all age/sex groups and across most sub-categories of expenditures, with hospital costs being the most heavily skewed (Deber, Forget, and Roos 2004).

One clear policy issue is whether efforts to control the cost curve are considering total, public, or provincial spending. What is sometimes called the "First Law of Cost Containment" stresses that the easiest way to contain costs is to shift them to someone else, but this is often penny wise and pound foolish. For example, if people cannot afford the drugs to control chronic diseases, there may be more hospital admissions, worse health outcomes, and higher total costs in the long run (Tamblyn et al. 2001). Patterns of spending by provincial governments may accordingly differ more than total expenditures of provinces, particularly if some cover services not required by the *Canada Health Act*.

Similar issues affect such common metrics as spending as a percentage of total provincial government program spending, which depends on what is counted in provincial or in other budgets. Health spending accounts for a higher proportion of the Ontario budget (41% in 2000 and 40% in 2010) than the Canadian average (36% in 2000 and 38% in 2010), but this partially reflects the legacy of policy decisions to shift some other costs (many not for health care) from the provincial to the municipal level, meaning that the denominator (provincial government spending) may not always represent the same thing across provinces.

Sustainability

Canada uses a mixture of models to finance care. In total, about 70% of Canada's total health expenditures are classified as public. Most of the publicly financed services use what the OECD refers to as a public contracting model (Docteur and Oxley 2003). This allows Canadian public insurers to use the market power of a single payer to control costs. The *Canada Health Act* defines such insured services in terms of where they are provided and by whom. This means that care that must be fully insured if provided in hospitals need not be publicly paid for if delivered in other locations by providers other than physicians. Changes in how and by whom care is delivered can thus imply changes in not only who pays but also what policy levers are available for cost containment. For example, in 2004 Ontario delisted coverage of outpatient physiotherapy and routine vision care. Similarly, several Ontario hospitals have been reducing rehabilitation services (Landry et al. 2009).

Ontario, like other Canadian provinces, has been fixated on questions of sustainability. Budgetary concerns and a substantial provincial deficit have led to particular attention to possibilities for innovation that could improve value for money (Health Care Innovation Working Group 2012). One widely cited report was from Ontario's Commission to Reform Ontario Public Services, chaired by Don Drummond, which made a series of recommendations (Ontario, Ministry of Finance 2012). Despite talk about sustainability, our examination of the data suggests that Romanow's conclusion still holds—publicly funded health care is as sustainable as we want it to be (Commission on the Future of Health Care in Canada 2002). Nonetheless, governments are concerned that growth in health expenditures has often outpaced economic growth, and that—to the extent that payments are service-based—these costs are difficult to cap. Clearly there is always scope for improvement, and several policy innovations have been attempted.

Policy reforms

Health economists have noted that health costs can be seen as the weighted average of service mix and cost and utilization for each service. Canada's reliance on a public contracting model for physicians and, to a large extent, hospital services has implications for the policy levers available to payers, since physicians have considerable flexibility in where and how they choose to practise and in which services they decide to provide (Deber et al. 2010). We focus on three areas of reform: hospitals, physicians, and long-term care.

Hospitals

Hospitals are expensive places to treat people, and one policy response has been to reduce the number of beds. A decade ago, CIHI data showed that, although hospitals were the largest category of national health expenditure, their costs were increasing less rapidly than other health spending, resulting in a drop in their share of national health expenditure from 45% in 1976 to 30% in 2002 (CIHI 2005). Even accounting for some reclassification (e.g., Ontario reclassified 10 psychiatric hospitals from residential facilities to hospitals), there was a substantial drop in the number of beds.

The most recent OECD data show that Canada had 3.2 hospital beds per 1,000 population in 2009, among the lowest internationally and down substantially from 6.8 in 1981 and 5.8 in 1991. Looking only at curative (acute) beds, Canada's reported figure for 2009 was 1.7 per 1,000. Ontario had fewer hospital beds per capita (2.4 per 1,000 population) than other provinces. The Ontario Hospital Association reported that the number of hospital beds staffed and in operation in the province had dropped from 49,391 in 1990 to 30,810 in 2010. The number of acute beds dropped from 33,403 to 18,355 over that period, but the decrease was even more striking for complex continuing care beds: from 11,435 to 5,798 (Ontario Hospital Association 2012).

Overall, this means that Ontario's hospital bed capacity has been cut by almost 40% since 1990, resulting in a definite reduction in the share of Ontario's health spending going to hospital costs. This was a desired goal, resulting in part from the work of the Health Services Restructuring Commission and reflecting changes in technology that allowed more care to be delivered outside hospital settings (Baumann et al. 1996; Sinclair, Rochon, and Leatt 2005). In Canada there has been a steady decline in hospital share of public-sector expenditures from 1976 until the late 1990s; it then became roughly stable in the past 10 years (CIHI 2011b). In 2011, per capita spending on hospitals by the Government of Ontario was $1,317, compared to $1,620 in the rest of Canada (see Table 9.1, above). Only Québec spent less ($1,298), and Newfoundland and Labrador spent the most ($2,502) (CIHI 2011b).

This reduction has been linked to Ontario's quite successful effort to shift care outside of hospitals where possible. CIHI reported that, after adjusting for age and sex, Ontario had the lowest rate of acute inpatient hospitalizations for 2010–11. Even from its low starting point in 1995–96, it dropped more than the national average over the 15-year period from 1995–96 to 2010–11. Ontario and Saskatchewan also reported the lowest length of stay (CIHI 2012a).

However, this successful effort has led to something of a backlash as advocacy groups point to difficulties with access and longer wait lists. Ontario, like many other provinces, employed global budgets as a mechanism for controlling overall costs. Decisions about how to use these budgets were left to individual hospitals. One result was unpopular decisions by particular organizations seeking to control costs that could be interpreted as impairing access. In turn this led to a policy emphasis on wait-time strategies, some of which were incorporated into the 2004 First Ministers' Accord; these often targeted particular services (such as diagnostic imaging, hip and knee surgery, and cataract surgery) that had been given lower priority by many hospitals. A key policy focus over the past decade throughout Canada has thus been wait-time and wait-list strategies, often based on the assumption that more is always better. Similarly, efforts to close hospitals and consolidate services have frequently led to local community resistance.

More recently, a related policy thrust—also underway in most provinces, particularly those with quality councils—is to move from a focus solely on reducing wait times to also considering the appropriateness of care (Deber 2008) and ensuring that treatments follow clinical guidelines for best practices. Ontario's 2010 *Excellent Care for All Act* expanded the mandate of Ontario's quality council, Health Quality Ontario, to include making recommendations about evidence-based delivery of care based on clinical guidelines, as well as to providing guidance to government on what things should cost.

Recently there has been a shift from global hospital budgets to activity-based payments. This has been portrayed by the provincial government as a way to seek more efficiency in care delivery per service, but there are also real risks to cost control in this policy direction, particularly if incentives to deliver more services are not linked to ensuring that they are appropriate (Sutherland 2011; Sutherland et al. 2011; Sutherland et al. 2013).

Physician costs, including primary-care reform

Primary care has been a particular focus of recent health reform in Ontario (Glazier and Redelmeier 2010; Hutchison et al. 2011). The stated goals have included improving access and quality, including increasing the number of physicians and encouraging primary-care providers to work in teams and provide after-hours care, and taking the pressure off hospital emergency departments.

Following the Barer-Stoddart Report of the early 1990s and policy decisions to reduce the number of physicians being trained, the pendulum swung to claims of physician shortages (Evans and McGrail 2008). One policy response from provincial governments in the past decade was to increase the number of physicians, both the number of domestic medical graduates and the number of international medical graduates. The number of active physicians per 100,000 population in Canada increased steadily, from 151 in 1980 to 186 in 1990, 188 in 2000, and 203 in 2010. Ontario growth was less pronounced, and less steady, than that in most other provinces. The number of physicians per 100,000 grew from 156 in 1980 to 191 in 1990, but dropped to 180 in 2000 before rising to 189 in 2010 (CIHI 2011c). Over the past five years this growth in the number of physicians in Canada has consistently outpaced population growth. As a result, Ontario, like most other provinces, has more physicians and is spending more on them. Trying to curb payments to physicians has thus become a major policy thrust of the Ontario government, although balanced against efforts to improve access, with the relative emphasis varying over time.

Over the past decade, Ontario has made significant investments in primary care, including encouraging less reliance on fee-for-service (FFS) payments to encourage primary-care providers to work in teams and provide after-hours services. As a result, 47.3% of Ontario physicians in family medicine were recipients of alternative clinical payments in 2009–10, considerably higher than in the other provinces (British Columbia, for example, reported 14.5%). In contrast, only 15.8% of Ontario specialists were in alternative plans, considerably lower than in the other provinces for which data are available (e.g., 21% in British Columbia and Québec, 27% in Saskatchewan).

In terms of distribution between family medicine and specialists, Ontario resembles the rest of Canada. In 2010 Ontario had about 92 family doctors per 100,000 population (compared to 103 for Canada) and 97 specialists (100 for Canada) (CIHI 2011c). This shift to alternative payment models means that it is more difficult to compare CIHI data about billings by province and/or by specialty. As an example, CIHI's data about billings captured information about Ontario family doctors for 62 physicians per 100,000 population (compared to 79 for the rest of Canada), and for Ontario specialists it captured data for 72 (compared to 67 for the rest of Canada). Some simple math reveals that Ontario billing data were relatively less likely than in the rest of Canada to capture the province's family doctors (62 out of 92, compared to 79 out of 103) but relatively more likely to capture specialists (72 out of 97, compared to 67 out of 100). This may in turn be related to the estimates already referred to about the relative likelihood that physicians in different provinces and different specialities would receive alternative clinical payments. Those differences may account in part for the higher reported average gross FFS payment per Ontario physician: for the subgroup that received at least $60,000 in payments, it was $237,330 for family medicine (compared to $236,346 for the rest of Canada) and for specialties it was $371,758 (compared to $326,825 for the rest of Canada).

An investigative report from Ontario's Institute for Clinical Evaluative Sciences (ICES), which stores and analyzes administrative data, examined payments to Ontario physicians from the Ontario Ministry of Health and Long-Term Care (MOHLTC) between 1992–93 and 2009–10 (Henry et al. 2012). ICES found that Ontario paid doctors approximately $8 billion in 2009–10, more than twice the amount they had received in 1992–93 (in unadjusted dollars). Note that these are not take-home wages, since physician payments include the costs of running a practice, including hiring other professionals where inter-professional teams are in use; clearly that differs by type of specialty and type of practice. The increase varied considerably by specialty, with the greatest going to family physicians. ICES concluded that the increase in physician costs was strongly related to two provincial government policies. The first was a decision to increase the number of physicians being trained, a result of the strongly held perception that there was a physician shortage, a trend that affected all Canadian jurisdictions. The second was a decision to change how, and how much, physicians were paid. The rationale was that changes in how physicians were organized—in particular, in how primary care was organized and delivered—would be essential to ensure that every Canadian had access to high-quality primary care (Hutchison et al. 2011).

In aggregate, the ICES study concluded that about 37% of the Ontario increase could be attributed to increases in physician supply and the remaining 63% to an increase in average payments per physician. However, this varied over time. The mean payment per physician remained fairly flat between 1992–93 and 2004–05, at or below the rate of inflation. The number of providers also contracted slightly between 1993–94 and 1999–2000, in part because of limitations on granting new billing numbers. Ontario also imposed a global ceiling on medical expenditures for three years, beginning in 1993–94, which involved "clawing back" physician billings by an across-the-board percentage if the total exceeded a cap (Archibald and Flood 2004; Barer, Lomas, and Sanmartin 1996). This approach was dropped in 1998 (Henry et al. 2012).

The 2004–05 agreement between the Ontario Medical Association (OMA) and the MOHLTC changed the process by which physician fees were determined. It provided additional payments to support the provincial wait-time strategy, and so in part reflected a planned increase in the number of services being provided, particularly by radiologists, nephrologists, and ophthalmologists. At the same time the number of physicians grew by about 5,000 in one decade, to about 26,000 in total. This was an intended result, as Ontario had seen a reduction in the number of family physicians and was concerned about access to care. Starting from about 1999, Ontario also deliberately changed the financial models, moving from fee-for-service to capitation-based and blended payment models for primary care (Glazier et al. 2009; Glazier, Zagorski, and Rayner 2012; Henry et al. 2012; Hutchison 2008; Lewis 2011). By 2012, about 70% of Ontario doctors were receiving some level of alternative funding, although about 70% of their earnings still came from FFS.

The provincial fiscal situation provoked some attention to these costs. In 2011 the provincial auditor general argued that value for money had not been demonstrated, with a particular focus on increased expenditures for family practitioners (Office of the Auditor General of Ontario 2011a, 2011b). The Drummond Report also recommended curbing physician costs, in part by placing less emphasis on FFS and more emphasis on salary or capitation (Ontario, Ministry of Finance 2012). In 2012 the Liberal provincial government announced that it wanted about 1.3 million public-sector workers in the province to agree to a two-year pay freeze to help trim a $15 billion deficit.

Against this background, negotiations with doctors and teachers went particularly badly. Negotiations between the government and the OMA, which represents 25,000 Ontario physicians, soon broke down. The provincial government responded by unilaterally cutting fees for hundreds of services by changing 37 items in the OHIP (Ontario Health Insurance Plan) fee schedule, with the expectation that this would save $338.3 million that year. The emphasis was on high-cost specialty services, particularly those delivered by cardiologists, radiologists, and ophthalmologists. One statistic the government emphasized was the fact that 407 specialists were billing OHIP more than $1 million each per year. The changes were made retroactive to April 1, 2012 (Talaga and Benzie 2012).

The OMA responded with anger, claiming that there would be longer waits (particularly in emergency departments and for test results) and that physicians would leave the province. The health minister, Deb Matthews, was not receptive. She claimed that "our doctors are the best paid in Canada," but her public remarks tended to equate physician billings with physician salaries. "Instead of another raise for doctors, we need a real wage freeze so we can invest in more home care," she told a press conference, and therefore, "I was left with no choice."

Each side used their own numbers and their own arguments. Matthews claimed that the physicians were seeking an additional $700 million and equated it to a 5% raise, or $20,000 per doctor. The OMA claimed that the demands represented a cut of $1 billion. Its representatives argued that they were willing to take a two-year fee freeze and to find another $250 million in savings. They also launched a $1.5 million advertising campaign to try to make their case. In June 2012 the OMA applied to the Ontario Superior Court of Justice, arguing that the government had not negotiated in good faith and that its behaviour constituted a violation of the Charter of Rights and Freedoms. In December 2012, both sides signed a physician services agreement that added "new priority investments" to the fee adjustments and stressed "new partnership initiatives aimed at modernizing the delivery of health care."

In reality, these cuts represented a combination of rationales. Some reflected changes in technology that meant that services could be completed more quickly than when the fee schedules were set. The newspapers quoted the minister as saying, "Specialties have seen tremendous windfall profits because of enhanced technology. We need to share in some of those productivity changes. It is only appropriate we update fees to reflect reality." As one example, payments for cataract surgery were to be cut to $397.75 from $441; one rationale was that such surgeries had taken two hours in the 1980s but could now be completed in 15 minutes, thanks to technological improvements. Similarly, fees for eye injections for retinal diseases were to be cut to $90 from $189 over four years.

Other cuts reflected suspicions that procedures were being overused (You et al. 2007; You et al. 2011). For example, payments for 250 different diagnostic radiology tests, such as X-rays, CT/MRI scans, and ultrasound, were to be reduced by 11% over four years. Fees were also to be cut for self-referrals, particularly since physicians who owned their own equipment appeared to be ordering more tests. Subsequently the Minister announced that she was open to modifying this when it was recognized that it could affect access in some geographical areas. Limitations were also placed on how many times per year certain services could be billed for (e.g., for retinal disease or glaucoma) (D'Aliesio 2012; Talaga and Benzie 2012). At the time of writing, the dispute was still going on.

Long-term care and home care

It has been increasingly suggested that care be shifted out of hospitals to home and community, and that this can be a cost saver (Deber 2009; Dumont-Lemasson, Donovan, and Wylie 1999; Health Council of Canada 2012; Hollander and Prince 2008). Moreover, a variety of people could benefit from home care. Care for potential clients can be categorized into *acute-care substitution*, which allows people to be safely discharged from acute hospitals; *long-term care (LTC) substitution*, which serves those who might otherwise be in LTC institutions; and *prevention/maintenance*, which keeps people healthy enough to remain out of institutions (Dumont-Lemasson, Donovan, and Wylie 1999). Those in the acute-care substitution category are often referred to as ALC (alternate levels of care) patients. Policymakers have repeatedly struggled with the provision of LTC, including the balance between facilities and community care and how various services should be financed and delivered. Such shifts move care beyond the requirements of the *Canada Health Act*. Depending on the jurisdiction, client group, and type of care, a varying share is paid publicly, but a sizeable share remains to be privately paid. A review of funding models has concluded that there is not yet good evidence on how best to reduce ALC (Sutherland and Crump 2011).

Unlike acute care, which is required for a relatively short time, LTC services are often required on a sustained basis. LTC may be delivered within specialized facilities (e.g., nursing homes or homes for the aged) or in the community (e.g., through in-home services, community support services, or supportive housing). Most community-based LTC services—often referred to as "home care"—are provided by family members, friends, and volunteers, with a strong role also for paid workers. One way of categorizing LTC is to distinguish between health care and social care; another is to distinguish among professional services (provided by nurses, rehabilitation professionals, etc.), personal care support (often provided by unregulated health-care workers), and social support. These categorizations may overlap, since the services classified as health care also tend to be clinical (e.g., medical care, nursing, rehabilitation) and to be delivered by trained health-care professionals and/or personnel under their supervision. Social care services include personal care, meals, day programs, transportation, and house-maintenance services, as well as support groups and/or respite care to assist informal caregivers (the family members and volunteers who provide care). Social care services are often delivered by less skilled workers and/or by volunteers. Depending on needs, such nonclinical assistance as adaptations for housing can also be helpful (Williams, Challis, Deber, et al. 2009; Williams, Lum, Deber, et al. 2009).

In general there are no good national data on home-care spending in Canada. CIHI has been seeking to capture data about home care but has decided to include only professional services and to omit social care, to be consistent with the OECD System of Health Accounts (CIHI 2007). However, limited data do exist. For example, most provinces submitted government home-care expenditures to CIHI between 1994–95 and 2003–04. The Canadian average per capita provincial/territorial spending for home care in 2003–04 was estimated at $91.15 (in 1997 dollars); Ontario was only slightly higher, at $98.74 (CIHI 2007). However, one study that surveyed some home-care recipients concluded that provincial spending represented a small portion of total home-care spending, with about 75% of Ontario's home-care costs that year being paid privately (Guerriere et al. 2008). However, subsequent policy initiatives have increased the emphasis on home care. From 2003–04 to 2008–09, Ontario government expenditures on home care, including both home health care and personal support, increased by more than 40%—from $1.22 billion to $1.76 billion (Office of the Auditor General of Ontario 2010).

In 2007 the Ontario MOHLTC announced its "Aging at Home" (AAH) strategy, whose stated objective was an investment of close to $1.1 billion over four years to allow seniors to stay healthy and live more independently in their own homes, through provision of an integrated continuum of community-based services. The program was delivered through Ontario's 14 regional health authorities (Local Health Integration Networks, or LHINs) and allowed for local variations in how the services were organized and delivered.

Subsequently, Ontario's home-care program has shifted in its focus. The Aging at Home program was initially intended to focus on LTC substitution, with elements of prevention/maintenance. However, efforts to control hospital costs moved the emphasis to acute-care substitution, particularly to decreasing the number of ALC patients and preventing unnecessary visits to hospitals. A series of programs with such names as "Home First" have been implemented. Good data about this change in priorities are not readily available, although it is reflected in some LHIN reports.

This change in emphasis was encouraged by reports that alleviating ALCs, sometimes referred to as "provision of continuing care in the most appropriate location," would help curb costs (Ontario Association of Community Care Access Centres, Ontario Hospital Association, and Ontario Federation of Community Mental Health and Addiction Programs 2010). For example, in 2011 Dr. David Walker was commissioned by the Ontario minister of health and long-term care to advise how to address ALC. His report, titled *Caring for Our Aging Population and Addressing Alternate Level of Care (ALC)*, was submitted that year; it called for targeted community investments in the LHINs to help support transitions from hospital to the "right" community services (Walker 2011). This focus on shifting care out of hospitals was echoed in the 2012 "Action Plan for Health Care" published by the MOHLTC; its aim was to ensure provision of care "as close to home as possible," as this "reduces pressure on emergency rooms and saves money" (Ontario 2012, 11).

Assessment and conclusion

Based on pan-Canadian data, it appears that Ontario spends relatively more on physicians and relatively less on institutional care than do the other provinces. Some of these differences in spending may be attributed to differences in classification of data across provinces and differences in classification over time within provinces. For instance, efforts to improve efficiency by transferring care from hospitals to the community underscore the importance of examining declines in hospital spending alongside increases in spending in other sectors that may be less well documented. However, some of the differences in spending that we observe are likely to reflect policy decisions that are unique to the province. In this paper we focused on policy initiatives in three sectors: hospitals, physicians, and long-term care.

On the basis of the decrease in bed numbers and the relative share of expenditures going to hospitals, one can conclude that Ontario has been quite successful in reducing the emphasis on hospital care. Additional "low-hanging fruit" may involve continuing efforts to introduce evidence-based best practices and prevent expensive illnesses, including attention to the determinants of health. More difficult efforts will include addressing how much providers are paid for treating particular conditions. Cost shifting by moving expenditures from public to private budgets is likely to be less helpful in bending the cost curve, particularly since such efforts may increase total costs rather than decrease them. In that connection, Ontario's policies are a mixed bag. Their stated goals include both short-term budgetary relief and longer-term efforts to bend down the cost curve and cap key budget lines, particularly for physician services.

Although at the time of writing managing a minority government meant that policy initiatives had been delayed, efforts to curb physician expenditures have been complicated by growth in population and in the number of physicians, meaning that a hard cap seems unlikely to succeed. The acrimonious negotiations with the OMA, including the court challenge that Ontario was bargaining in bad faith, were also less than helpful in developing more evidence-based practice, although progress is being made, in part through working with providers to implement changes in hospital-funding formulas by linking them to clinical guidelines. The shift from hospitals to home and community appears to be working relatively well, although careful attention to how best to target services to those who need them, and to ensure that costs are not simply shifted onto individuals, will be crucial.

Acknowledgements

The authors thank Christopher Kuchciak, Ruolz Ariste, and Geoff Ballinger, CIHI, for clarifying data, and Owen Adams, Adalsteinn Brown, Sarah Caldwell, Michael Hillmer, and Guillermo Sandoval for helpful comments. They bear no responsibility for the inferences drawn in this paper.

References

Archibald, T., and C. M. Flood. 2004. "The Physician Services Committee: The Relationship between the Ontario Medical Association and the Ontario Ministry of Health and Long-Term Care." IRPP Working Papers no. 2004–03. Montreal: Institute for Research and Public Policy. http://archive.irpp.org/wp/archive/medicare_basket/wp2004-03.pdf.

Barer, M. L., J. Lomas, and C. Sanmartin. 1996. "Re-minding Our Ps and Qs: Medical Cost Controls in Canada." *Health Affairs* 15, no. 2: 216–34. http://dx.doi.org/10.1377/hlthaff.15.2.216.

Baumann, A. O., L. O'Brien-Pallas, R. Deber, G. Donner, D. Semogas, and B. Silverman. 1996. "Downsizing in the Hospital System: A Restructuring Process." *Healthcare Management Forum* 9, no. 4: 5–13. http://dx.doi.org/10.1016/S0840-4704(10)60756-9.

CIHI (Canadian Institute for Health Information). 2005. *Hospital Trends in Canada: Results of a Project to Create a Historical Series of Statistical and Financial Data for Canadian Hospitals over Twenty-Seven Years.* Ottawa: CIHI. https://secure.cihi.ca/free_products/Hospital_Trends_in_Canada_e.pdf.

———. 2007. *Public-Sector Expenditures and Utilization of Home Care Services in Canada: Exploring the Data.* Ottawa: CIHI. https://secure.cihi.ca/free_products/trends_home_care_mar_2007_e.pdf.

———. 2011a. "Health Care Cost Drivers: The Facts." Ottawa: CIHI. https://secure.cihi.ca/free_products/trends_home_care_mar_2007_e.pdf.

———. 2011b. "National Health Expenditure Trends, 1975–2011." Ottawa: CIHI. https://secure.cihi.ca/estore/productFamily.htm?pf=PFC1671&lang=en&media=0.

———. 2011c. "Supply, Distribution and Migration of Canadian Physicians, 2010." Ottawa: CIHI. https://secure.cihi.ca/estore/productFamily.htm?pf=PFC1680&lang=en&media=0.

———. 2012a. "Highlights of 2010–2011 Inpatient Hospitalizations and Emergency Department Visits." Ottawa: CIHI. https://secure.cihi.ca/estore/productFamily.htm?pf=PFC1840&lang=en&media=0.

———. 2012b. *Hospital Cost Drivers Technical Report: What Factors Have Determined Hospital Expenditure Trends in Canada?* Ottawa: CIHI . http://www.cihi.ca/CIHI-ext-portal/pdf/internet/hospital_costdriver_tech_en.

Commission on the Future of Health Care in Canada. 2002. *Building on Values: The Future of Health Care in Canada.* Ottawa: Queen's Printer. http://publications.gc.ca/collections/Collection/CP32-85-2002E.pdf.

D'Aliesio, R. 2012. "Specialists Brace Clinics for Impact of McGuinty's Fee Cuts." *Globe and Mail*, 8 June.

Deber, R. 2008. "Access without Appropriateness: Chicken Little in Charge?" *Health-care Policy* 4, no. 1: 12–18. http://archive.irpp.org/wp/archive/medicare_basket/wp2004-03.pdf.

———. 2009. "Canada." In *Cost Containment and Efficiency in National Health Systems: A Global Comparison*, edited by J. Rapoport, P. Jacobs, and E. Jonsson, 15–39. Weinheim, Germany: Wiley-VCH.

Deber, R., A. Baumann, B. Gamble, and A. Laporte. 2010. "Supply and Demand of Health Workers in an Economic Downturn." Paper presented at 12th Annual International Medical Workforce Collaboration, New York. http://rcpsc.medical.org/publicpolicy/imwc/2010-IMWC12/IMWC10deber.pdf.

Deber, R., E. Forget, and L. Roos. 2004. "Medical Savings Accounts in a Universal System: Wishful Thinking Meets Evidence." *Health Policy* 70, no. 1: 49–66. http://dx.doi.org/10.1016/j.healthpol.2004.01.010.

Docteur, E., and H. Oxley. 2003. "Health-Care Systems: Lessons from the Reform Experience." OECD Health Working Papers no. 9. Paris: OECD. https://www1.oecd.org/els/health-systems/22364122.pdf.

Dumont-Lemasson, M., C. Donovan, and M. Wylie. 1999. *Provincial and Territorial Home Care Programs: A Synthesis for Canada.* Ottawa: Health Canada; http://www.hc-sc.gc.ca/hcs-sss/pubs/home-domicile/1999-pt-synthes/index-eng.php.

Evans, R. G., and K. M. McGrail. 2008. "Richard III, Barer-Stoddart and the Daughter of Time." *Healthcare Policy* 3, no. 3: 1–11.

Glazier, R. H., J. Klein-Geltink, A. Kopp, and L. M. Sibley. 2009. "Capitation and Enhanced Fee-for-Service Models for Primacy Care Reform: A Population-Based Evaluation." *Canadian Medical Association Journal* 180, no. 1): E72–81. http://dx.doi.org/10.1503/cmaj.081316.

Glazier, R. H., and D. A. Redelmeier. 2010. "Building the Patient-Centered Medical Home in Ontario." *Journal of the American Medical Association* 303, no. 2): 2186–87. http://dx.doi.org/10.1001/jama.2010.753.

Glazier, R. H., B. M. Zagorski, and J. Rayner. 2012. *Comparison of Primary Care Models in Ontario by Demographics, Case Mix and Emergency Department Use, 2008–09 to 2009–10.* Toronto: ICES. http://www.ices.on.ca/Publications/Atlases-and-Reports/2012/Comparison-of-Primary-Care-Models.

Guerriere, D. N., A. Y. M. Wong, R. Croxford, V. W. Leong, P. McKeever, and P. C. Coyte. 2008. "Costs and Determinants of Privately Financed Home-Based Health Care in Ontario, Canada." *Health and Social Care in the Community* 16, 2: 126–36. http://dx.doi.org/10.1111/j.1365-2524.2007.00732.x.

Health Care Innovation Working Group. 2012. *From Innovation to Action: The First Report of the Health Care Innovation Working Group.* Toronto: Council of the Federation. http://www.councilofthefederation.ca/en/publications/.

Health Council of Canada. 2012. *Seniors in Need, Caregivers in Distress: What Are the Home Care Priorities for Seniors in Canada?* Toronto: Health Council of Canada. http://www.healthcouncilcanada.ca/rpt_det_gen.php?id=348.

Henry, D. A., S. E. Schultz, R. H. Glazier, R. S. Bhatia, I. A. Dhalla, and A. Laupacis. 2012. "Payments to Ontario Physicians from Ministry of Health and Long-Term Care Sources, 1992–93 to 2009–10." Toronto: ICES. http://www.ices.on.ca/Publications/Atlases-and-Reports/2012/Payments-to-Ontario-Physicians.

Hollander, M., and M. J. Prince. 2008. "Organizing Health Care Delivery Systems for Persons with Ongoing Care Needs and Their Families: A Best Practices Framework." *Healthcare Quarterly* 11, no. 1: 44–54. http://dx.doi.org/10.12927/hcq.2013.19497.

Hutchison, B. 2008. "A Long Time Coming: Primary Healthcare Renewal in Canada." *Healthcare Papers* 8, no. 2: 10–24. http://dx.doi.org/10.12927/hcpap.2008.19704.

Hutchison, B., J.-F. Levesque, E. Strumpf, and N. Coyle. 2011. "Primary Health Care in Canada: Systems in Motion." *Milbank Quarterly* 89, no. 2: 256–88. http://dx.doi.org/10.1111/j.1468-0009.2011.00628.x.

Landry, M. D., N. A. Eldarrat, S. R. Raman, and T. Dyck. 2009. "'Penny-Wise, Pound-Foolish': The Commodification of Physiotherapy Services in an Era of Precarious Demand." *Physiotherapy Research International* 14, no. 1: 1–5. http://dx.doi.org/10.1002/pri.426.

Law, M. R., A. Ystma, and S. G. Morgan. 2011. "The Short-Term Impact of Ontario's Generic Pricing Reforms." *PLoS Medicine* 6, no. 7: 1–4. doi: 10.1371/journal.pone.0023030.

Lewis, S. 2011. *What Ontarians (and Their Auditor General) Should Be Asking about Physician Pay: Essays*. Toronto: Longwoods. http://www.longwoods.com/content/22687.

Office of the Auditor General of Ontario. 2010. "Home Care Services." In *Annual Report of the Office of the Auditor General of Ontario*, 113–31. Queen's Printer for Ontario. http://www.auditor.on.ca/en/reports_en/en10/304en10.pdf.

———. 2011a. "Funding Alternatives for Family Physicians." In *Annual Report of the Office of the Auditor General of Ontario*, 150–70. Queen's Printer for Ontario. http://www.auditor.on.ca/en/reports_en/en11/306en11.pdf.

———. 2011b. "Funding Alternatives for Specialist Physicians." In *Annual Report of the Office of the Auditor General of Ontario*, 150–70. Queen's Printer for Ontario. http://www.auditor.on.ca/en/reports_en/en11/307en11.pdf.

Ontario. 2012. *Ontario's Action Plan for Health Care: Better Patient Care through Better Value from Our Health Care Dollars*. Toronto: Government of Ontario. http://www.health.gov.on.ca/en/ms/ecfa/healthy_change/docs/rep_healthychange.pdf.

Ontario. Ministry of Finance. 2012. *Public Services for Ontarians: A Path to Sustainability and Excellence*. Toronto: Ontario Ministry of Finance. http://www.fin.gov.on.ca/en/reformcommission/.

Ontario Association of Community Care Access Centres, Ontario Hospital Association, and Ontario Federation of Community Mental Health and Addiction Programs. 2010. *Ideas and Opportunities for Bending the Health Care Cost Curve: Advice for the Government of Ontario*. http://www.oha.com/KnowledgeCentre/Library/Documents/Bending%20the%20Health%20Care%20Cost%20Curve%20(Final%20Report%20-%20April%2013%202010).pdf.

Ontario Hospital Association. 2012. "Health System Facts and Figures: Beds Staffed and in Operation, Ontario 1990 to 2010." Accessed 18 October 2012. http://www.healthsystemfacts.com/Client/OHA/HSF_LP4W_LND_WebStation.nsf/page/Beds+staffed+and+in+operation+Ontario+1990+to+large.

Sinclair, D., M. Rochon, and P. Leatt. 2005. *Health Care: Riding the Third Rail—The Story of Ontario's Health Services Restructuring Commission, 1996–2000*. Montreal: Institute for Research on Public Policy.

Sutherland, J. M. 2011. *Hospital Payment Mechanisms: An Overview and Options for Canada*. Reports on Cost Drivers and Health System Efficiency no. 4. Ottawa: CHSRF. http://www.cfhi-fcass.ca/Libraries/Hospital_Funding_docs/CHSRF-Sutherland-HospitalFundingENG.sflb.ashx.

Sutherland, J. M., M. L. Barer, R. G. Evans, and R. T. Crump. 2011. "Will Paying the Piper Change the Tune?" *Healthcare Policy* 6, no. 4: 14–21. http://www.ncbi.nlm.nih.gov/pmc/articles/PMC3107112/.

Sutherland, J. M., and R. T. Crump. 2011. *Exploring Alternative Level of Care (ALC) and the Role of Funding Policies: An Evolving Evidence Base for Canada.* Ottawa: Canadian Health Services Research Foundation. http://www.cfhi-fcass.ca/SearchResultsNews/11-09-20/29f5b70f-e94f-4986-9455-231888e40f4a.aspx.

Sutherland, J. M., R. T. Crump, N. Repin, and E. Hellsten. 2013. "Paying for Hospital Services: A Hard Look at the Options." Commentary no. 378. Toronto: C. D. Howe Institute. http://www.cdhowe.org/pdf/Commentary_378.pdf.

Talaga, T., and R. Benzie. 2012. "Deb Matthews Slashes Fees for OHIP Services to Save $338 Million." *Toronto Star*, 7 May.

Tamblyn, R., R. Laprise, M. Abrahamowicz, J. A. Hanley, S. Scott, N. Mayo, J. Hurley, R. Grad, E. Latimer, R. Perreault, P. McLeod, et al. 2001. "Adverse Events Associated with Prescription Drug Cost-Sharing among Poor and Elderly Persons." *Journal of the American Medical Association* 285, no. 4: 421–29. http://dx.doi.org/10.1001/jama.285.4.421.

Walker, D. 2011. *Caring for Our Aging Population and Addressing Alternate Level of Care.* Ottawa: Minister of Health and Long-Term Care. http://www.health.gov.on.ca/en/common/ministry/publications/reports/walker_2011/walker_2011.pdf.

Williams, A., D. Challis, R. Deber, J. Watkins, K. Kuluski, J. Lum, and S. Daub. 2009. "Balancing Institutional and Community-Based Care: Why Some Older Persons Can Age Successfully at Home While Others Require Residential Long-Term Care." *Healthcare Quarterly* 12, no. 2: 95–105. doi: 10.12927/hcq.2009.3974.

Williams, A. P., J. Lum, R. Deber, R. Montgomery, K. Kuluski, A. Peckham, J. Watkins, A. Williams, A. Ying, and L. Zhu. 2009. "Aging at Home: Integrating Community-Based Care for Older Persons." *Healthcare Papers* 10, no. 1: 8–21. http://dx.doi.org/10.12927/hcpap.2009.21218.

You, J. J., D. A. Alter, K. Iron, P. M. Slaughter, A. Kopp, R. Przybysz, D. Thiruchelvam, L. Devore, and A. Laupacis. 2007. *Diagnostic Services in Ontario: Descriptive Analysis and Jurisdictional Review.* Toronto: ICES. http://www.ices.on.ca/Publications/Atlases-and-Reports/2007/Diagnostic-services-in-Ontario.

You, J. J., J. Gladstone, S. Symons, D. Rotstein, A. Laupacis, and C. M. Bell. 2011. "Patterns of Care and Outcomes after Computed Tomography Scans for Headache." *American Journal of Medicine* 124, no. 1: 58–63.e1. http://dx.doi.org/10.1016/j.amjmed.2010.08.010.

ten

Québec: Sustainability—Perception and Reality

FRANÇOIS BÉLAND AND CLAUDE GALAND[1]

... imperious necessity seemed to dictate that a yearly increase of produce
should if possible be obtained at all events; that in order to affect this
first great and indispensable purpose, it would be advisable to make
a more complete division of land, and to secure every man's property
against violation by the most powerful sanctions ... The institution
of marriage, or at least of some express or implied obligation on every
man to support his own children, seems to be the natural result of these
reasonings in a community under the difficulties that we have supposed.
— Thomas R. Malthus (1888, 277–79)

Introduction

Calls for controlling health-care expenditure (HCE) in Québec are deeply
embedded in the history of public financing of health care. In 1968, seven
years after Québec implemented its public hospital insurance plan with federal cost sharing, the Government of Québec was instrumental in promoting national task forces on the costs of health services (Canadian Museum
of Civilization 2012; Gaumer 2008, 147). In 1985, the Commission
d'enquête sur les services de santé et les services sociaux, also known as the
Rochon Commission, studied the organizational and financial issues facing the health and social services public system. The Commission was
mandated by the minister of health and social services, Guy Chevrette,
in a Parti Québécois government. The Commission concluded that HCE
increased from 1975 to 1985 at a rate somewhat greater than the gross
domestic product (GDP) and at the same rate as total government spending (Québec 1988, 324, 388). However, cost pressures were forecast to
increase HCE over inflation by 3.5% annually from 1985 on (Québec 1988,
644). The Commission rejected private financing as a solution, including
user fees (Québec 1988, 657). However, the tax increases of the 1960s and

---

1 We are grateful to Rebecca Rupp for her much-appreciated editorial work and advice.

1970s were no longer seen as an option by the Québec government in the 1980s. The Commission recommended that fiscal policies be directed at the triad that resonates today in the context of globalization: economic recession, competitive fiscal policy, and deficit reduction (Québec 1988, 391).

The Rochon Commission set the stage for future debates on sustainability of public HCE in Québec. In 1990, the Liberal minister of health and social services, Marc-Yvan Côté, presented a global reform for health and social services. Claiming to be inspired by the Rochon Commission Report (MSSS 1990), the reform identified the need to control health-care costs in view of HCE's increasing government revenue share, the brutal decrease in federal transfers for medicare to provinces, and the consequences of the 1989–92 recession for debt charges. The reform was to be based on a new principle: patients (referred to as "consumers" in the policy statement) should share responsibility for the costs they generate. The proposal was to add the expenditures for health services provided by the public system to individual taxable incomes, with a means-tested maximum. In 1991, premiums and user charges were added to this proposal, as well as provisions for delisting of "non-necessary" medical and hospital services (MSSS 1991).

Additional reports from working groups and commissions were preoccupied with financial sustainability. For example, the Arpin working group (Arpin et al. 1999) reported on the private sector's potential contribution to health care, this time to Pauline Marois, the Parti Québécois government's minister of health and social services. The Arpin Report rejected any form of out-of-pocket contributions from users for necessary medical and hospital services, but suggested that services considered necessary should be revised on a continual basis.

The topic of public HCE sustainability was raised again by the Clair Commission in its report to Minister Marois in 2001 (Québec 2000). The level and growth rate of public HCE were reaching critical levels, according to the Commission, echoing the context and terms used by the Rochon Commission. The Québec government was faced with high deficits, high taxes, and decreasing federal transfers for health. The system's sustainability would be jeopardized in the event of an economic recession. The Clair Commission also called for continual revision of "necessary" medical and hospital services, with delisting as a consequence. Long-term care was also to be financed through a social security mechanism.

None of the proposals of the different working groups and commissions touching on changes to direct or indirect patient contributions was adopted. All the proposals asked for changes to the 1984 *Canada Health Act*, none of which were enacted. Instead, the Ministry of Health and Social Services (Ministère de la santé et des services sociaux, or MSSS) acted on structural and organizational features of the system, which cul-minated in the 2003 Couillard reform. General hospitals, nursing homes (*centres hospitaliers de soins de longue durée*, or CHSLDs), and community health and social services centres (*centres locaux de services communautaires*, or CLSCs) were integrated into 95 *centres de santé et de services* (CSSSs) throughout Québec (Levine 2005; MSSS 2004). The CSSSs were man-dated with responsibility for health and social services delivery to the population living in their respective catchment areas. The allocation of financial resources was to be determined on a capitation basis.

The financial components of the Couillard model were never fully implemented; however, aspects of the proposed structural, organizational, and clinical models were adopted. Nevertheless, concerns over the sus-tainability of HCE have continued to intensify since then. A flurry of reports from working groups from the MSSS and the Ministry of Finance (Castonguay, Marcotte, and Venne 2008; Gagné et al. 2009; Ménard et al. 2005) has appeared in recent years, complemented by budgetary documents specifically addressing the issue (Finances Québec 2007a, 2010a). These more recent reports all share one common assumption: public HCE is unsustainable in the medium to long term unless fundamental changes are made in the way health-care services are financed. These changes usually involve the introduction of some form of privatization of service deliv-ery, private insurance schemes, and user fees and premiums for publicly financed services. The analyses and conclusions of these recent government working group reports are in line with claims that cost pressures are used to promote the ideology of the inevitability of private financing of health care (Evans et al. 2000; Evans and Vujicic 2005) and introduce the need for a two-tier system (Boothe and Carson 2003; Hirsch 2005; Pammolli, Riccaboni, and Magazzini 2008; Petretto 2010).

The debate on the non-sustainability of public HCE has strong ideological and political components (Evans and Vujicic 2005). In one sense, the goal of sustainability and the mechanisms to adapt health systems to sources of pressures are elusive (Prada et al. 2004), yet sustainability cannot be assessed without some idea of what it is and how it can be measured. *Sustainability* has been variously defined by assumptions about increasing demand for health care (Appleby and Harrison 2006), HCE growth rates that jeopardize public budgets (Van Elk, Mot, and Franses 2009), and the increasing mismatch between HCE growth and fiscal resources (Boothe and Carson 2003).

Evans and Vujicic (2005) offer a simple definition: sustainability involves comparison of rates of change in growth rates (Di Matteo and Di Matteo 2011). However, in Evans and Vujicic's (2005) terms, analyses of sustainability require taking into consideration the institutional framework in which sustainability and growth rates are to be deliberated. Even though the wealth of a nation is one of the dimensions to consider (Marchildon and Di Matteo 2011), the analysis cannot be confined to comparison of HCE and GDP growth rates (Di Matteo and Di Matteo 2011; Pammolli, Riccaboni, and Magazzini 2008). Components of the institutional framework in which the sustainability issue has been considered in Québec were suggested by both the Rochon and Clair commissions. In addition to GDP, these components include the provincial government's own sources of revenue (OSR), the federal Canada Health Transfer, accumulated deficit and debt charges, and the disturbing effect of economic recessions. Also, both commissions pointed to differences in the pressures generated by health services covered by medicare (physician services and hospitalization) and by other services, mainly prescribed drugs and long-term care.

In this chapter, sustainability will be assessed by comparing growth rates in HCE with growth rates in GDP and with Québec government OSR, deficit and debt charges, and federal health transfers. Also, we will take into account Evans and Vujicic's (2005) comments on the rhetorical use of total HCE figures to conclude that medicare is not sustainable, and Orosz and Morgan's (2004) recommendation to consider the functional distribution of components of HCE and their changes over time. Growth rates for total HCE and for medicare- and non-medicare-covered services will be tracked and compared with indicators of growth rates for GDP, Québec government OSR, annual deficits, and debt charges. The Québec government's ability to maintain sustainability of the public health system in the face of internal and external challenges and using medicare institutional framework, or "institutional ingenuity" (Evans and Vujicic 2005), will be examined, as well as the interplay among the institutional components of public health care over time. Thus, sustainability will not be assessed here in terms of relative changes in HCE and other separately considered components. Sustainability is considered to be the result of a set of historically elusive and fuzzy equilibria and disequilibria and periods of balanced and unbalanced growth rates. The efforts of government authorities to use many or a few degrees of the freedom they have, under various pressures from inside and outside the health-care system, are also considered.

Fiscal sustainability: Québec's point of view

The increasing share of public HCE in relation to government financial resources is a major issue in the debate on sustainability of medicare in Québec. A *share* is simply a ratio—a numerator (here, government health spending) over a denominator (financial resources). This simple ratio hides a complex issue: how are governmental program spending and financial resources defined? The values and trends of this ratio and the conclusions derived affect public policy. Department documents, government working group reports, commission reports, and press coverage all contain examples of how trends in the ratio of public spending on health care to governmental financial resources have been used to bias the debate on sustainability and to influence policy options.

Dramatic conclusions on the sustainability of public financing of health care have been drawn from total government program spending estimates in Department of Finance (Finances Québec) or Treasury Board (Conseil du trésor) budgetary documents and health-care spending estimates from the MSSS total budget. For example, the Bédard Report, mandated by the MSSS, proposed changes to the health-care system based on an analysis of trends in expenditures for both health and social services (Bédard et al. 2002, 3). The Clair Commission concluded that it was necessary to limit the growth of government spending on health and social services, based on their increasing share of program spending—from 35.3% in 1990 to 39.8% in 2000, with a projection of 50.0% in 2010–11 (Québec 2000, 147). An influential document in the public debate on the sustainability of public financing of health care, the Ménard Report used the same premise as the Clair Commission in its analysis of trends in health and social services, estimating its share of program spending at 32% in 1984–85 and 43% in 2004–05 (Ménard et al. 2005, 17). In response to the Supreme Court judgment on the *Chaoulli* case (*Chaoulli v. Québec* 2005), the MSSS initiated a consultation process with the publication of "Garantir l'accès: un défi d'équité, d'efficience et de qualité" (MSSS 2006). Analyses of trends in health-care spending were reported in terms of MSSS expenditure compared to governmental program spending, showing an increase from 31.9% in 1985–86 to 43.1% in 2005–06. In all these reports, as in the 2008 Castonguay Report to the Québec government, health is defined as including both health and social services (Castonguay, Marcotte, and Venne 2008, 3).

Though Canadian Institute for Health Information (CIHI) data was not used in any of these documents to estimate government health-care expenditure, it was not completely ignored in government documentation. Finances Québec (2007a, 2007b) used CIHI estimates on private health spending in an analysis of health-care spending in Québec, as well as MSSS expenditures to estimate government health spending, as reflected in the Castonguay Report (Castonguay, Marcotte, and Venne 2008, 25). However, in that report, the authors recommended a specific annual account for government health-care spending (p. 268). In 2009, Finances Québec asked a group of four economists to examine government spending and revenue and make recommendations for preparation of the 2010 budget (Gagné et al. 2009). The figures on health-care expenditure and the projections of its share of program spending were drawn from MSSS expenditure and program spending figures in budgetary documents; health-care spending was shown to have increased from 30% to 45% from 1980 to 2009. However, another, much lower estimate of health-care spending was obtained by comparing Québec and Ontario 2008–09 program spending, using data from Statistics Canada's Financial Management System (FMS). The figures for Québec indicated that health-care spending was $23.17 million; total program spending, including debt charges, was $86.082 million, yielding a share of 27% for health care (Gagné et al. 2009, 15), compared to 44% obtained for the same year from Finances Québec budgetary documents. This discrepancy was never raised in the Finances Québec reports.

These documents have had considerable influence in the public debate on the sustainability of government spending on health care. Health care's increasing share of program spending has been used extensively to persuade the public that changes in health-care financing, organization, and delivery must be implemented.

Data from the CIHI annual report on trends in health-care expenditure have also been reported in the public domain, but they have essentially been ignored in the debate on sustainability. Bourgault-Côté (2006a) reported in Le Devoir that according to CIHI, health care's share of program spending was 31.7% in Québec. On 29 October 2010, Le Devoir (2010) reported the CIHI figure as 33.1%. It doesn't seem to have occurred to anyone that these figures were not compatible with those used by the working groups and government documents for 2005 and 2009 (41.3% and 43.1% respectively). CIHI data were also used in a front-page article in La Presse (Noël 2007), on health-care costs and aging. The article was followed by a debate in the op-ed section (Béland 2007; Godbout et al. 2007) and an editorial (Pratte 2007). CIHI data were used again in a brief presented to the National Assembly of Québec's Commission des affaires sociales (Béland 2006). Dr. Philippe Couillard, then minister of health and social services, declared that he was convinced by the brief that government health spending was sustainable now and in the future (Bérubé 2006; Bourgault-Côté 2006b). He was castigated by columnists (David 2006), who were unconvinced by Couillard's conversion. However, the coverage in Le Devoir and La Presse, as well as Couillard's conversion, were soon forgotten, and the public debate on sustainability continued on its usual course.

Using program and health-care spending data from CIHI instead of Finances Québec budgetary documents is not merely rhetorical. Figure 10.1 shows trends in the share of health-care expenditure (HCE) compared to program spending, using both CIHI and Finances Québec data. A cursory look at Figure 10.1 will show how the two curves lead to completely different readings of sustainability of government health-care spending in Québec. There are fairly consistent differences from 1975 to 1996, but starting in 1999, the two datasets began to diverge dramatically: the CIHI curve hovers around 30%, while the curve using Finances Québec data surges ever upward. Of course, using CIHI figures would not generate spectacular news headlines or dramatic public debate. Though the Québec health-care system has problems that induce legitimate angst and worry, the sustainability debate cannot flourish with flat curves such as CIHI's in Figure 10.1. Indeed, the financial sustainability issue could have been supplanted by questions raised by Bertholot in Daoust-Boisvert (2011) on whether or not Québec spent enough on health care, at least in comparison with the much higher spending in other provinces.

The MSSS is responsible for health and social services, and social services accounted for an average of 12% of MSSS expenditure. Expenditure on health care is also part of the budgets of other department and government bodies (MSSS 2011). Thus only a small part of the difference between CIHI and Finances Québec estimates of the share of health-care spending compared to overall program spending can be attributed to using MSSS expenditures for health spending in the numerator. This difference, then, has to come from the denominator.

Up to 2009, CIHI used Statistics Canada's Financial Management System (FMS) estimates for federal, provincial, and territorial total and program spending. In FMS, public administrations are composed of all government-sector entities included in the public accounts, plus agencies and funds that perform government functions (Statistics Canada 2009, 7). "Public administration" includes ministries, departments, autonomous and non-autonomous funds, pension funds, and public organizations for education and health and social services. The Canada/Québec Pension Plan (CPP/QPP) and government business enterprises are excluded, as "they operate in the market place, often in competition with privately owned organizations" (Statistics Canada 2009, 14). Statistics Canada gives figures for two entities: first, federal or provincial government, and second, "general" federal or provincial government, or "general government." The latter excludes non-autonomous pension funds and autonomous sources of income and associated spending for public organizations providing education and health and social services.

Figure 10.1 Health-care expenditures (HCE) as percentage of program spending: estimates from CIHI and Finances Québec

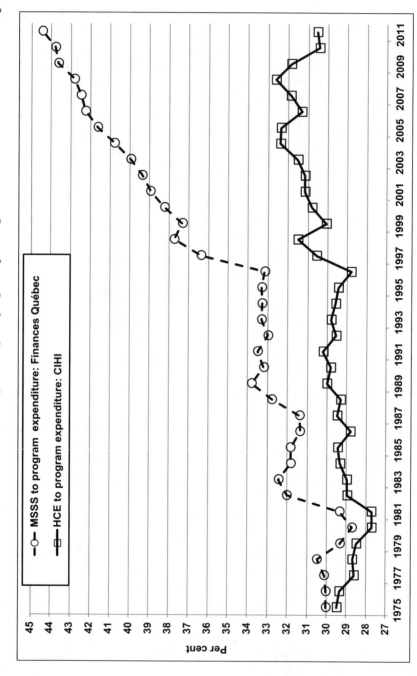

Sources: Finances Québec 2012, 7, Table 6; CIHI 2012, Table D.4.5.1 and App. D.1.

Table 10.1 Provincial program spending: ratios of provincial budgetary estimates to FMS's "general" and "provincial" government categories, fiscal year 2008–2009

Group	Province	Budgetary Documents: FMS "General"	Budgetary Documents: FMS "Provincial"
Outliers	Québec	76.4%	66.0%
Ratios <95%	Newfoundland and Labrador	93.0%	87.6%
	Prince Edward Island	93.8%	85.9%
	Saskatchewan	93.9%	86.2%
	Alberta	94.8%	87.9%
Ratios 95%–100%	Nova Scotia	97.1%	85.9%
	British Columbia	99.6%	88.6%
	Ontario	97.5%	87.9%
Ratios >100%	New Brunswick	100.5%	87.7%
	Manitoba	110.9%	100.8%

Sources: Statistics Canada, CANSIM, Tables 380–0001 and 380–0002; Finance Canada, Tableaux de référence financiers, http://www.fin.gc.ca/frt-trf/2011/frt-trf-11 -fra.asp (accessed 27 July 2012).

Items included in FMS for "provincial government" and "general government" are not coterminous with those considered in provincial government budgetary documents (Statistics Canada 2009, 7). New Brunswick and Manitoba figures exceeded FMS estimates in 2008–09 (see Table 10.1), but Québec is the real outlier. Finances Québec "general funds" tables are valued at 76.4% of FMS figures for "general government" and 66.0% for "provincial government" (Finances Québec 2012, 7). Clearly the denominator used by CIHI is much bigger than the denominator used by Finances Québec in estimating health care's share of program spending. Figure 10.2 shows these variations in program spending estimates from 1974–75 to 2010–11 for Finances Québec and for FMS "general government" and from 1998–99 to 2008–09 for FMS "provincial government."

FMS and Finances Québec data start to fan out in 1997, with program spending estimates from the FMS following sharper curves.[2] Notably,

---

2 Figures from Finances Québec budgetary documents are the same here as those obtained from reference tables from Finance Canada, at http://www.fin.gc.ca/frt-trf/2011/frt-trf-11-fra.asp.

Figure 10.2 Three different estimates of program spending, Québec (1997 dollars)

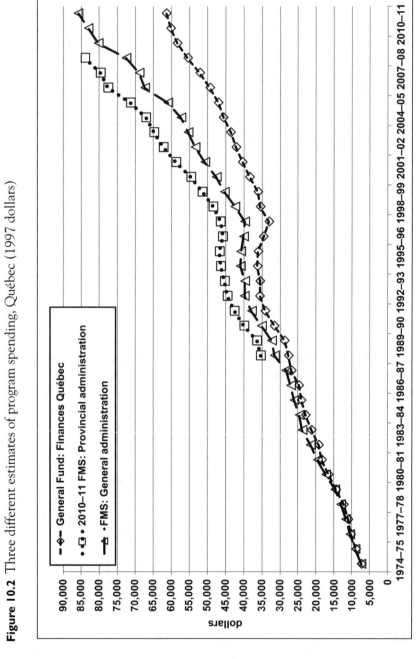

Sources: Statistics Canada, CANSIM, Tables 380–0001 and 380–0002; Finances Québec 2012, 7, Table 6.

Finances Québec lowered estimated program spending compared with FMS, starting the same year the Bouchard government introduced the "zero deficit" law requiring a balanced budget.

Finally, accounting rules and structural changes in public administration often introduce significant differences in annual reports on budgetary transactions from different sources. For example, using the adjusted figures for 2010–11 (Finances Québec 2012, 7) instead of the non-adjusted figures (Finances Québec 2010a, I.9), HCE share of program spending jumps from 42.7% to 44.5%, without the MSSS having spent a penny more.

The debate on financial sustainability of public HCE is about the ability of the public administration to sustain these expenditures, given the full range of its responsibilities, the accompanying revenues from all sources, and expenditures on all items (Vaillancourt and Perrault 2007). Clearly estimates from the MSSS, Finances Québec, and the Conseil du trésor do not stand up to these criteria and should not be used to examine the sustainability of provincial government expenditures for health in Québec.

The FMS reported revenue and spending on a large subset of public administration activities. "General government" as a category excludes spending and income from health, social services, and public educational institutions. Only FMS "federal/provincial government" figures include the full set of public administration responsibilities. However, these figures are available only for fiscal years 1988–89 to 2008–09. CIHI provides data on HCE, government program, and total spending from 1975 to 2012 (CIHI 2012). CIHI figures for the fiscal years 1988–89 to 2008–09 correspond to those found in Statistics Canada's Table 385–0002 for "general government." Figures for the 1974–75 to 1983–84 period are the same as those found in the Statistics Canada FMS historical dataset (1992), though there are small discrepancies between CIHI and FMS figures for 1984–85 to 1987–88. Thus CIHI data allow interprovincial comparisons, and CIHI is the most comprehensive and reliable data source for examining the sustainability of public HCE in Québec over 37 years.

Government health-care expenditure is all about GDP—or is it?

Baseline: GDP growth in Canada and Québec

From 1975 to 1981, GDP in Canada was growing in real terms. Implicit price indexes for the provinces are available in Statistics Canada's CANSIM only from 1981 on. However, as the Canadian and Québec nominal GDPs were growing at the same rate, Québec real GDP probably experienced the same growth rate as in Canada as a whole. From 1981 to 2009, Québec and Canada experienced three recessions (1981–82, 1989–92, and 2008) and an economic slowdown in 2001 (Cross 1996, 2005). The Canadian economy grew at a higher rate than Québec's following the 1981–82 and 1989–92 recessions. After the 2001 economic slowdown, a persistent decrease in GDP growth rate is observed, again more pronounced in Québec than in Canada as a whole. Evans and Vujicic (2005) show a similar trend since the end of the 1970s, with GDP in Canada falling during times of recession and not fully recovering following recessions. Also of note, the 2008 recession was more severe in Canada than in Québec.

Québec nominal GDP per head was 84% of Canadian GDP in 1975. It increased to 90% of Canadian GDP before the 1989–92 recession but subsequently fell back to its 1975 level of 84%.

GDP and HCE growth rates

The pattern of cumulative growth rate for government HCE in Québec is very similar to Québec's GDP pattern: five slowdown phases are shown in Figure 10.3, all following a recession or economic downturn. The 1974–75 recession was followed in 1976 by a reduced HCE growth rate in all the provinces. HCE growth rates fell in Québec after the 1981–82 recession but not in Canada; however, the 1992–96 "big drop" hit all of the provinces. Only Québec experienced reduced growth rate following the 2001 business cycle slowdown. Finally, 2009 showed a repeat of the dominant pattern following the 2008 recession.

Growth in all provincial government HCE and Québec government HCE is parallel only in the aftermath of the 1989–91 recession. Otherwise, Canada's curve is always steeper than Québec's, resulting in Québec's being among the provinces with the lowest per capita provincial government spending on health care. It is noteworthy that differences between Québec and all provincial government cumulative HCE growth rates reflect the differences in their GDP growth rates. Of course, GDP cumulative growth rates are lower than those of HCE.

Are HCE components equal?

As shown above, analyses of the non-sustainability of government HCE in Québec and proposals to introduce changes in financing health care have used MSSS expenditure data and Finances Québec figures for government

Figure 10.3 Health-care expenditure cumulative growth rates (1997 dollars; recession impact series emphasized)

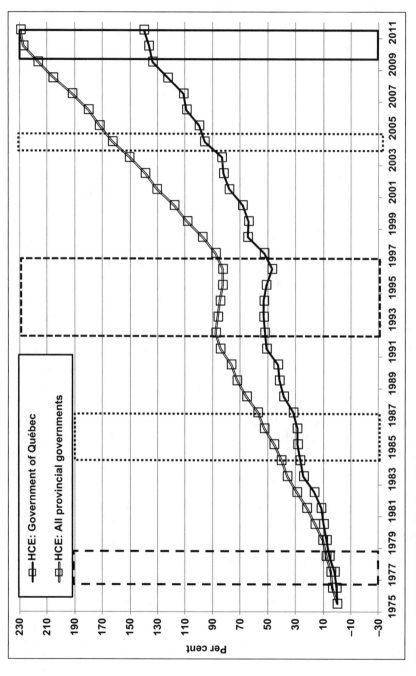

Sources: CIHI 2011, Tables B.1.1 and D.4.5.1.

program spending estimates. In particular, Finances Québec proposals to introduce user fees for medical and hospital services, and a pool tax dedicated to health care, have been justified on the basis of trends in the share of MSSS expenditure of total program expenditure over the past 30 years, and on a catastrophic projection of both over the next 25 years (Finances Québec 2010b). Thus, the rationale for an apocalyptic view of spending trends for medical and hospital care, and for the introduction of user fees for medicare-covered services, is based on expenditure for all health care—acute and long-term care, services included in medicare and those excluded, and so forth. But do expenditures on medicare- and non-medicare-covered services show the same trend? And are they both related to GDP growth rates?[3]

In Figure 10.4, the share of total HCE to GDP shows three blips from 1981 to 2011, associated with recessions. A decrease in the share of medicare-covered services can also be seen in 1975–76 as a remnant of the 1974–75 recession. Total HCE share of GDP regressed to 1970s figures after each recession up until 2000. But something started happening in 2000: there is a continuous increase of HCE share up until the 2008 recession. Also, as a consequence of the recession, HCE increased in 2009 in terms of GDP. The only noticeable exception is 1999, for undocumented reasons but possibly due to implementation of the Treasury Board and MSSS retirement plan offered to health-care providers in 1997.

Trends for expenditure on medicare and non-medicare services followed divergent paths from 1975 until 1996. In the first case the trend edged downward, with increases and decreases in times of recession. In the second case, the changes were much less abrupt. Only from 2000 to 2008 did expenditure for medicare and non-medicare services work in parallel. Since 2008, cuts in HCE have hit non-medicare services harder than medicare services.

GDP and HCE: How about a lag? Give me two or three years!

A proposal to limit the increase in government HCE to the GDP annual growth rate appeared in several policy statements and government working

---

3 In 2007, the MSSS and CIHI jointly revised their estimates of HCE, limiting their review to from 1997 on (CIHI 2007). Though total HCE did not change with this revision, the main items affected were spending on hospitals and on long-term care institutions. We will assume that trends in medicare and non-medicare expenditures were not affected by the changes in either the 1975–96 or the 1997–2011 series. However, a break in the plotted series is used in Figure 10.4 as a reminder that figures for health-care costs between series cannot be compared in dollars.

Figure 10.4 Health-care expenditure as percentage of GDP and medicare and non-medicare expenditures (recession series emphasized)

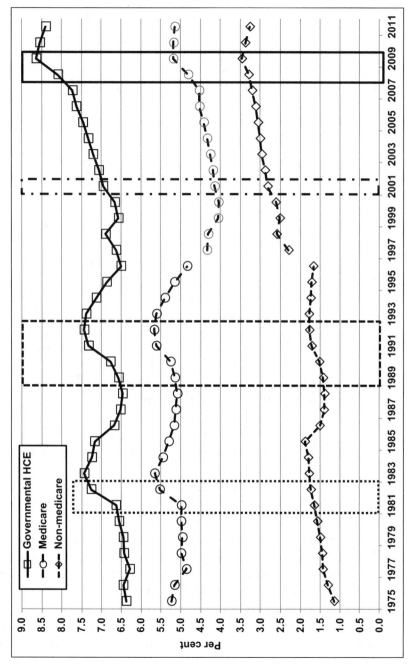

Sources: CIHI 2011, D.4.5.1 and App. A.1; Finances Québec 2012, 17, Table 14.

group reports (Castonguay, Marcotte, and Venne 2008, 262–63; Ménard et al. 2005, 101). Even though expenditure on medicare-covered services grew at a rate similar to the GDP's from 1981 to 1986—1.8% compared to 1.6%—and at respectively 3.0% versus 2.3% thereafter, the hypothesis was that contemporaneous rates of growth were unsustainable. Ironically, this same proposal became the basis of the new federal policy on the Canada Health Transfer to the provinces, with a 3% floor in nominal terms starting in 2017. A closer look at trends in GDP and HCE may help give a better picture of how they are related.

In Figure 10.5, GDP cumulative growth rates are projected with a lag of three years over cumulative growth rates for total HCE and medicare. In this figure, the recession and HCE series collapse into each other. The shape of the GDP curve follows closely the curve for total HCE until 2004, at which point HCE continues to grow at 1997–2003 rates while GDP growth rate decreases.

Total HCE growth rates slowed down in 1984, three years after the 1981–82 recession began. The same pattern is observed in 1992, three years after the 1989–92 recession. But the cuts starting in 1992 were deep and continued for four years after the recession ended. Thus expenditures for medicare increased at more or less the same rate and with the same pattern as GDP, with a three-year lag. Understandably, provincial health-care system financing cannot be redirected by sleight of hand. It seems that it takes two to three years for successive Québec governments to see the results of implementation of financial restraints. The Québec government does not seem to have the same ability with non-medicare services (curve not shown); user fees, copayments, premiums, private insurance, and other forms of out-of-pocket contributions are added to government spending for these services. Also, private initiatives and funding are encouraged through explicit policies (MSSS 2006).

It is remarkable to note that not only HCE growth rates but also HCE spending grew during times of recession, and it experienced reduced growth in both rates and real terms following recessions. Thus, two series are emerging from trends in GDP and HCE. The first is associated with recession, the second with the aftermath of recession. During times of recession, GDP growth is pared down, and provincial governments cannot adjust HCE instantly when a recession begins. Their share of GDP increases as a function of both increases in real terms of HCE (the numerator) and decreases in GDP (the denominator). After each recession, HCE decreased in constant dollars, but, as shown below, cuts are seen only in medicare-covered services. Thus two series associated with economic recessions have to be taken into account:

Figure 10.5 Health-care expenditure, medicare, and GDP cumulative growth rates, with three-year lag (1997 dollars; recession and recession impact series emphasized)

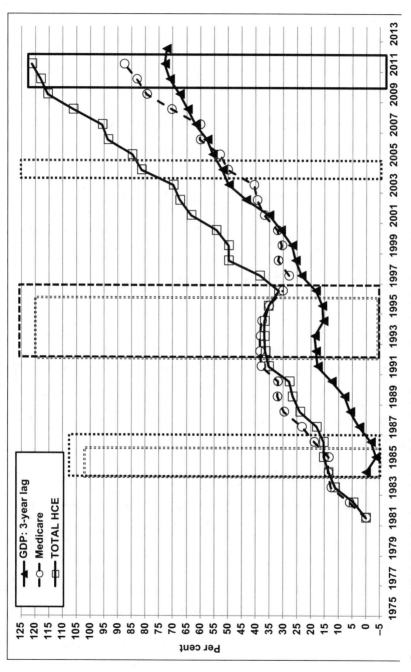

Sources: CIHI 2011, D.4.5.1, App. A.1, and App. B.1; Statistics Canada CANSIM, Table 384-0013 (adjusted so 1997=100).

(1) the recession series, built from data on economic recessions, and (2) the series on the impact of recessions on HCE. Not taking into account the lag in adjustment of HCE to GDP artificially reduces their correlation.

Government health-care expenditure is all about fiscal policies—or is it?

Where does the money come from? What does Québec do with it?

Budgetary documents from Finances Québec report on two sources of government revenue: own-source revenues (OSR) and total. And to obtain the total amount of money available, annual deficits should be added. Figure 10.6 plots them from 1975 to 2011 for "general government" (CIHI 2011; Statistics Canada 2009). As OSR are much larger than total federal transfers and annual deficits, they have been plotted separately on different scales. Following the 1974–75 recession, Québec government OSRs did not experience growth, while the annual deficit increased year after year, leaving the government in a difficult situation in the face of the severe 1981–82 recession (Cross 1996). However, total federal transfers increased in 1981–82, only to decrease after the recession. OSR showed positive growth rates between the 1981–82 and 1989–92 recessions, and in 1987 a surplus appeared. This story was repeated around the 1989–92 recession, except for a reduction in total federal transfers in 1991. Again in the aftermath of this recession, OSR increased and annual deficits were reduced. However, in 1996, the federal government abruptly cut transfers to the provinces. In a sense, the Québec government made up for the loss with increasing OSR. From 1999 on, the trends for OSR plateau as a result of a series of tax reduction measures introduced by the Québec government. Béland (2008) reported an extract from Finances Québec annual budgetary documents linking the reductions or moderate increases of OSR to tax reduction measures. For example, in 2001–02, a 2.1% decrease in OSR was expected by Finances Québec (Finances Québec 2001, 2.5); the 2001 economic slowdown and the reduced GDP growth rates that followed may also have had an effect. However, from 2004 on, federal transfers made up for the loss of OSR. Starting in 2006, a combination of tax reduction policies and the 2008 recession resulted in a three-year plateau (Finances Québec 2007b, C.13). Since 2009, the trend for OSR has been up, while total federal transfers have been flat and annual deficits have remained.

Figure 10.6 Own sources of revenue, total federal transfers, and annual deficit (1997 dollars; recession series emphasized)

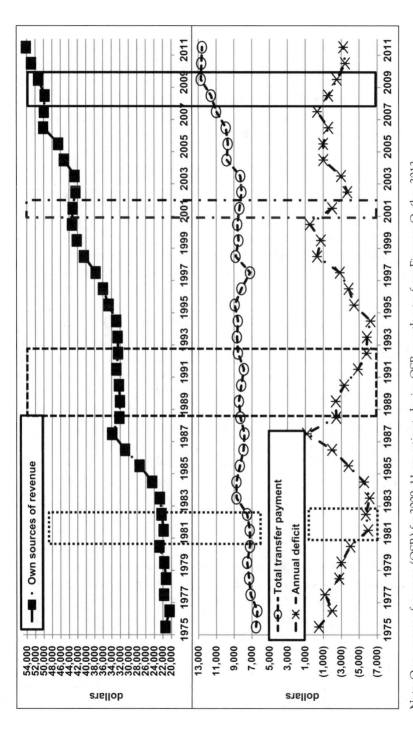

Note: Own sources of revenue (OSR) for 2009–11 are estimated using OSR growth rates from Finances Québec 2012.
Sources: Statistics Canada CANSIM, Tables 385-0002 and 384-0013 (adjusted so 1997=100); Statistics Canada FMS historical data, Tables H1–H4; Finances Québec 2012.

What is Québec doing about it?

For the purpose of analysis, total government expenditure will be divided into three components: HCE, items other than health ("non-HCE"), and debt charges. In Figure 10.7, these components are plotted from 1975 to 2011 as a share of total expenditure, with the annual deficit plotted at the bottom. Expenditure on non-HCE was graphed on a smaller scale than the other items to show variations in the series.

HCE share of total expenditure varied in a range of 25% to 32%, with higher figures during recessions and lower or stable figures immediately after recessions. The share of non-HCE showed a much larger range of variation, working counter-cyclically. Increases in both HCE and non-HCE in times of recession are associated with increases in annual deficits. Cumulative deficits have an impact on debt charges; they represent 5% of total expenditure in 1975, increasing to 12.2% in 2002 and diminishing slowly thereafter.

Expenditures for the same items are associated with fluctuations in business cycles and counter-cyclic policies. Nonetheless, some peculiarities are worth mentioning. First, expenditure for items other than health care increased (in 1997 dollars) from $27.311 million to $35.816 million, and growth rates remained flat. Meanwhile, HCE increased from $12.484 million to $18.585 million. Also, the Québec government responded to the 2008 recession with significant increases in expenditure for items other than health, while the rate of increase for HCE was reduced starting in 2009. Thus, any concerns about government expenditure being crowded out by HCE have to take into account the counter-cyclical policies implemented by government authorities. High expenditures on items other than health in times of recession are usually followed by periods of either lower real expenditures or, at a minimum, reduction in growth rates.

HCE, OSR, debt charges, and the CHT

Trends in HCE and expenditure for medicare-covered services are associated with the Québec government's OSR and a three-year lag. But OSR also reflects fiscal policies. Part of the 2000–03 and 2006–08 plateaus in OSR is attributable to 1999 and 2006 tax cuts. The fact that negative trends in HCE growth rates go beyond recessions is associated with the lasting effect of a recession on OSR. The exception is the 2001 economic slowdown, where OSR was also affected by tax cuts.

Debt charges are related to HCE as well. Debt charges tend to increase after a recession and then recede, the exception being the aftermath of the 1974–75 recession, a period when annual deficits increased continuously.

Figure 10.7 Total health-care and non-health expenditure, deficit, and debt charges as percentage of total spending (recession series emphasized)

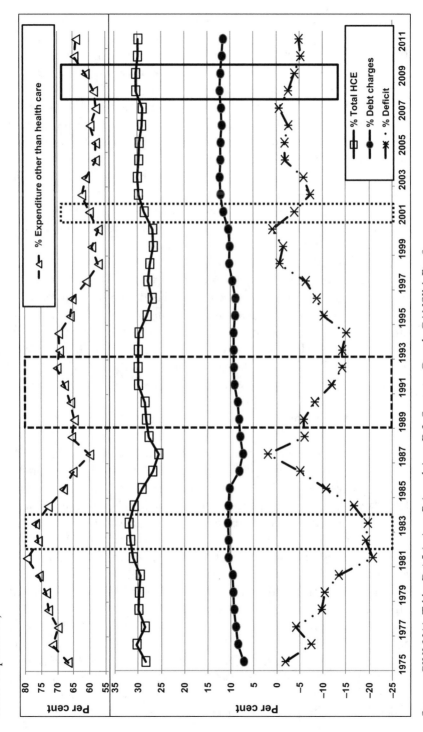

Sources: CIHI 2011, Tables D.4.5.1, App. B.1, and App. D.2; Statistics Canada CANSIM, Fig. 8.

As both OSR and federal transfers did not increase during the 1975–80 period, HCE growth was partly financed by borrowing at historically high interest rates. Beginning in 1997, debt charges stopped increasing and HCE began a positive trend. With the 2008 recession, debt charges started to grow again, accelerating annual deficits.

Both CHT and previous federal health transfer payments (hereafter both designated as CHT) are related to HCE. In Figure 10.8, only spending on medicare-covered services is compared with the CHT, taking into consideration only the "medically necessary" services that are referred to in the *Canada Health Act*: medical, hospital, and diagnostic services. The transfer payments were reduced from 1975 to 1976 and remained at the 1977 level for the next five years. They increased during the following four years (1983–86), including the years when HCE experienced the impact of the 1981–82 recession. The trends in expenditure for medicare strictly followed CHT trends during this period.

Expenditure for medicare was hard hit following the 1989–92 recession, under pressure from steadily decreasing CHTs during the same period— CHT reductions represented a third of the medicare cutbacks. Medicare growth rates were generally positive from 1997 to 2011, and CHT increased in three steps. The first threshold is linked with the 2003 federal-provincial agreement on the CHT, and the second threshold occurred in 2006, which saw a halt to the sharp increase.

Putting it all together

The 1974–75 recession was characterized by inflation rates in the 15% to 20% range that lasted until 1981. In fact, from 1975 to 1981 the growth of debt charges ($1.576 billion) surpassed (in 1997 dollars) the growth in HCE ($1.031 billion) and OSR ($406 million). In this period, expenditure on items other than health care and the deficit grew at higher rates than those observed in the 1989–92 and 2008 recessions and the 2001 economic slowdown. Nevertheless, HCE and expenditure on medicare services followed paths that would repeat after each recession in the following 36 years: growth rates for medicare services decreased after recessions and growth rates for total HCE experienced a slowdown.

Inflationary pressures of the 1970s were eased with the 1981–82 recession. The interplay, during and after recessions, of debt charges, spending on items other than health, OSR, annual deficits, and CHT components with HCE and expenditures for medicare services components can be seen in full for the first time with the 1981–82 recession. Spending on items other than health and annual deficits are at an all-time high in times of

Figure 10.8 Expenditures on medicare and Canada Health Transfers (1997 dollars; recession impact series emphasized)

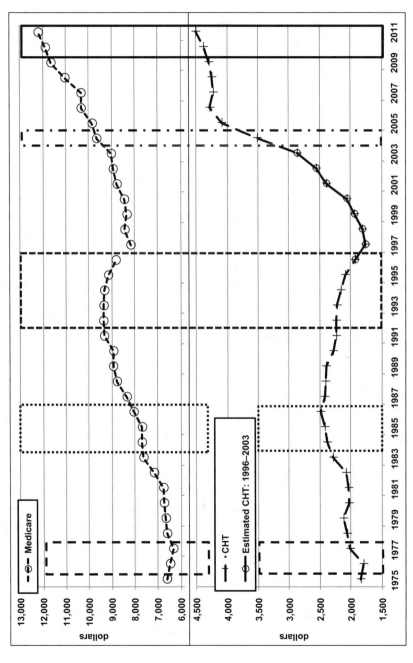

Sources: Statistics Canada CANSIM, Fig. 8; Finance Canada 2012 (CHT table).

recession, and HCE and expenditure on medicare increase in real terms. Following a recession, HCE and expenditure for medicare display the 1975–77 pattern: slow or negative growth for HCE, negative growth for medicare. Spending on items other than health and the annual deficit recedes and debt charges increase. The CHT begins to fall. Idiosyncratic historical events may occur to modify some of these parameters. For example, in the aftermath of the 1981–82 recession, the Québec government made up for the loss due to falling CHT with its OSR, which was growing at an unprecedented rate.

The ability of the Québec government to face the consequences of catastrophically falling federal health transfers was ultimately thwarted by the 1989–92 recession. All the components—HCE, expenditure on medicare and on items other than health, debt charges, annual deficits, and OSR—played the same role in the 1989–92 recession as in the 1981–82 recession and its aftermath. The historically specific event here was a continual drop in federal health transfers, resulting in a historic drop in expenditure on medicare services. In the mid 1990s the MSSS mandated regional authorities to cut health and social expenditures. In Montréal, the MSSS fixed the cuts at $190 million over three years. Montréal regional health authorities embarked on an ambitious initiative, including a formal consultative process, that resulted in redistribution of financial resources towards ambulatory care and home care and in the closing of hospital beds (Roy et al. 2000).

Similar to the 1986 to 1991 period, growth rates of HCE and expenditure on medicare have been on a positive course since 1997. However, increased CHTs rallied OSR positive growth rates, reducing annual deficits and setting debt charges and spending on items other than health on a more or less flat course. The surge in the CHT was not the only idiosyncratic element in that period. With increasing OSR and a triumphant neo-liberal political agenda, the Québec government, led by the Parti Québécois, introduced tax cuts in 1999, some of which were implemented by the Liberal Party in the 2000s. HCE and medicare-covered services were saved from deep cuts in 2003–06 by ever-expanding CHTs. In 2007, when the CHT stopped growing, OSR came to the rescue.

From economic determinism to institutional ingenuity

A "neo-Malthusian" interpretation of the impact of GDP—the wealth of the nation—and business cycles on public HCE is that the emperor has no clothes on! Let the law of inverse growth of population and resources undo what governments will not do—but this is only a partial understanding of Malthus's point. Malthus was convinced that nature is harsh and that human action can make it even harsher (Evans and Vujicic 2005). However, in Malthusian terms, two social institutions—private property and marriage—can impose discipline on man in such a way "that a yearly increase of produce should if possible be obtained at all events" (Malthus 1888, 279). The point here is not to sustain the moral, ideological, and political agenda of Malthus but to emphasize that human beings have the potential to use their ingenuity in building social institutions in the face of powerful determinants (Parsons 1937, 102–7). In this sense, both the sustainability and the non-sustainability of public HCE are sensitive to moral, ideological, and political choice. Of course, institutional ingenuity can head in more than one direction, and it can take more than one path.

Québec has chosen to use institutional ingenuity to address the health-care cost curve, and this choice has taken many forms. First, every 10 years or so, a *commission d'études sur les services de santé et de services sociaux*, a governmental working group, has been set up to examine the cost issue. In the early days recommendations on costs, financing health care, and patient contributions were ignored. Recently, recommendations to implement user fees (Castonguay, Marcotte, and Venne 2008, 241–57; Gagné et al. 2010, 72–74) were retained by the Liberal government but then discarded (Finances Québec 2010b, 26–29). However, a pool tax implemented in 2010 projected a contribution of $945 million to health services financing in the fiscal year 2013–14 (Finances Québec 2010b, 22–26). The Parti Québécois government choose to amend but maintain the pool tax. Initiatives to change health agency budgetary rules or organizational arrangements have also been suggested; some initiatives were implemented, others were not.

The budgetary constraints from 1992 to 1996, decided by the Treasury Board, are another example. Regional health and social service authorities implemented MSSS-mandated restraints by two methods: cuts prorated on agency budgets or estimated savings from expected performance gains, and zero-based budgeting. Eventually the MSSS had to take charge of the cumulative deficits resulting from the implemented restraints (Bédard et al. 2002, 26).

In 1997, at the end of a period of deep HCE cuts, the Parti Québécois government proposed an accelerated retirement program for civil servants and health-care providers, in concert with the unions. Some 1,500 physicians and 4,000 nurses retired, with subsequent savings; in 1998–99 the Auditor General estimated the forgone remuneration to retirees in the health-care sector at $144 million (Vérificateur général du Québec 1999, 179). However, replacement rates seem to have been higher in the health-care sector than in other sectors, and no figures for total savings are available. The estimates of total savings for the accelerated retirement program gave rise to a heated debate between J. Léonard, then Treasury Board minister, and the Auditor General. Léonard estimated the global savings at $1 billion in 1998–99 (Québec, Assemblée Nationale 1999), while the Auditor General's figure was $435 million (Vérificateur général du Québec 1999). The Auditor General estimated the net savings over nine years to be $155 million, taking into consideration the necessary replacement of health-care retirees.

Various proposals to change the budgetary processes, mainly for hospitals, have been examined. In 1977, budgetary rules were tentatively revised to adjust hospital budgets according to budget types designed on the basis of a hospital classification system. This initiative collapsed, given the complexity of the method, problems with hospital classification, and a tight government budgetary situation (Lemay et al. 2012). Bédard and his committee members (2002) proposed a combination of population-based and diagnostic group–based methodology; this proposal has not been implemented. More recently, activity-based methods proposed (Gagné et al. 2010, 66; Lemay et al. 2012; Ouellette 2007) were planned for implementation in 2013. In 2003 the restructuring of the Québec health and social care system around 95 CSSSs was supposed to bring about a major change in the budgetary process, based on population-adjusted figures (MSSS 2004); this budgetary reform was never completed (MSSS 2012). At the time of this writing, the Lean Six Sigma methodology is being actively promoted by the MSSS, the Treasury Board, and Finances Québec (Québec Conseil du trésor 2012; Finances Québec 2010b). This approach actively pursues change in governance and clinical processes to increase performance, with the clear goal of cost control and reduction. Associated with the zero-deficit policy, a 10% reduction in administrative costs has been fixed by law (Québec 2010, 9). Finally, Finances Québec has fixed the annual increase in HCE from fiscal years 2011–12 to 2013–14 at 5.0% (Finances Québec 2010b). The pool tax dedicated to health was justified to guarantee this level of increase in HCE throughout the period.

The initiatives listed above have been short-listed from a longer collection. The exact impacts on cost and expenditure of those that have been implemented have not been evaluated as far as we know. Some initiatives addressed the micro-management level, as in the Lean Six Sigma approach. Others were effective at the macro level, such as the Treasury Board cuts in 1992–96 and the 1997 retirement plan. Macro-level initiatives are associated with recessions, diminishing returns of OSR, and increasing debt charges, and these initiatives were successful in controlling HCE.

The "fundamentals" of the basic model seem to work as a cycle: (1) recession; (2) its effect on OSR, deficit, and debt charges; (3) increases in expenditure on items other than health; (4) reduction in HCE growth rates; and (5) exit point. The Government of Québec took on macro-level initiatives—often decided by the Treasury Board and/or Finances Québec—to control HCE as in the above cycle. In recession times, expenditure on items other than health goes up, and HCE follows the same course in the first years. Deficits go up, as well as debt charges. Reduction of the HCE growth rate appears two to three years after inception of the recession. Following this period, increases in the HCE growth rate resume.

Idiosyncratic events modify the course of these so-called fundamentals, working in the same direction or in an opposing direction. In the 1981–82 recession, the CHT worked in the same direction as GDP and OSR, but cuts in the CHT continued way beyond the recession and the increasing debt charges added up. The Québec government found itself in a very difficult situation that led to deep cuts in health and social services, mainly in medicare-covered services. From 1997 to 2001, GDP, OSR, debt charges, and the CHT were all going in the right direction, and HCE followed the same course. Reductions in OSR growth rates were expected with the 2001 break and change of regime in GDP growth. But the slowdown effect of the 1999 and 2003 tax breaks on OSR had to be considered, such that real OSR was reduced up until 2006. However, the CHT was on a continuous upswing, and since debt charges were under control, the Québec government was able to finance HCE at the level it did.

HCE has, predictably, experienced slow growth following the 2008 recession. The idiosyncratic event is that both medicare- and non-medicare-covered services saw a slowdown in their respective growth rate, with no indication, at least for now, of a negative growth curve for medicare. Also, expenditure on items other than health stopped increasing, while a zero deficit was planned for the fiscal year 2012–13 (Finances Québec 2010c, A.13) and OSR is on a positive course. However, debt charges are increasing, zero deficits have been pushed to fiscal year 2014–15 (Finances Québec 2013), and CHT rules have been unilaterally changed by the federal government. In 2016–17, the CHT will grow at no more than the nominal GDP growth rate, with a lower limit of 3%. Can HCE growth expect to be renewed in the aftermath of reduced growth following recession? This remains to be seen in the face of economic uncertainty, the consequences of the Québec government's ability to maintain OSR, and the expected reduction in growth of the CHT.

Provincial government HCE in Québec hovered around 29% of program spending from 1975 to 1996, and 31% since then. From 1998 to

2008, aging accounted for 22% of growth in HCE and population growth for 10% (Marchildon and Di Matteo 2011). Inflation is estimated to have contributed 32%, leaving 36% for other cost drivers such as technology, increases in service utilization, and other items. Getzen (2006) has shown that macro-level constraints determine total HCE when fixed by regional or national authorities, while micro-level initiatives are used to allocate resources and improve efficacy and efficiency. Their impact on costs is minimal. However, institutional ingenuity is not limited to micro-level initiatives. The comparison of HCE growth rates in Québec and Canada (Figure 10.3) shows that Québec rates were much more sensitive to recessions than Canadian rates, while in the longer run, HCE share of program spending was almost flat in Québec but not in Canada. This flat scheme occurred in the face of a rapidly aging population and pressures from other cost drivers. Thus there is no inevitable reduction of HCE growth rates with recession, nor an ever-increasing HCE share in program spending. The Québec government chose to act to bend the cost curve at the macro level, sometimes implementing drastic cost-cutting measures while at other times using money made available by stable debt charges and increases in OSR and the CHT. Macro-level initiatives do work … sometimes.

References

Appleby, J., and A. Harrison. 2006. *Spending on Health Care: How Much Is Enough?* London: King's Fund.

Arpin, R., A. Côté, A. d'Amours, R. Larouche, J. E. Morin, and F. Turenne. 1999. *La complémentarité du secteur privé dans la poursuite des objectifs fondamentaux du système public de santé au Québec.* Québec: Ministère de la santé et des services sociaux. Accessed 30 November 2012. http://publications.msss.gouv.qc.ca/acrobat/f/documentation/1999/99_653/rapport.pdf.

Bédard, D., R. Bastien, B. Brown, J. P. Chicoine, M. Laroche, and R. Rouleau. 2002. *La budgétisation et la performance financière des centres hospitaliers : Rapport du Comité sur la réévaluation du mode de budgétisation des centres hospitaliers de soins généraux et spécialisés.* Québec: Ministère de la santé et des services sociaux.

Béland, F. 2006. "Les dépenses de santé au Québec: la bataille des chiffres." Brief presented to the Assemblée Nationale du Québec, Commission des affaires sociales, Québec, 24 March 24. Accessed November 30, 2012. http://meteopolitique.com/Fiches/sante_malade/analyse/Jean_Yves_Proulx/08/08.pdf.

———. 2007. "'Une vision apocalyptique.'" *La Presse*, 2 August.

———. 2008. "Les dépenses de santé au Québec: Une énigme ou un signal d'alarme?" In *Le privé dans la santé : Les discours et les faits*, edited by F. Béland, A.-P. Contandriopoulos, A. Quesnel-Vallée, and L. Robert, 171–205. Montréal: Presses de l'Université de Montréal.

Bérubé, G. 2006. "Perspectives : Fausse alerte." *Le Devoir*, 17 August.

Boothe, P., and M. Carson. 2003. "What Happened to Health-Care Reform?" Commentary no. 193. Toronto: C. D. Howe Institute.

Bourgault-Côté, G. 2006a. "La santé coûte moins cher au Québec que dans le ROC." *Le Devoir*, 2 November.

———. 2006b. "Financement du réseau de la santé : Couillard revendique le droit de changer d'idée." *Le Devoir*, 23–24 September.

Canadian Museum of Civilization. 2012. *Les groupes de travail nationaux sur le coût des services de santé, 1968–1969*. Ottawa: Canadian Museum of Civilization. Accessed July 25, 2012. http://www.museedelhistoire.ca/cmc/exhibitions/hist/medicare/medic-6h04f.shtml.

Castonguay, C., J. Marcotte, and M. Venne. 2008. *Rapport du groupe de travail sur le financement du système de santé : En avoir pour notre argent*. Québec: Ministère des finances et Ministère de la santé et des services sociaux. http://www.groupes.finances.gouv.qc.ca/financementsante/fr/rapport/pdf/RapportFR_FinancementSante.pdf.

Chaoulli v. Québec (Attorney General). 2005. 1 S.C.R. 791, 254 D.L.R. (4e) 577, 2005 CSC.

CIHI (Canadian Institute for Health Information). 2007. "National Health Expenditure Trends, 1975–2007." Ottawa: CIHI.

———. 2011. "National Health Expenditure Trends, 1975–2011." Ottawa: CIHI.

———. 2012. "National Health Expenditure Trends, 1975–2012. Ottawa: CIHI.

Cross, P. 1996. "Alternative Measures of Business Cycles in Canada: 1947–1992." *Canadian Economic Observer*. Cat. no. 11–010-XPB. Ottawa: Statistics Canada.

———. 2005. "Long-Run Cycles in Business Investment." *Canadian Economic Observer*. Cat. no. 11–010-XPB. Ottawa: Statistics Canada.

Daoust-Boisvert, A. 2011. "Santé: les dépenses croissent moins." *Le Devoir*, 4 November.

David, M. 2006. "Les vieux trucs." *Le Devoir*. 29 August, A3.

Le Devoir. 2010. "Les dépenses en santé au Québec: Les plus faibles au Canada." 29 October.

Di Matteo, L., and R. Di Matteo. 2011. *Viabilité financière des systèmes publics de santé du Canada et politiques stratégiques quant au déséquilibre budgétaire*. Ottawa: Fondation canadienne de la recherche sur les services de santé.

Evans, R. G., M. L. Barer, S. Lewis, M. Rachlis, and G. L. Stoddart. 2000. *Private Highway, One-Way Street: The Deklein and Fall of Canadian Medicare?* Vancouver: Health Policy Research Unit.

Evans, R. G., and M. Vujicic. 2005. "'Political Wolves and Economic Sheep: The Sustainability of Public Health Insurance in Canada." In *The Public–Private Mix for Health Care*, edited by A. Maynard, 117–40. Abingdon, UK: Radcliffe.

Finances Québec. 2001. *Budget 2001–2002: Plan budgétaire*. Québec: Gouvernement du Québec.

———. 2007a. *Budget 2007–2008: Relever le défi du financement de la santé*. Québec: Gouvernement du Québec.

———. 2007b. *Budget 2007–2008: Plan budgétaire*. Québec: Gouvernement du Québec.

———. 2010a. *Budget 2010–2011: Plan budgétaire*. Sect. 1, *Données historiques*. Québec: Gouvernement du Québec.

———. 2010b. *Budget 2010–2011: Vers un système de santé plus performant et mieux financé*. Québec: Gouvernement du Québec.

———. 2010c. *Budget 2010–2011: Plan budgétaire*. Québec: Gouvernement du Québec.

———. 2012. *Budget 2012–2013: Données historiques*. Québec: Gouvernement du Québec.

———. 2013. *Mise à jour économique et financière*. Québec: Gouvernement du Québec, http://consultations.finances.gouv.qc.ca/media/pdf/2014-2015/COMFR_20131128.pdf.

Gagné, R., P. Fortin, L. Godbout, and C. Montmarquette. 2009. *Le Québec face à ses défis: Des services publics étendus; une marge de manœuvre étroite; de nouveaux défis à relever.* Comité consultatif sur l'économie et les finances publiques. Québec: Ministère des finances. http://consultations.finances.gouv.qc.ca/media/pdf/ le-quebec-face-a-ses-defis-fascicule-1.pdf.

———. 2010. *Le Québec face à ses défis: Une voie durable, pour rester maîtres de nos choix.* Comité consultatif sur l'économie et les finances publiques. Québec: Ministère des finances; http://consultations.finances.gouv.qc.ca/media/pdf/le-quebec-face-a-ses -defis-fascicule-3.pdf.

Gaumer, B. 2008. *Le système de santé et de services sociaux du Québec: Une histoire récente et tourmentée 1921–2006.* Québec: Les presses de l'Université Laval.

Getzen, T. 2006. "Aggregation and the Measurement of Health Care Costs." *Health Services Research* 41, no. 5: 1938–54. http://dx.doi.org/10.1111/j.1475-6773 .2006.00558.x.

Godbout, L., M. Arseneau, S. St-Cerny, and P. Fortin. 2007. "Un élan insoutenable." *La Presse,* 21 July.

Hirsch, D. 2005. *Facing the Cost of Long-Term Care: Towards a Sustainable Funding System.* York, UK: Joseph Rowntree Foundation.

Lemay, A., F. Lemoyne, C. Paradis, L. Vincent, and L. Bouchard. 2012. *Allocation des ressources aux établissements de santé et de services sociaux : Pistes et balises pour implanter le financement à l'activité.* Montréal: Association québécoise d'établissements de santé et de services sociaux.

Levine, D. 2005. "Healthcare Revolution: Quebec's New Model of Healthcare." *Healthcare Quarterly* 8, no. 4: 38–46. http://dx.doi.org/10.12927/hcq.2013.17690.

Malthus, T. R. 1888. *An Essay on the Principle of Population.* 9th ed. London: Reeves and Turner.

Marchildon, G., and L. Di Matteo. 2011. *Health Care Cost Drivers: The Facts.* Ottawa: CIHI.

Ménard, J., D. Adam, J. S. Bernard, J. P. Chicoine, M. Clair, J. M. Dumesnil, H. Elbaz, J. P. Hotte, M. C. Martel, N. Neamtan, et al. 2005. *Pour sortir de l'impasse: La solidarité entre nos générations.* Comité de travail sur la pérennité du système de santé et de services sociaux du Québec. Québec: Ministère des finances et Ministère de la santé et des services sociaux. http://www.bibliotheque.assnat.qc.ca/01/ MONO/2005/07/818789/Tome_1_ex_1.pdf.

MSSS (Ministère de la santé et des services sociaux). 1990. *Une réforme axée sur le citoyen: La réforme Côté—La réforme de la santé et des services sociaux Québec.* Québec: MSSS.

———. 1991. *Les services de santé et les services sociaux au Québec: Un financement équitable à la mesure de nos moyens.* Québec: MSSS.

———. 2004. *L'intégration des services de santé et des services sociaux : Le projet organisationnel et clinique et les balises associées à la mise en œuvre des réseaux locaux de services de santé et de services sociaux.* Québec: MSSS.

———. 2006. *Garantir l'accès: un défi d'équité, d'efficience et de qualité.* Québec: MSSS. http://msssa4.msss.gouv.qc.ca/fr/document/publication.nsf/0/e90f534d231477858 52571150053f04e?OpenDocument

———. 2011. *Comptes de la santé, 2009–2010 à 2011–2012.* Québec: MSSS.

———. 2012. *Mode d'allocation des ressources 2012–2013.* Québec: Service de l'allocation des ressources, MSSS.

Noël, A. 2007. "Le régime aurait la santé pour absorber le choc du vieillissement." *La Presse,* 12 July.

Orosz, E., and D. Morgan. 2004. *SHA-Based National Health Account in Thirteen OECD Countries: A Comparative Analysis.* Health Working Papers no.16. Paris: OECD.

Ouellette, P. 2007. *Efficience et budgétisation des hôpitaux et autres institutions de santé au Québec.* Québec: Groupe de travail sur le financement du système de santé.

Pammolli, F., M. Riccaboni, and L. Magazzini. 2008. *The Sustainability of European Health Care Systems: Beyond Income and Ageing.* Dipartimento di scienze economiche WPS no. 52. Verona: Università degli studi di Verona.

Parsons, T. 1937. *The Structure of Social Action.* New York: Free Press.

Petretto, A. 2010. *On the Fuzzy Boundaries between Public and Private in Health Care Organization and Funding Systems.* Dipartimento di scienze economiche WP no. 09/2010. Firenze: Università degli studi di Firenze.

Prada, G., G. Roberts, S. Vail, M. Anderson, E. Down, C. Fooks, A. Howatson, K. Grimes, S. Morgan, K. Parent, et al. 2004. *Understanding Health Care Cost Drivers and Escalators.* Ottawa: Conference Board of Canada.

Pratte, A. 2007. "Les erreurs de calcul." *La Presse*, 3 August.

Québec. 1988. *Report : Commission d'enquête sur les services de santé et les services sociaux, Québec* [Rochon Commission]. Québec: MSSS.

———. 2000. *Les solutions émergentes: Report et recommandations—Commission d'étude sur les services de santé et les services sociaux* [Clair Commission]. Québec: MSSS.

———. 2010. *Projet de loi no. 100: Loi mettant en œuvre certaines dispositions du discours du budget du 30 mars 2010 et visant le retour à l'équilibre budgétaire en 2013–14 et la réduction de la dette.* Présenté le 12 mai 2010, 39ième législature de l'Assemblée nationale, 1ière session, 2010. Québec : Éditeur officiel du Québec.

Québec. Assemblée Nationale. 1999. Conférence de presse de M. Jacques Léonard, ministre d'État à l'administration et à la fonction publique : Réaction à la partie du rapport du Vérification général touchant le Programme de départs volontaires, 9 December. Accessed 29 November 2012. http://www.assnat.qc.ca/fr/actualites -salle-presse/conferences-points-presse/ConferencePointPresse-603.html.

Québec. Conseil du trésor. 2012. *Budget de dépenses 2012–2013.* Vol. 5, *Message de la président du Conseil du trésor et renseignements supplémentaires.* Québec: Conseil du trésor.

Roy, D., R. Choinière, P. Tousignant, R. Pineault, N. Lauzon, and M. Mongeaon. 2000. *Rapport annuel 2000 sur la santé de la population : Impact de la transformation du réseau montréalais sur la santé.* Montréal: Direction de la santé publique, Régie régionale de la santé et des services sociaux de Montréal-Centre.

Statistics Canada. 1992. *Financial Management System (FMS).* Ottawa: Industry Canada.

———. 2009. *Financial Management System (FMS).* CS68–0023/2009E-PDF. Ottawa: Industry Canada.

Vaillancourt, F., and L. M. Perrault. 2007. *Le financement des services de santé au Québec: Le compte santé et son financement.* Groupe de travail sur le financement de la santé. Québec: Gouvernement du Québec.

Van Elk, R., E. Mot, and P. H. Franses. 2009. *Modelling Health Care Expenditures: Overview of the Literature and Evidence from a Panel Time Series Model.* CPB Discussion Paper 121. The Hague: Netherlands Bureau for Economic Policy Analysis.

Vérificateur général du Québec. 1999. *Rapport à l'Assemblée nationale pour l'année 1998–1999.* Vol. 2. Québec: Gouvernement du Québec.

eleven

British Columbia: Cost Control in the Country of the Red Queen

KIMBERLYN M. McGRAIL AND ROBERT G. EVANS[1]

"Well, in our country," said Alice, still panting a little, "you'd generally get to somewhere else—if you run very fast for a long time, as we've been doing."

"A slow sort of country!" said the Queen. "Now, here, you see, it takes all the running you can do, to keep in the same place. If you want to get somewhere else, you must run at least twice as fast as that!"
—Lewis Carroll, *Through the Looking-Glass*

Introduction

Modern health-care systems in high-income countries are, without exception, predominantly financed, directly or indirectly, from the public sector. Where this reality encounters strong ideological resistance, as in the United States, there is much public posturing and a great deal of effort wasted in futile debate, fantastical policy proposals, and very expensive institutional workaround frameworks to conceal the reality. But the health-care system is nonetheless predominantly publicly financed.[2]

It is also true that modern health-care systems display, for both good and bad reasons, a powerful inherent drive towards expenditure growth, a dynamic that Aaron Wildavsky memorably labelled the "Law of Medical Money" (Wildavsky 1977). Very simply, this "law" asserts that health-care systems will use all resources made available to them. It follows that in all

---

1 Our thanks to Dawn Mooney for creating the figures. This chapter uses data developed by the British Columbia Ministry of Health's Planning and Innovation Division. We are grateful to the Division and to the Ministry for their generosity in sharing these data.
2 The reality is obscured where, as in the United States and to a lesser extent Canada, "tax expenditures"—tax concessions—offset about a third of the cost of "private" health insurance. This public contribution in the form of forgone revenue is not always included along with public expenditure, thus understating the public share. More indirectly, a government may mandate enrolment in private insurance under strictly regulated conditions and premiums—*de facto* public coverage but "off budget."

modern states, governments at different levels are forced continually to wrestle with the politically demanding process of restraining the growth of the health-care system and to manage its tendency to absorb an ever-growing share of government budgets and of the national economy.

The phrase "bending the cost curve" is a currently fashionable short-hand for the collectivity of these efforts by public and private actors, portraying them as attempts to shift the trajectory of health-care cost escalation, if not downward, then at least to a more gentle upward slope. It originates in the United States, the country that over time has been the most spectacularly unsuccessful in this endeavour. While the phrase itself is a catchy one, we need to be careful not to import American experience and perceptions of the problem along with the label that Americans have attached to it. What is interesting, and instructive, is that public policies in different countries meet with varying success at different times. The range of national (and sub-national) experiences, and especially their shifts over time, provides a wealth of demonstrations that bending the cost curve *is* possible, and to a significant degree (Kizer, Demakis, and Feussner 2000; Priest, Rachlis, and Cohen 2007).

More than technical solutions

Bending the cost curve cannot, however, be achieved solely through institutional gadgetry. The problems may have technical solutions, but implementing those solutions often—perhaps always—requires political decisions. As a matter of basic accounting, a country's total health expenditures must be precisely equal to the total of incomes earned by those supplying resources to the health sector: doctors, nurses, pharmacists, administrators, and support staff, but also employees, managers, and shareholders of firms that develop and sell pharmaceuticals and supplies, provide construction services, or assemble the public and private financing of health services. Bending the cost curve requires the political will—and capacity—to thwart the income expectations and aspirations of at least some of these groups (Evans 1997).

Identifying total expenditure and total incomes is the source of the powerful and frequently effective political opposition to efforts to bend the cost curve. Here the clash of interests comes out into the open, because if one really proposes to bend the cost curve there is no way of avoiding the question of how many members of different occupations should be able to draw incomes from the sector, or how much they should earn. Everyone may in principle be in favour of controlling expenditures, but only as long as that expenditure control does not affect their own part of health-care delivery.

Opposition to cost containment can take many forms, not excluding backroom lobbying and, in some cases, simple bribery.[3] The more overt political strategies to resist bending involve undermining the legitimacy of the objective itself, as well as proposing various alternative mechanisms for shifting and expanding the financing base to keep the overall flow of expenditures growing through less noticeable or controllable channels. It is for all these reasons that potentially cost-reducing innovations (of which there have been many) rarely if ever result in overall reductions in expenditure, in British Columbia or elsewhere.

Obviously, cost containment is not the only objective. If it were, payers would simply control their outlays, and ultimately costs would be shifted to patients. But we have not seen governments anywhere reducing their commitment to (largely) publicly funded health-care systems. This is because there is in fact a dual objective: the hope is to bend the cost curve without threatening the present or future health of the population served. The objective of bending the curve thus embodies a simultaneous implicit assertion of the potential for significant reductions in present or future health expenditure without compromising patient or, more broadly, population health (Berwick, Nolan, and Whittington 2008). There is ample evidence to support this implicit assertion, but equally there is ample scope for controversy as to both the potential for such savings and the mechanisms through which they might be achieved.

A focus on British Columbia

Every student of health services research is aware that in all modern health-care systems, a small proportion of the population uses a large proportion of services in any given year, and also over time. For example, a long history of research in the United States shows that the 5% or so of Medicare recipients who die in any given year consume 25% to 30% of all Medicare expenditures (Riley and Lubitz 1993; Scitovsky 2005). In British Columbia, the top 5% of users have been shown to use 30% all of physician services (Reid et al. 2003). More important, these users were also shown to have chronic (and often complex) conditions, and thus this concentration of spending is maintained if we look at lifetime rather than annual costs

---

3 In British Columbia there have been rumours in past years of attempted bribes by the pharmaceutical industry and physical threats related to the laboratory industry, though none of these have been substantiated. In the United States, criminal convictions and fines in the billions of dollars are now common for pharmaceutical firms and private hospital chains (Laurance 2012).

Figure 11.1 Total and provincial government per capita health-care spending, Canada and British Columbia, 1975–2011

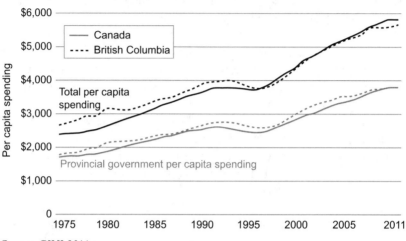

Source: CIHI 2011a.

(Forget et al. 2008; Hanley and Morgan 2009). Heavy use of health care is driven by high levels of need; thus any idea that cost escalation results from unnecessary or "frivolous" use by "consumers" is a free-market economist's fantasy. Unfortunately, it does not follow that all the services received by those in need are in fact necessary.

As can be seen in Figure 11.1, total health-care spending in British Columbia in 2011 was projected to be $5,450 per capita, less than the Canadian average of $5,811 (CIHI 2011a). Provincial government spending was $3,603, or 66% of this total; the Ministry of Health estimates that more than 80% of hospital, physician, and pharmaceutical expenditures are on people with chronic conditions (BC Ministry of Health 2012a). This suggests that it might be possible to bend the cost curve by focusing efforts on populations that have higher average expenditures, and that is the focus the BC Ministry of Health chose to pursue, starting in 2010 (BC Ministry of Health 2012b). This direction is described as critical because of the concentration of spending but also because the population is aging and prevalence of chronic disease is increasing. One specific policy direction is to provide as much care as possible outside hospitals and long-term care institutions, the most expensive forms of care in the system.

This chapter addresses the health-care cost experience in British Columbia, the influence of specific population groups on health-care costs as well as the potential of a focus on high users to bend the cost curve, and the specific approach BC is taking to achieve its policy objectives. We start with an analysis of national health expenditures data, move to a more detailed analysis of BC spending on specific population groups, and end with a provincial framework for implementing and evaluating innovations that are intended to bend the cost curve and improve quality of care in British Columbia.

Health-care spending in British Columbia

When general price levels are rising over time and the population served is both growing and aging, stabilizing nominal expenditure levels amounts to de facto reductions in financing. The proper focus of attention for "bending" is the trend in "real" (i.e., inflation-adjusted) expenditures per capita, with some additional adjustment for the effect of changing age structure.

Figure 11.1 shows per capita constant-dollar expenditures for both total and provincial government expenditures in Canada and British Columbia. The level and trend for both overall and provincial government expenditures track very closely; over this long sweep of time, BC expenditures move from just above to just below the national average. But BC, like Canada as a whole, experienced a relentless increase in per capita spending. Provincial government spending (in 2011 dollars) doubled from just under $1,800 per capita in 1975 to just under $3,800 in 2011, an average rate of 2.1% per year sustained over 36 years.

A portion of this per capita increase is associated with the changing age structure of the population. Older people have, on average, poorer health and greater needs for health care. This has consistently been estimated to account for increases of less than 1% per year, though greater for some services (e.g., long-term institutional care) than for others (e.g., physicians' services) (CIHI 2011b; Evans et al. 2001; McGrail et al. 2011; Morgan and Cunningham 2011). Applying this rate of 1% per year since 1975—which is almost assuredly an overstatement over that long time span—produces an estimate of provincial government per capita expenditures in 2011 of less than $2,600, or $1,200 less than the actual. This translates to $5.5 billion in spending by the provincial government in 2011 that cannot be attributed to population growth or population aging.[4] This additional spending must come from some combination of health care–specific price increases (beyond general inflation) and expanding service use. Everywhere

---

4 It would perhaps be most desirable to age-standardize to calculate this effect. But age standardization requires age-specific patterns of utilization, which CIHI estimates only back to 1996.

in Canada and, indeed, across all OECD nations, the population is receiving an ever-increasing amount of health-care services, and these increases cannot be explained by demographics.

The apparently parallel experiences in British Columbia and Canada begin to diverge, however, when we consider the distribution of total spending among different sub-sectors of the health-care system. In 2011 it appears that the provinces and territories in Canada have distinct health-care systems (Table 11.1). For example, health-care spending devoted to "other institutions," which is dominated by long-term care facilities (nursing homes), ranges from 7.4% of all health-care spending in Alberta to 10.6% in New Brunswick, 13.9% in Québec, and 19.3% in Yukon Territory. Spending on hospitals also varies considerably, from 23.1% of the total in Yukon to 26.1% in Québec to 31.5% in BC, 38.7% in Newfoundland and Labrador, and 40.4% in the Northwest Territories. The proportion of health-care spending devoted to hospitals is in fact positively correlated with overall per capita spending: the greater the dependence on acute care, the more likely that overall expenditures will be higher ($r^2 = 0.48$). This suggests that there may indeed be ways to keep people out of acute care, and through that shift to moderate the escalation of health expenditures.

These differences suggest that provinces took quite varying paths from the start of medicare in the early 1970s to their current patterns of spending. Figure 11.2 focuses on provincial government spending in British Columbia and Canada, and even more specifically on a few categories of spending: hospitals, "other institutions," physicians, prescription drugs, and "other health spending." The first four are of interest because they are the largest of the spending categories. The "other health spending" category is included because it is where home health-care spending is buried, along with health research and other miscellaneous items. Since the focus of this chapter is on services provided outside hospitals, it is essential to include this category, though it is a catchall and interpretations must be drawn carefully.

Some patterns in health spending are distinctive to British Columbia. Hospital expenditures per capita were lower than the national average before 2001 but then started to catch up and eventually exceeded the national average. In effect the "recovery" from the federal government's clampdown on transfer payments (Marchildon 2004; McIntosh 2004), which hit hospitals particularly hard, had a bit more bounce in BC. Expenditures on physicians are consistently somewhat higher in BC, though that difference diminishes substantially by 2009. Drug spending began to fall behind the national average in 1993, and more particularly

Table 11.1 Percentage distribution of health-care spending by sector and province, 2011

Province	Hospitals	Other Institutions	Physicians	Other Professionals	Drugs	Capital	Public Health	Administration	Other Health Spending	Total
NL	38.7	14.6	12.4	5.8	15.0	4.0	3.1	3.2	3.3	100
PE	29.8	11.8	11.8	8.1	15.5	4.4	5.2	8.5	4.9	100
NB	33.1	10.6	12.4	9.6	17.6	3.7	3.4	3.8	5.9	100
NS	32.2	12.6	12.6	9.2	18.1	2.0	3.2	4.9	5.2	100
QC	26.1	13.9	13.1	9.2	19.7	5.6	4.0	3.4	5.1	100
ON	27.3	8.7	15.9	11.8	16.2	3.9	7.5	2.7	6.1	100
MB	30.6	12.1	12.6	9.0	13.1	4.1	7.0	2.9	8.5	100
SK	27.7	12.7	13.1	10.1	14.5	3.7	9.2	2.8	6.4	100
AB	34.6	7.4	14.0	11.8	13.3	5.5	5.7	2.4	5.4	100
BC	31.5	8.1	11.7	11.7	12.9	4.9	6.8	3.6	8.8	100
YT	23.6	19.3	9.0	7.9	9.0	5.6	14.9	3.4	7.3	100
NT	40.4	7.7	11.2	6.6	6.9	3.6	8.4	2.5	12.8	100
NU	36.3	6.6	11.1	4.5	5.6	8.8	10.1	6.3	10.7	100

Source: CIHI 2011a, Tables D.1 and D.2.

Figure 11.2 Provincial government per capita health-care spending by sector, Canada and British Columbia, 1975–2011 (2011 dollars)

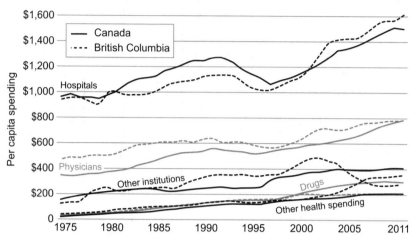

Source: CIHI 2011a.

after 2001. By 2011, provincial government spending in BC was more than $90 per capita below the national average. For a population of almost 4.6 million, this amounts to savings of more than $400 million.

The most distinguishing changes over time in British Columbia are the downward curve for spending on "other institutions" after 2003, both in absolute terms and relative to trends in Canada overall, and the corresponding upward curve in "other health spending." BC's public funding of nursing homes and some home nursing care began in 1978 (Hollander and Pallan 1995), which can be seen in a quick rise in the spending at that time. Publicly funded home-based services were expanded beyond nursing care in 1981; this may explain both the increase in that year in "other health spending" and the shift down in "other institutions" over the next few years. After this, BC's per capita spending on other institutions remains consistently above the national average all the way to 2005. When spending in this area starts to decrease there is a countervailing increase in per capita spending on "other health spending." In fact, the two lines cross in 2007, after which spending on "other institutions" is below "other health spending," and much below the national average.

One should be cautious about placing too much weight on these trends, given the murkiness of the categories. The "other health spending" category is, after all, dominated by health research, not home health services. Nevertheless, the data paint a picture of a particular policy environment that is moving away from institutional care and focusing instead on community-based services, and doing so in a way that appears to be different from other parts of the country. Moreover, this picture is consistent with the declared policy intent of the BC government, which has in fact been trying to emphasize non-facility-based care. Perhaps the clearest example of this is the pledge the BC Ministry of Health made in 2001 to build 5,000 new nursing-home beds. The promise was made because it was recognized that bed supply had fallen well behind the force of population aging. Beds had to be built simply to keep pace with the greater number of elderly residents of the province. Over time, however, this promise morphed into replacing rather than adding new beds, and to building assisted-living units rather than nursing-home beds (Cohen, Tate, and Baumbusch 2009; Hunter 2009). British Columbia was in fact the first province in Canada to regulate and publicly fund assisted living, which is presented as a middle option between living independently in the community and living in facilities that provide 24/7 nursing coverage (McGrail et al. 2010). This sort of living arrangement can help support the independence of older adults, and the facilities are also significantly cheaper to build, operate, and regulate.

It is not possible to use these data to make conclusions about the correctness of policy, because they tell us nothing about the distribution of care within the community, the quality of services provided, or the outcomes for the patients who receive (or do not receive) services. But it is possible to conclude—within the limits of the less-than-perfect data available—that British Columbia has taken a different path than other provinces to spending in these sectors of health care.

Spending on population groups

Research over many years and in many countries has shown wide variations in care patterns across geographic areas, and that these variations have significant cost consequences. The most extensive and most recent evidence, from the United States, shows that higher spending does not result in different outcomes, measured from either the patient or the provider perspective (Fisher et al. 2003a, 2003b; Fowler et al. 2008). The implication is that there are population groups that can be expected to need and to use significant health-care resources, but just how much or how many services are needed is not fixed. In fact, the presence of geographic variations suggests that the provision of care is influenced to a large degree by local custom and habits of providers, which are in turn influenced by the local supply of health-care resources (Fisher and

Wennberg 2003; Wennberg 2010). There is a potential opportunity, then, to improve care and limit costs if it is possible to influence these local patterns of practice.

While much of the most comprehensive research on clinical variations has come from the United States, such variations have also been demonstrated in Canada (Hanley, Janssen, and Greyson 2010; McGrail, Schaub, and Black 2004; Morgan, Cunningham, and Hanley 2010; Roos and Roos 1981; Roos et al. 1986; Tu et al. 2006). We present analyses based on a unique dataset constructed by the BC Ministry of Health. The Planning and Innovation Division of the Ministry uses linked individual-level administrative data to create an analytic file that is available in a semi-public form. The construction of the dataset was influenced by the "bridges to health" model developed by Lynn and colleagues (2007). That model, and consequently the Ministry of Health data, first identifies clearly delineated population groups or segments, defining the groups by similar needs for health-care services. This dataset includes 14 mutually exclusive and exhaustive population segments, ranging from non-users of services up through people in palliative care at the end of life. Detailed definitions of these groups are included the appendix to this chapter. Where individuals fall into more than one category—for example, under maternity care and low-complexity chronic conditions— they are placed in the category representing the higher expected use of services.

As of early 2012, the data created by the Ministry were available for fiscal years 2002–03 through 2008–09. In 2008–09 they included about $9 billion in government health-care expenditures, out of a total of nearly $16 billion in public-sector expenditures and a little more than $22 billion in health-care spending overall (CIHI 2011a). We use these data to provide a population-segment analysis of health-care expenditures and to estimate the potential impact of bending the cost curve for both lower and higher expenditure groups.

Figure 11.3 shows the distribution of the population across the 14 health segments in both 2002–03 and 2008–09. In both years, about 14% of the population were non-users—they had no contact at all with the health-care system. In both years the single largest group was the "healthy" population segment, which had limited contact with the health-care system and no major or ongoing diagnoses. These two groups combined represented half or more of the population in both years, but the healthy group declined from 42% to 36% of the total between 2002–03 and 2008–09. The shift in general was from the healthy (and low-cost) group to the low-, medium-, and high-complexity chronic condition groups.

Figure 11.3 Percentage distribution of BC population by population health segment, 2002–2003 and 2008–2009

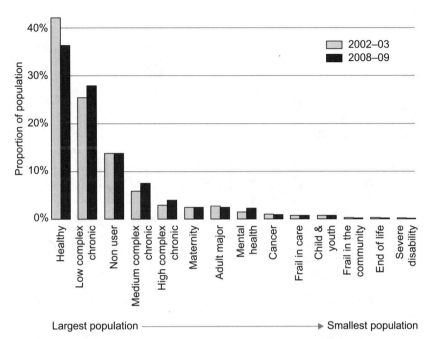

Source: Dataset developed by Planning and Innovation Division, British Columbia Ministry of Health.

As expected, the different population segments have very different average cost profiles. Figure 11.4 shows both total expenditures (on the left axis) and average costs per capita (on the right axis) for each population segment, with segments ordered from left to right by descending population size. (The non-user group does not appear on this chart because they generate no health-care expenditures.) The "healthy" group—36% of the total population—had a very low cost per capita (about $200) and as a consequence accounted for about $350 million in total expenditures: less than 4% of the total captured in these data. Given the small amount of that total, clearly changing service use for this group would have limited potential impact on overall expenditures. Similarly, the "severe disability" group generated very high expenditure per capita (more than $40,000 per year) but was such a small population (barely registering in Figure 11.3) that the overall spending on this group was less than 1% of the total. There may be good reasons to improve services for this group, but measures targeting expenditure

Figure 11.4 Total and per capita spending by population health segment, British Columbia, 2008–2009

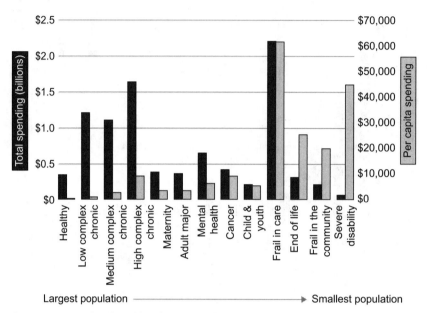

Source: Dataset developed by Planning and Innovation Division, British Columbia Ministry of Health.

reduction for it clearly cannot significantly influence overall health-care expenditures.

The two groups that accounted for the largest share of health-care expenditures were the "frail in care" (meaning in nursing homes) and "high complex chronic condition" population segments. Together these groups accounted for less than 5% of the population but more than 40% of total expenditures (again, the caveat is that the percentage is of the $9 billion in expenditures captured in this dataset). The "frail in care" group is significant because of the marrying of high per capita costs (more than $60,000 per annum) and a sufficient population size (more than 35,000) to create large overall expenditures. The "high complex chronic condition" group had a lower cost per capita (less than $10,000) but, as seen in Figure 11.3, this was a reasonably large (more than 175,000) and growing group.

About half of the "high complex chronic condition" group are people who are 75 and over. In 2008–09 there were nearly 90,000 individuals aged 75 and over in this group (2% of the total population), with total health-care spending of more than $860 million, or nearly 10% of the total (Table 11.2). The per capita expenditures for this group were $9,668, but once again, averages

Table 11.2 Size of and expenditures on "high complex chronic condition" population segment aged 75 years and over, 2002–2003 and 2008–2009

	2002–03	2008–09	% change
High complex chronic conditions, age 75+	60,916	89,101	46.3%
Total population age 75+	279,250	327,264	17.2%
"High complex" as % of total	21.8%	27.2%	24.8%
Total per capita costs	$9,371	$9,668	3.2%
Total costs	$570,860,431	$861,408,800	50.9%
Expenditures (% of population 75+ static)		$690,181,249	

Source: Dataset developed by Planning and Innovation Division, British Columbia Ministry of Health.

Figure 11.5 Per capita spending by local health area, "high complex chronic condition" population segment aged 75 years and over, 2008–2009

○ Local health area

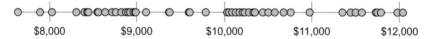

Source: Dataset developed by Planning and Innovation Division, British Columbia Ministry of Health.

can be misleading. Figure 11.5 shows per capita spending on this population segment by local health area in British Columbia. Even within this relatively homogeneous population segment there were wide variations in expenditures per capita, from less than $8,000 to more than $12,000. A reduction of $1,000 in the average per capita spending on this group would result in savings of nearly $90 million overall. A reduction of all regions to the average of the lowest would push this estimate up to about $150 million. This is a large number, but it represents only 1% to 1.5% of total expenditures.

There are limitations to this analysis, one of which is that the dataset captures only 56% of provincial government health-care expenditures. The unallocated spending (which ranges from non-fee-for-service physician payments to cancer care to emergency department services and public health) may not be distributed across population groups in the same way as the allocated spending. More important, however, there is a limitation in how we might interpret these data. The above calculation of $90 million (or $150 million) represents potential one-time savings. Bending the cost curve requires more than this. It requires not just spending less but also modifying the relentless increase in per capita health-care spending seen in Figure 11.1. It may make sense to pursue bending the curve in targeted high-need and high-utilization groups first, but changing population-level expenditure patterns will require population-wide changes in how and when people use services and how many services they use. Efforts in specific population groups can easily be offset by the introduction of new technology or new drugs or the identification of entirely new potential patient groups.

We can, in fact, see this effect by expanding the information in Figure 11.3. Table 11.2 provides some detail on the "high complex chronic condition, age 75 plus" group, comparing 2002–03 with 2008–09. While the per capita costs within this group grew at a modest < 4% (inflation-adjusted) over these years, the size of the group itself increased by an extraordinary 25%. If this group had remained at its 2002–03 share of the total population (i.e., allowing for population aging but not "population sickening"), expenditures would have been $170 million lower than they were. In other words, the change in the distribution of the population across health segments appears to swamp any "savings" we might get by reducing variations in spending within the segment. Bending the curve for one population segment may not even be as good as running to stay in the same place.

The current approach to innovation in British Columbia

The BC Ministry of Health's current policy directions are outlined in their government service plan (BC Ministry of Health 2012b) and in a document summarizing their "innovation and change" agenda (BC Ministry of Health 2012a). The overall goals of this agenda are parallel with the Institute for Healthcare Improvement's "Triple Aim": improved population health, quality clinical service, and a sustainable publicly funded health-care system. Three overarching "key results areas" are identified that are intended to help achieve these objectives: effective health promotion and prevention, high-quality hospital services, and integrated primary and community care. For the latter, the objectives are to provide as much care as possible in the community (keeping people out of acute care and long-term facility-based care) and to focus on services used by people with chronic conditions, particularly the frail or soon-to-be-frail elderly.

Essentially, the label "integrated primary and community care" is an umbrella term for several changes intended to achieve all three aspects of the Triple Aim, including bending the cost curve. This initiative is in its very early stages, so it is impossible to say whether it will have the desired effect. It is nevertheless a current priority reform area and is described in broad terms

Figure 11.6 Collaborative relationships involved in integrated primary and community care

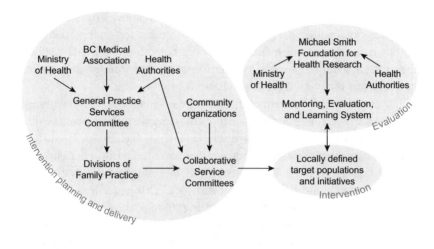

here. The current initiative is built on several changes dating back several years, starting with creation of the General Practices Services Committee (GPSC) in 2004 "to support the provision of full-service family practice and improve patient care" (General Practice Services Committee 2009).

The GPSC is a joint committee of the BC Ministry of Health, the BC Medical Association, and the Society of General Practitioners of BC; representatives from British Columbia's health authorities attend meetings as guests of the committee. It has received more than $800 million in funding since its inception (General Practice Services Committee 2011). Some of its larger initiatives include fee-for-service incentive payments intended to encourage physicians to provide "full-service" family practice; the Practice Support Program, which provides training and resources with learning modules on topics that include practice management, mental health care, and end-of-life care; and the development of networks of community-based physicians called Divisions of Family Practice. The latter are intended to provide a strong collective voice for family physicians and a forum for coordinated work on local health-care priorities. The divisions are a way of encouraging collective projects of GPs in communities without requiring a structural change either in the way they are paid (i.e., no move away from the dominance of fee-for-service) or how they work on a day-to-day basis (most are still in solo or small group practices).

The more recent integrated primary and community care initiative is meant to develop even more partnerships—among the Ministry of Health, the Divisions of Family Practice, BC's health authorities, and local service providers, including community groups such as Meals on Wheels (see Figure 11.6). Local "collaborative service committees" of health authorities, community groups, and providers are meant to work together to identify target population groups, choose and structure interventions, implement the changes, and evaluate the outcomes. This attempt to capitalize on a collective recognition of the need for change combines top-down system management with a more bottom-up approach to identification of specific issues or population groups of interest and specific interventions targeted to those populations.

The evaluation component of the initiative is a unique part of this arrangement, and it is yet another partnership, this time with the Michael Smith Foundation for Health Research (MSFHR). The Michael Smith Foundation is British Columbia's research-funding agency and has a history of close and cooperative work with the Ministry of Health, for example, through its Health Services Research and Policy Support Network. This new partnership takes the cooperation one step further, from setting strategic directions and providing funding to one of direct involvement in evaluation. During 2011, the MSFHR developed what it calls the Monitoring, Evaluation and Learning System, or MELS. The form of this system is still evolving, but at present it includes funding to hire a lead evaluator and two community evaluators in each of BC's five geographic health authorities; identification of a suite of indicators and a mechanism for their production that will help local initiatives monitor the initial and immediate impacts of their programs (e.g., emergency department visits, new residential care placements); plans for collection of primary data from patients, their caregivers, and providers; and a steering committee, including academics, that will help oversee the system, the data collection, and the use of the data. The whole system is still evolving, although the lead evaluators have been in place since mid 2012.

Conclusions

The desire to control health-care expenditures and bend the cost curve is unique neither to British Columbia nor to Canada. Similar strategic priorities, however, do not preclude tactical differences. The tactical appraoch in BC is to focus more heavily on high-needs patient groups that are also high utilizers of health-care services and who thus account for higher-than-average expenditures. The intent is to rationalize care for these groups to avoid, as much as possible, both admissions to acute care and permanent moves to long-term care (nursing homes). Part of this is to be achieved by providing public funding for less intensive facility-based care such as assisted living, but a still greater emphasis is being placed on community supports to enable people to remain in their homes for as long as possible. In this sense, the BC experiments are trying to address one cost driver—population aging. Changing the trajectory of care for high-use older populations is one potential way to mitigate the impact of that driver. Holding all other factors constant, changes in the age structure of the BC population are projected to increase health expenditures per capita by about 1% per year. Changing the relative use of higher-use groups might help counteract at least part of this increase and thus bend the cost curve.

While reasonable in themselves, however, these experiments do not address the much larger and seemingly relentless increases in utilization at every age. Diagnostic imaging and laboratory testing have increased for the whole population, not just among the old and infirm (McGrail et al. 2011). The increases are indeed most rapid among that sub-population, but the cost impact of the more general increase is much greater. Similarly, the use of more—and more expensive—drugs has been occurring across the population as a whole, not just among the most vulnerable (Morgan and Cunningham 2011). These population-wide changes are being driven in part (perhaps in large part) by the availability of new techniques and technology; they may be only tangentially related, if at all, to any changes in population health status or outcomes.

Despite the limitations, British Columbia is engaged in some interesting policy initiatives. Improving care for people who are high users has the potential to improve quality and control costs. Keeping people out of acute care and nursing homes and providing alternative supports in the community are goals shared by patients, their families, and health-care system managers. However, BC is pursuing this agenda within the same environment as everyone else, and without fundamentally altering the basic structure of the health-care system. Physicians in BC are still largely autonomous self-employed providers working in fee-for-service practices, and it is physician decisions that drive at least 60% of health-care expenditures, in particular, physician payments, hospital care, and pharmaceuticals (CIHI 2011a).

Ultimately, the biggest challenge every health-care system faces is that the curve its paymasters are trying to bend is not exogenous. There is no clear and mutually agreed-upon *need* in the population, just as there is wide variation in response to patients when they present for care. Meanwhile there is a basket of policies put in place by a broad group of stakeholders, and their effects on costs do not all pull in the same direction. Downward cost pressure comes from serious attempts to improve care pathways, prevent errors and duplication, and reduce the need for high-end acute services. Upward pressure comes from the continual drive to increase capacity in its many forms, such as diagnostic imaging equipment, beds, and physician supply.

In this policy environment, as in the country of the Red Queen, would-be curve benders have to run as fast as they can just to stay in the same place. Significant bending of the curve will require something more, including the political willingness to challenge those providers and groups in the health system that would benefit from bending the curve up rather than down. Whatever their public rhetoric, many of the most powerful actors are committed to objectives and strategies for keeping the escalation going, or even for bending the curve upwards rather than downwards. And those actors and their strategies are "co-evolving" in response not only to changing needs and medical technologies but also to public policies. There is no one who controls the rudder or who can persuade (much less coerce) everyone to row in the same direction. The different rowers are all trying to get to different places.

British Columbia's attempts to improve and rationalize the situation of the elderly, infirm, and chronically ill—the high-cost users—are commendable. They may well do some good, as may other reform efforts in other provinces. But to get anywhere in the country of the Red Queen, you have to run twice as fast as you can. Globally uncoordinated policies arising from competing agendas are unlikely to be compatible with bending the cost curve.

References

Berwick, D. M., T. W. Nolan, and J. Whittington. 2008. "The Triple Aim: Care, Health, and Cost." *Health Affairs* 27, no. 3: 759. http://content.healthaffairs.org/content/27/3/759.short.

British Columbia Ministry of Health. 2012a. *Innovation and Change Agenda: Detailed 2010–2013 Health System Strategy Map*. Victoria: Ministry of Health. https://www.thinkhealthbc.ca/downloads/the-plan.en.pdf.

———. 2012b. *2012/13–2014/15 Service Plan*. Victoria: Ministry of Health.

CIHI (Canadian Institute for Health Information). 2011a. National Health Expenditure Database. Ottawa: CIHI. http://www.cihi.ca/CIHI-ext-portal/internet/en/document/spending+and+health+workforce/spending/spending+by+geography/spend_nhex.

———. 2011b. *Health Care Cost Drivers: The Facts*. Ottawa: CIHI.

Cohen, M., J. Tate, and J. Baumbusch. 2009. *An Uncertain Future for Seniors: BC's Restructuring of Home and Community Health Care, 2001–2008*. Vancouver: Canadian Centre for Policy Alternatives.

Evans, R. G. 1997. "Going for the Gold: The Redistributive Agenda behind Market-Based Health Care Reform." *Journal of Health Politics Policy and Law* 22, no. 2: 427–65. http://jhppl.dukejournals.org/content/22/2/427.abstract.

Evans, R. G., K. M. McGrail, S. G. Morgan, L. M.. Barer, and C. Hertzman. 2001. "Apocalypse No: Population Aging and the Future of Health Care Systems." *Canadian Journal on Aging* 20 (Suppl. 1): 160–91. http://ideas.repec.org/p/mcm/sedapp/59.html.

Fisher, E. S., D. E. Wennberg, T. A. Stukel, D. J. Gottlieb, F. L. Lucas, and E. L. Pinder. 2003a. "The Implications of Regional Variations in Medicare Spending. Part 1: The Content, Quality, and Accessibility of Care." *Annals of Internal Medicine* 138, no. 4: 273–87. http://annals.org/article.aspx?volume=138&issue=4&page=273.

———. 2003b. "The Implications of Regional Variations in Medicare Spending. Part 2: Health Outcomes and Satisfaction with Care." *Annals of Internal Medicine* 138, no. 4: 288–98. http://annals.org/article.aspx?articleid=71607.

Fisher, E. S., and J. E. Wennberg. 2003. "Health Care Quality, Geographic Variations, and the Challenge of Supply-Sensitive Care." *Perspectives in Biology and Medicine* 46, no. 1: 69–79. http://www.ncbi.nlm.nih.gov/pubmed/12582271.

Forget, E. L., L. L. Roos, R. B. Deber, and R. Walld. 2008. "Variations in Lifetime Healthcare Costs across a Population." *Healthcare Policy/Politiques de santé* 4, no. 1: e148–67. http://www.pubmedcentral.nih.gov/articlerender.fcgi?artid=2645209&tool=pmcentrez&rendertype=abstract.

Fowler, F. J., P. M. Gallagher, D. L. Anthony, K. Larsen, and J. S. Skinner. 2008. "Relationship between Regional Per Capita Medicare Expenditures and Patient Perceptions of Quality of Care." *Journal of the American Medical Association* 299, no. 20: 2406–12. doi:10.1001/jama.299.20.2406. http://www.ncbi.nlm.nih.gov/pmc/articles/pmc2438036.

General Practice Services Committee. 2009. "Backgrounder." http://www.gpscbc.ca/system/files/GPSC_Backgrounder.pdf.

———. 2011. *General Practice Services Committee 2010–2011 Annual Report*. Vancouver: General Practice Services Committee of British Columbia.

Hanley, G. E., P. A. Janssen, and D. Greyson. 2010. "Regional Variation in the Cesarean Delivery and Assisted Vaginal Delivery Rates." *Obstetrics and Gynecology* 115, no. 6: 1201–8. doi:10.1097/AOG.0b013e3181dd918c. http://www.ncbi.nlm.nih.gov/pubmed/20502291.

Hanley, G. E., and S. Morgan. 2009. "Chronic Catastrophes: Exploring the Concentration and Sustained Nature of Ambulatory Prescription Drug Expenditures in the Population of British Columbia, Canada." *Social Science and Medicine* 68, no. 5: 919–24. doi:10.1016/j.socscimed.2008.12.008.

Hollander, M. J., and P. Pallan. 1995. "The British Columbia Continuing Care System: Service Delivery and Resource Planning." *Aging* (Milan, Italy) 7, no. 2: 94–109. http://www.ncbi.nlm.nih.gov/pubmed/7548269.

Hunter, J. 2009. "New Beds for Seniors Fall Far Short of Promise, Health Minister Acknowledges." *Globe and Mail*, April. http://www.theglobeandmail.com/news/british-columbia/new-beds-for-seniors-fall-far-short-of-promise-health-minister-acknowledges/article1195738/.

Kizer, K. W., J. G. Demakis, and J. R. Feussner. 2000. "Reinventing VA Health Care: Systematizing Quality Improvement and Quality Innovation." *Medical Care* 38, no. 6 (Suppl.): I7–16.

Laurance, J. 2012. "Drug Giants Fined $ 11bn for Criminal Wrongdoing." *The Independent*, 20 September. http://www.independent.co.uk/life-style/health-and-families/health-news/drug-giants-fined-11bn-for-criminal-wrongdoing-8157483.html.

Lynn, J., B. M. Straube, K. M. Bell, S. F. Jencks, and R. T. Kambic. 2007. "Using Population Segmentation to Provide Better Health Care for All: The 'Bridges to Health' Model." *Milbank Quarterly* 85, no. 2: 185–208. doi:10.1111/j.1468-0009.2007.00483.x. http://www.ncbi.nlm.nih.gov/pubmed/17517112.

Marchildon, G. P. 2004. *Three Choices for the Future of Medicare*. Ottawa: Caledon Institute of Social Policy. http://www.caledoninst.org/Publications/PDF/466ENG.pdf.

McGrail, K. M., R. G. Evans, M. L. Barer, K. J. Kerluke, and R. McKendry. 2011. "Diagnosing Senescence: Contributions to Physician Expenditure Increases in British Columbia, 1996–97 to 2005–06." *Healthcare Policy/Politiques santé* (Montrouge, France) 7, no. 1: 41–54.

McGrail, K. M., M. B. Lilly, M. J. McGregor, A.-M. Broemeling, K. Salomons, S. Peterson, R. McKendry, and M. L. Barer. 2010. *Who Uses Assisted Living in British Columbia? An Initial Exploration.* Vancouver: University of British Columbia Centre for Health Services and Policy Research.

McGrail, K. M., P. Schaub, and C. Black. 2004. *The British Columbia Health Atlas.* 2nd ed. Vancouver: University of British Columbia Centre for Health Services and Policy Research. http://www.chspr.ubc.ca/pubs/atlas/be-health-atlas-second-edition.

McIntosh, T. 2004. "Intergovernmental Relations, Social Policy and Federal Transfers after Romanow." *Canadian Public Administration/Administration publique du Canada* 47, no. 1: 27–51. http://doi.wiley.com/10.1111/j.1754–7121.2004.tb01969.x.

Morgan, S. G., and C. Cunningham. 2011. "Population Aging and the Determinants of Healthcare Expenditures: The Case of Hospital, Medical and Pharmaceutical Care in British Columbia, 1996 to 2006." *Healthcare Policy/Politiques de santé* 7, no. 1: 68–79. http://dx.doi.org/10.12927/hcpol.2011.22525.

Morgan, S. G., C. M. Cunningham, and G. E. Hanley. 2010. "Individual and Contextual Determinants of Regional Variation in Prescription Drug Use: An Analysis of Administrative Data from British Columbia." *PLoS ONE* 5, no. 12: 6. http://www.ncbi.nlm.nih.gov/pmc/articlerender.fcgi?artid=3012101&tool=pmcentrez&rendertype=abstract.

Priest, A., M. Rachlis, and M. Cohen. 2007. *Why Wait? Public Solutions to Cure Surgical Waitlists.* Vancouver: Canadian Centre for Policy Alternatives.

Reid, R., R. G. Evans, M. L. Barer, S. B. Sheps, K. Kerluke, K. M. McGrail, C. Hertzman, et al. 2003. "Conspicuous Consumption: Characterizing High Users of Physician Services in One Canadian Province." *Journal of Health Services Research and Policy* 8, no. 4: 215–24. doi:10.1258/135581903322403281.

Riley, G. F., and J. D. Lubitz. 1993. "Trends in Medicare Payments in the Last Year of Life." *Health Services Research* 45, no. 15: 565–76. doi:10.1111/j.1475-6773.2010.01082.x.

Roos, N. P., G. Flowerdew, A. Wajda, and R. B. Tate. 1986. "Variations in Physicians' Hospitalization Practices: A Population-based Study in Manitoba, Canada." *American Journal of Public Health* 76, no. 1: 45–51. http://www.ncbi.nlm.nih.gov/pmc/articlerender.fcgi?artid=1646401&tool=pmcentrez&rendertype=abstract.

Roos, N. P., and L. L. Roos. 1981. "High and Low Surgical Rates: Risk Factors for Area Residents." *American Journal of Public Health* 71, no. 6: 591–600. http://dx.doi.org/10.2105/AJPH.71.6.591 http://www.ncbi.nlm.nih.gov/pmc/articlerender.fcgi?artid=1619829&tool=pmcentrez&rendertype=abstract.

Scitovsky, A. 2005. "The High Cost of Dying: What Do the Data Show?" *Milbank Quarterly* 83, no 4: 825–41. doi:10.1111/j.1468-0009.2005.00402.x.

Tu, J. V., W. A. Ghali, L. Pilote, and S. Brien. 2006. *Canadian Cardiovascular Atlas: A Collection of Original Research Papers.* Toronto: Pulsus Group and Institute for Clinical Evaluative Sciences. http://books.google.com/books?id=IDVNSAAACAAJ&pgis=1.

Wennberg, J. E. 2010. *Tracking Medicine: A Researcher's Quest to Understand Health Care.* Oxford: Oxford University Press. http://books.google.ca/books?id=IDVNSAAACAAJ&pgis=1&redir_esc=y.

Wildavsky, A. 1977. "Doing Better and Feeling Worse : The Political Pathology of Health Policy." *Daedalus* 106, no. 1: 105–23.

Appendix: Population segment definitions

This information is taken verbatim from Excel files provided by the British Columbia Ministry of Health. It defines the 14 population segments in the aggregated dataset used in our analyses. The Health System Matrix divides the BC population each year into 14 population segments, each with different health states ranging from "healthy" to "end of life," based on their highest need for health care in the year. People are assigned to population segments based on data held by the Ministry, including chronic conditions registries, diagnoses from physician MSP fee-for-service billings and hospitalizations, PharmaCare programs, and use of home and community care services. After each person is assigned to one or more population segments, based on the definitions of each segment, they are uniquely assigned to the one population segment that represents their highest need for health care in the year. See the Ministry's "Unique Assignment" worksheet for further information.

Population Segment	High Level Definition	UNIQUE ASSIGNMENT: People with multiple health conditions are assigned to one population segment based on their most significant health conditions. See "Unique Assignment to PS" worksheet to see hierarchy for assignment.
PS00 Non User	BC residents of any age who used no publicly funded health care services in the year and did not have any health conditions which would assign a person to a higher acuity population segment.	After assigning people to population segments PS14 End of Life to PS04 Low Complex Chronic Conditions, the remaining 54% of the BC population were non-users, healthy, or people who had other major health conditions. People who used no publicly funded services in the year were assigned to the Non-Users population segment.
PS01 Healthy	BC residents of any age who were low users of publicly funded services, and did not have any health conditions which would assign a person to a higher acuity population segment.	After assigning people to population segments PS14 End of Life to PS04 Low Complex Chronic Conditions, the remaining 54% of the BC population were non-users, healthy, or people who had other major health conditions. Of this group, the Healthy population comprises all BC residents who used up to $1,500 of physician services and up to $1,000 of prescription drugs (PharmaNet expenditures which includes both government paid and out-of-pocket / extended benefits prescription drugs); did not use any other health care services; and were alive at the end of the year.
PS02 Adult Major Age 18+	BC residents age 18 years and older with major health conditions other than those which assign a person to a higher acuity population segments.	After assigning people to population segments PS14 End of Life to PS04 Low Complex Chronic Conditions, the remaining 54% of the BC population were non-users, healthy, or people who had other major health conditions. Of this group, the Adult Major Health Conditions population comprises all adults age 18 years or older who used more than $1,500 of physician services; or used more than $1,000 of prescription drugs (PharmaNet expenditures which includes both government paid and out-of-pocket / extended benefits prescription drugs); or used any other health care services; or died during the year.

Population Segment	Short Definition	Detailed Definition
PS03 Child and Youth Major	BC residents under the age of 18 with major health conditions other than those which assign a person to a higher acuity population segments.	After assigning people to population segments PS14 End of Life to PS04 Low Complex Chronic Conditions, the remaining 54% of the BC population were non-users, healthy, or people who had other major health conditions. Of this group, the Child and Youth Major Health Conditions population comprises all children and youth under age 18 years who used more than $1,500 of physician services; or used more than $1,000 of prescription drugs (PharmaNet expenditures which includes both government paid and out-of-pocket / extended benefits prescription drugs); or used any other health care services; or died during the year. The population also includes newborns who did not fit the Maternity population segment definition for "healthy newborns." The newborns in the Child And Youth Major Health Conditions population segment are defined as a newborn hospitalization with any hospital case mix group other than singleton vaginal delivery (CMG576) or normal newborns in multiple or Caesarean delivery (CMG 577); or who had an atypical length of stay in hospital; or used any of the 16 flagged interventions; or had 1+ special care unit days.
PS04 Low Complex Chronic Conditions	People with osteoporosis, diabetes, hypertension, osteoarthritis, depression or asthma, and do not have high or medium co-morbidities.	People with osteoporosis, diabetes, hypertension, osteoarthritis, depression or asthma, and do not have high or medium co-morbidities. This definition is based on the Ministry's Chronic Condition Management Registries which identify people who have had specific chronic conditions diagnoses recorded in physician MSP fee for service billings, or hospitalizations, or have used specific prescription drugs, in the current or any previous years. People with chronic conditions have been divided into high, medium or low complexity chronic condition groups. People in the low complex chronic conditions population segment are in one or more CCM registries for osteoporosis, diabetes, hypertension, osteoarthritis, depression or asthma, and do not have any of the chronic conditions or specific co-morbidities which would identify them in the high or medium complex chronic condition population segments.

(Continued)

Population Segment	High Level Definition	
		UNIQUE ASSIGNMENT: People with multiple health conditions are assigned to one population segment based on their most significant health conditions. See "Unique Assignment to PS" worksheet to see hierarchy for assignment.
		People with pre-dialysis chronic kidney disease, chronic obstructive pulmonary disease, angina, rheumatoid arthritis, or have had a acute myocardial infarction (heart attack), coronary artery bypass graft, or percutaneous cardiac intervention, or other medium complex combination of comorbidities.
PS05 Medium Complex Chronic Conditions	People with pre-dialysis chronic kidney disease, chronic obstructive pulmonary disease, angina, rheumatoid arthritis, or have had a acute myocardial infarction (heart attack), coronary artery bypass graft, or percutaneous cardiac intervention, or other medium complex combination of comorbidities.	This definition is based on the Ministry's Chronic Condition Management Registries which identify people who have had specific chronic conditions diagnoses recorded in physician MSP fee for service billings, or hospitalizations, or have used specific prescription drugs, in the current or any previous years. People with chronic conditions have been divided into high, medium or low complexity chronic condition groups.

People in the medium complex chronic conditions population segment are in one or more CCM registries for chronic kidney disease (excluding those in the dialysis registry), chronic obstructive pulmonary disease, angina, rheumatoid arthritis, acute myocardial infarction (heart attack), or cardiac intervention (coronary artery bypass graft or percutaneous cardiac intervention), or have medium complex co-morbidities: osteoporosis and osteo-arthritis); osteoporosis and hypertension; diabetes and depression; or osteoarthritis and hypertension; and do not have any of the chronic conditions or specific co-morbidities which would identify them in the high complex chronic condition population segment. |
| PS06 Mental Health & Substance Use | People with severe mental health or substance use conditions. | People with mental health or substance use issues were identified by diagnoses; because there is no available measure of severity, it was assumed that only people with severe mental health or substance use issues would require hospitalization. Also, these conditions are considered to be chronic (i.e., long duration). Therefore the definition of this population segment was based on people hospitalized for mental health and substance use issues in the current year or anytime in the previous four years. |

PS07 Maternity & Healthy Newborns	Women who were pregnant or delivered in the current year, and their healthy newborns.	Women who received maternity or obstetric services from a physician (MSP FFS billing) or a hospital in the year. Because services to newborns might be recorded under the mother's personal health number for the first few weeks, healthy newborns are also included in this population segment. Healthy newborns are defined as normal newborns in singleton vaginal deliveries (CMG576), normal newborns in multiple or Caesarean deliveries (CMG 577), who had a typical length of stay in hospital, did not use any of the 16 flagged interventions, and had no special care unit days.
PS08 Frail In The Community	People who are living in the community and require assistance with activities of daily living.	People who are living in publicly funded Assisted Living units or living in their own homes receiving publicly funded home support. Eligibility for publicly funded Assisted Living and Home Support is based on health authority assessments of the person's physical and cognitive state.
PS09 Severe Disability	People with severe disabilities who are receiving Home and Community Care publicly funded services.	This population is made up of two groups.1) People who live in their own homes with home support provided through the HCC Community Services for Independent Living (CSIL) program. This is primarily people with severe physical or mental challenges who are capable of living independently. 2) People in the HCC Acquired Brain Injury program. Because this definition is based on a narrow range of HCC clients, it likely understates the true size of the severe disability population. Those who are not included will be assigned to other population segments based on the available health care utilization data.
PS10 High Complex Chronic Conditions	People who have dementia, cystic fibrosis, congestive heart failure, are on dialysis for chronic kidney disease, have had a stroke or organ transplant, or a complex combination of chronic conditions.	This definition is based on the Ministry's Chronic Condition Management Registries which identify people who have had specific chronic conditions diagnoses recorded in physician MSP fee for service billings, or hospitalizations, or have used specific prescription drugs, in the current or any previous years. People with chronic conditions have been divided into high, medium or low complexity chronic condition groups. People in the high complex chronic conditions population segment are in one or more CCM registries for dementia, cystic fibrosis, congestive heart failure, dialysis, stroke or organ transplant, or have complex co-morbidities: angina and chronic obstructive pulmonary disease (COPD); heart attack and pre-dialysis chronic kidney disease; rheumatoid arthritis and osteoporosis; diabetes; hypertension, and osteo-arthritis)

(Continued)

Population Segment	High Level Definition	UNIQUE ASSIGNMENT: People with multiple health conditions are assigned to one population segment based on their most significant health conditions. See "Unique Assignment to PS" worksheet to see hierarchy for assignment.
PS11 Cancer	People who were diagnosed with cancer in the year or previous year.	People who had a diagnosis of a malignant, non skin cancer on a physician fee for service billing or hospitalization. Care provided by the BC Cancer Agency (BCCA) is not reported to the Ministry databases; therefore the definition includes patients with a cancer diagnosis in the previous year, before beginning care with the BCCA.
PS12 Frail In Care (In Residential Care)	People with complex care needs who are in long term residential care.	People with complex care needs who are permanent residents in publicly funded residential care. These facilities include extended care wings of acute care facilities, and stand alone facilities. Facilities may be owned by the health authority or contracted by the Health Authority.
PS13 End Of Life	People who received health care services specifically for palliative care	People who received palliative care services from physicians (MSP FFS billing for palliative care), PharmaCare (registered in PharmaCare Plan P), Home and Community Services (HCC clients with designated palliative care), or Hospitals (hospitalized specifically for palliative care).
PS ALL POPULATION	All Population Segments	

twelve

Alberta: Health Spending in the Land of Plenty

STEPHEN DUCKETT

Introduction

With a population of just under 3.8 million people, Alberta is Canada's fourth-largest province. It has a young population: at 36, its median age is considerably younger than in the other provinces (the Canadian median age is 39.9). Alberta also has a smaller proportion of its population over 65: 10.8%, compared to the Canadian average of 14.4%.

Alberta is the wealthiest of the provinces, with a median family income of $83,560 in 2009 (Canada: $68,410). Provincial per capita GDP in 2009–10, the latest year for which data are available, is also the highest of the provinces ($67,756). However, Alberta's economic base is narrow and exposed to fluctuations in oil and gas prices; its per capita GDP has declined 10% since 2007–08 (see Figure 12.1), following a significant downturn in the oil and gas industry. In contrast, overall Canadian GDP declined only about 1.5% over this period. Alberta's economic volatility exposes the province's health sector to the vicissitudes of oil and gas prices to the detriment of long-term budget planning

Provincial administrations in Alberta are conservative in ideological orientation and long lasting, with only three changes of the party in government since Alberta became a province in 1905 (Alberta Liberal Party to United Farmers of Alberta in 1921, to Social Credit in 1935, to Progressive Conservative in 1971) and most elections leading to a substantial majority for the governing party. Even the shift from Social Credit to Progressive Conservative in 1971 could be argued to be a continuation of the ideological mix of individualism, populism, and provincial autonomy so deeply embedded in Alberta's political culture (Wesley 2011), and both Social Credit and the Progressive Conservatives exhibited moral conservatism (Denis 1995). This stability of government was associated with stability of leadership in the health sector: there were only two health ministers for the province over the period 1923 to 1957, and two deputy ministers between 1912 and 1952 (Lampard 2009).

One-party dominance has led to the current Progressive Conservative Party's covering a broad ideological spectrum, from extreme economic free-marketer to "Red Tory." However, the overall government orientation

Figure 12.1 Gross domestic product per capita, Canada and Alberta (current dollars)

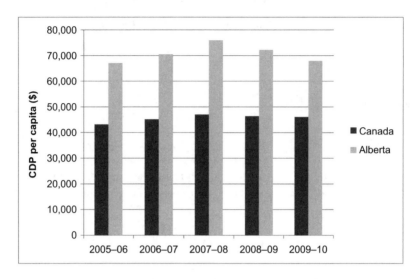

emphasizes economic liberalism. According to the Fraser Institute, Alberta is one of the "most free" economies in North America (on one measure it tops the list) based on indicators of (low) tax, (low) labour regulation, and (small) size of government (Ashby, Bueno, and McMahon 2012).

Wealth and political stability have not translated into either better health status or better health care for Albertans. Measured on health system performance, wealthy Alberta is the poor cousin, and the most expensive in terms of per capita provincial government health spending (after adjusting for the province's younger-than-average population). This chapter illustrates this dismal conclusion through an analysis of health spending trends, using a variety of metrics on input costs and data on health outcomes. Alberta has pursued several mostly unsuccessful strategies to "bend the cost curve," and the chapter concludes with speculation about potential reasons for the province's poor health system performance.

Health spending trends

Figure 12.2 shows health expenditure trends from 1996 to 2008 for Alberta and the average of other Canadian provinces. Comparison is made with other provinces rather than the entire rest of Canada because territorial health expenditure is quite different, given demographic factors associated with low population density.

Figure 12.2 Provincial government health expenditures, Alberta and other provinces, 1996–2008 (2002 dollars)

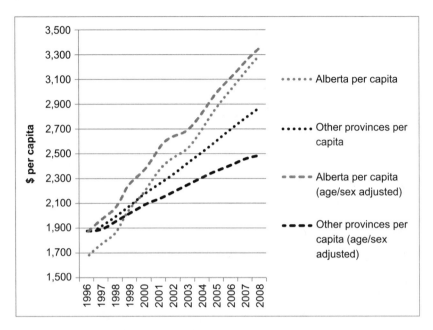

In 1996 Alberta's provincial government per capita health expenditure was about 12% below that of the other provinces. By 2008, however, Alberta was spending about 15% more per person. In just over a decade, per capita expenditure doubled in Alberta, compared to an increase of about 50% in other provinces. The province's wealth provided the capacity to spend more, and Alberta's political environment created the conditions that led to conversion of potential spending on health into reality.

Relative to other provinces, Alberta has a younger population that is not aging as rapidly. Adjusting for age and gender of its population, Alberta would be expected to have lower levels of expenditure and lower expenditure growth than other provinces. But age/gender standardization causes Alberta's expenditure growth to diverge further from the other provinces. Since the mid 1990s, Alberta's provincial government health expenditure growth rate has been above the growth rate in other provinces (see Figure 12.3). Since 2000, average spending growth in Alberta has been around 10%, compared to 7% in other provinces.

Alberta diverges from pan-Canadian patterns in three significant areas of spending: hospitals, other institutions, and—related to the previous two—capital.

Figure 12.3 Change in provincial government health expenditure (two-year moving average), 1994–1996 to 2010–2012 (current dollars)

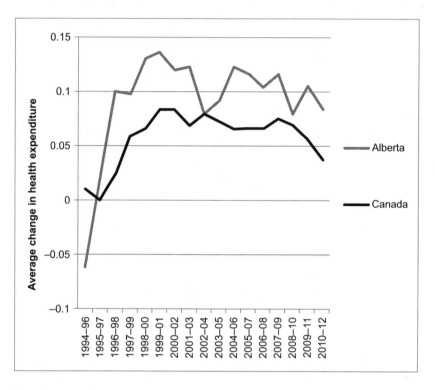

Spending on hospitals and other institutions

All provinces have attempted to bend the health cost curve over the past few decades by constraining hospital expenditure via bed rationalization and closing small hospitals. Here policies have been able to be implemented in parallel with clinical practice changes and changes in community transport patterns. New anesthetic agents and the use of laparoscopic techniques have shifted many procedures from lengthy in-hospital stays to same-day admissions and discharges, and they trim days off the recovery period for procedures that still require an overnight stay. New pharmaceuticals are also speeding up hospital treatment of medical admissions. In turn, these changes reduce the number of beds required to serve a population.

The viability of smaller rural hospitals can be challenged by such changes, particularly as people are able to travel farther for shopping and other activities. The Prairie provinces in particular have embarked on strategies to reduce beds that serve local rural populations, in addition to reductions in the number of rural hospitals.

Figure 12.4 Share of provincial government health expenditure, hospitals and other institutions, Alberta and other provinces, 1996–2011

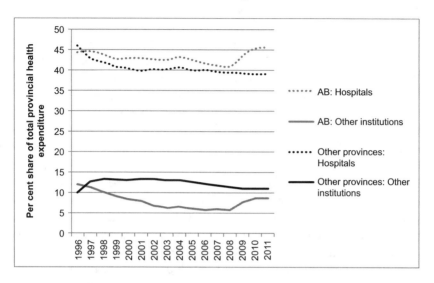

Figure 12.4 shows the impact of strategies designed to constrain hospital expenditure on the share of total provincial health expenditure accounted for by hospital spending. Hospitals are accounting for a declining share of total provincial health spending across Canada, but Alberta shows a different pattern. Although the starting point for the share of health spending accounted for by hospitals in 1996 was similar between Alberta and the other provinces (45% versus 46%), the other provinces saw a sharp decline in the 1990s followed by a slower decline from 2000 onward. The average spending share in other provinces is now 39%. Alberta showed a slower but nevertheless steady decline up to 2008, followed by a sharp increase in 2008 and 2009, so spending share is now back to 1996 levels.

The 2008–09 increase occurred in the context of the oil and gas industry collapse in Alberta. Health-sector employment in Alberta is highly exposed to movements in this industry (Bloom, Duckett, and Robertson 2012; Duckett, Bloom, and Robertson 2012). This expenditure share increase may have resulted from being able to fill long-vacant staff positions in health services as household income from oil and gas industry employment evaporated, combined with weak expenditure controls in the first year of the newly created Alberta Health Services (AHS).

Figure 12.4 also shows the quite different (implicit) strategy followed in Alberta with respect to investment in "other institutions" such as residential aged care. As in the rest of Canada, Alberta's population is aging, albeit at a slower rate—from 1996 to 2011 the median age in Canada increased by 13%, from 35.3 to 39.9, while the increase in Alberta was 8%, from 33.4 to 36.0. This would argue for a policy to increase "other institutional" spending and an increased proportion of provincial expenditure allocated to this function. In contrast, Alberta disinvested significantly in this area, with its spending share halving from 12% in 1996 to 5.7% in 2008 before increasing again to 8.6% in 2011. In other provinces, spending share on other institutions increased from 1996 (10.3%) to a peak of 13.2% in 2002 before declining to around 11.2% from 2008 onward.

Capital spending

Alberta has a higher level of capital spending than other provinces, both as a share of total provincial spending and per capita (see Figure 12.5). Its capital spending trends are similar to other elements of health expenditure, with Alberta having a lower level of spending in the mid 1990s than other provinces but sharply diverging thereafter. Capital spending was reined in at the time of the oil and gas downturn (2008–09). Since 2000, Alberta has spent an average of 7% of provincial government health expenditure on capital, 2 percentage points higher than the other provinces' average.

Figure 12.5 Capital spending as share of provincial health spending and per capita, Alberta and other provinces, 1995–2011

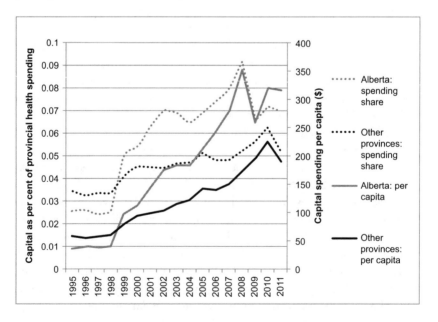

By 2008 the gap in funding had grown so much that Alberta's per capita capital spending was almost twice that of other provinces.

Capital spending both drives and is driven by other spending. Capital expansion drives additional operating spending when the buildings are complete. A larger capital stock (more hospitals, or more beds) also requires a greater level of expenditure to keep hospital and long-term care facilities both modern and safe. Until 2009 the funding ministries did not estimate or budget for additional operating expenses when new capital was approved; instead they responded to such requests as part of commissioning decisions. This funding approach provided an incentive for regional health authorities to seek additional capital as a means of growing their funding allocations.

A higher share of spending on hospital care and a higher capital outlay are associated with higher hospital utilization. In 2009–10, for example, Alberta's age/gender-adjusted hospital utilization rate was 8,442 beds per 100,000 population, 10% above the national average.

Health share of provincial spending

As in other provinces, Alberta's health expenditure is consuming an increasing proportion of total provincial government budgets (see Figure 12.6). Alberta's high relative growth rates (and lower tax policies) have led to a health

Figure 12.6 Health spending as share of total provincial government spending, 1996–2010

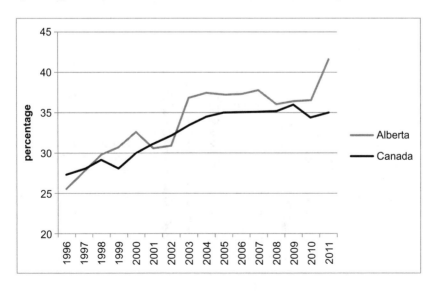

expenditure share that is slightly higher in Alberta than the all-Canada average. In 2011, provincial government health spending in Alberta accounted for 5.9% of provincial gross domestic product (GDP), up from 4.1% in 1995—a 42% increase. But Alberta's health GDP share is still well below the national average of 7.5% for provinces and territories because of Alberta's higher GDP per capita.

Budget control

The health system in Alberta has not been subject to rigorous budget control, as evidence from estimates and outcomes shows in Figure 12.7. The budget estimate is the allocation to health made at the start of the fiscal year; it is revised during the year as additional spending is approved or adjusted. The spending outcome is announced in the subsequent year's budget papers (technically an "expected outcome," as budget documenta-tion occurs before audit).

Comparison of spending outcomes to either initial or revised bud-gets reveals that health-sector budget adherence is not good. Over the full period in Figure 12.7, actual spending was about 1.5% above the initial budget allocation, reducing to 1.3% above the revised allocation. However, for the four years before the creation of AHS, budget adherence was worse—averaging 4% above initial allocation and 3% above revised allocation—compared to the post-2008 period, when average spending outcomes were marginally below allocations on both measures.

Figure 12.7 Alberta provincial health budget estimates and outcomes, 2004–2011

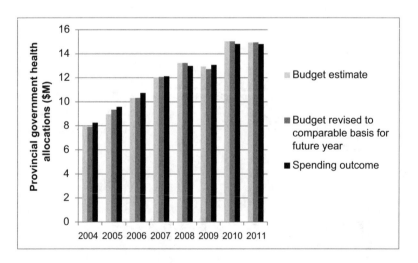

Over the entire period, year-on-year growth in budget allocations (initial compared to revised base of prior year) was 7.6%. The high growth in spending seen in Alberta was thus in part a predicted outcome and in part regular overspending against allocated budgets by the health ministry and health authorities.

Inputs and other drivers

One reason that Alberta is more expensive than other provinces is that the province's hospitals are less efficient than the average Canadian hospital (see Figure 12.8). In 2009, for example, the average cost per patient treated in Alberta's hospitals, taking into account case mix, was 12% greater than the Canadian average. On average, over the three-year period 2007–09 it cost 15% more to treat a patient in Alberta compared to the cost of similar treatment in the average Canadian hospital.

The Canadian Institute for Health Information (CIHI) publishes four hospital productivity measures: total hours worked per case mix–adjusted weighted patient treated for clinical laboratory services, diagnostic imaging, pharmacy, and nursing (see Figure 12.9). For the three smaller services, the pattern of reported productivity is mixed, possibly because of reporting artifacts caused by different patterns of outsourcing. Of the nine data points, Alberta shows poorer productivity on four and better on five. The total of hours worked in the three services averaged across the three years is

Figure 12.8 Cost per weighted case, Alberta and Canada, 2007–2009

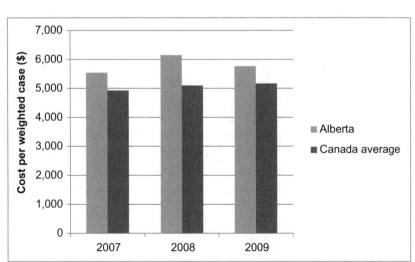

Figure 12.9 Comparative hospital productivity measures, Alberta and Canada, 2007–2009

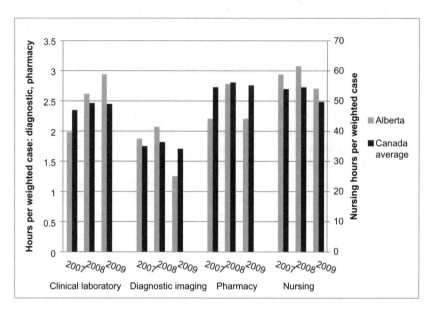

approximately the same (6.7 hours in Alberta, compared to the Canadian average of 7 hours per weighted patient treated).

Nursing productivity in Alberta is well behind other provinces; an average of 58 hours of nursing time is provided for each patient, compared to 53 hours for the same patient in the average Canadian hospital. The influence of poorer nursing productivity is compounded by salary differentials (see Figure 12.10). At $32.99 per hour, a newly graduated nurse in Alberta is paid more than in any other province except Saskatchewan, and 26% above the (unweighted) average for the other provinces. A similar picture emerges at the top of the scale, where a nurse in Alberta is paid 31% more than the average in other provinces.

Physician costs in Alberta are generally higher than in the rest of Canada (see Figure 12.11). Alberta has the highest average cost for family medicine consultations and visits—32% higher than the next-most expensive province and a similar differential to the Canadian average. The same pattern is true of internal medicine consultation and visits (14% higher than New Brunswick, 51% above the Canadian average) and for the cost of surgical procedures (22% above Québec, 30% above the Canadian average). Alberta is not the most expensive province in terms of the cost of

Figure 12.10 Hourly pay rates of general-duty registered nurses, by province, 2012

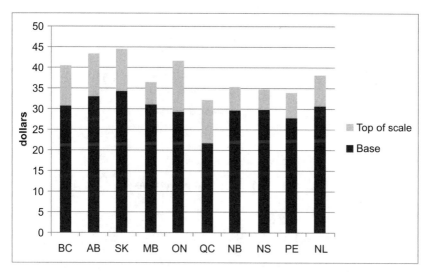

Source: Canadian Federation of Nurses Unions, http://www.nursesunions.ca/sites/default/files/2011.07.contract_comparison.e.pdf (accessed 18 June 2012).

surgical consultations—British Columbia is about 5% more expensive—but surgical consultations in Alberta are, on average, still 40% more expensive than the Canadian average.

Comparing the total average incomes of physicians is complex, as there are different patterns of take-up of alternative payment plans across Canada, and because of the need to take into account part-time working arrangements. The more tightly defined metric of average fee-for-service income (for physicians who bill more than $60,000 per annum) shows a similar pattern to that shown for cost per visit, with Alberta being more generous and more expensive than every other province for the three groups examined.

Outcomes

Alberta's higher spending might be seen as worthwhile if it had commensurately better outcomes, but it does not. Although wider social and economic determinants have a significant impact on longevity, health systems can also be judged on this metric. In 2000–02, life expectancy at birth in Alberta was on par with the Canadian average at 79.6 years, but

Figure 12.11 Cost per visit and average annual gross fee-for-service income (physicians earning >$60,000 per annum), by specialty and province, 2009–10

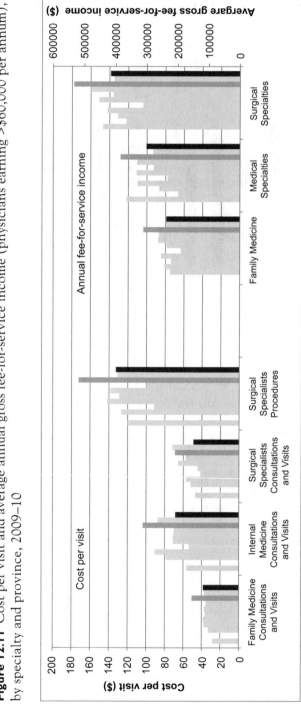

Note: Provinces are ordered east to west. Alberta: medium grey; Canada average: dark grey.

by 2007–09 it had slipped marginally behind (80.7 years, compared to 81.1 years). Alberta's life expectancy at age 65 was marginally better in 2000–02 than the Canadian average (19.3 compared to 18.9) but that advantage has now been lost (both stood at 20.2 years in 2007–09). Significantly more potentially avoidable years of life were lost in Alberta per 100,000 population in 2007 (3,870) than the Canadian average (3,428).

The Canadian Institute for Health Information publishes several broad measures of health system performance, covering domains such as accessibility, appropriateness, and patient safety over recent time periods. A total of 58 data points are available. The Alberta experience is not statistically significantly different from the average Canadian experience on any data point; for 30 of the observations, the Alberta experience is better than the Canadian average, and for 28 it is worse. Survival rates for leading cancers are worse in Alberta than in other provinces for which data are available (Coleman et al. 2011), and Alberta does not have any advantage on a range of other outcome indicators (Duckett, Kramer, and Sarnecki 2012).

Strategies for bending the curve

Despite the very different outcomes in terms of spending levels, Alberta's spending constraint strategies have been similar to those of other provinces, at least at the rhetorical level: structural change, privatization, and an emphasis on primary care. The three strategies start from different assumptions:

- Structural change is based on the assumption that changes in governance, for example, by integrating hospitals and primary-care services or reducing the number of governance points, will lead to better resource allocation decisions.
- Privatization strategies operate on the implicit but often unproved assumption that private provision is inherently more efficient than public provision. It also provides an opportunity for private profit.
- Structural change is often hoped to lead to a greater emphasis on primary care, but this strategy of creating alternatives to hospital care can also be pursued provincially.

Of the three strategies, structural change and privatization have been the focus of most change in Alberta.

Structural change

Like most other provinces (the notable exception being Ontario), Alberta has seen a dramatic consolidation of administrative structures over the past two decades. Prior to 1988 there were two health ministries, one for hospitals and medical care and one for community health, and almost 200 separate public administrative entities: 128 hospital boards, 40 long-term care boards, 25 public health boards, and two province-wide entities (for cancer and mental health). A minor rationalization occurred in 1988 with consolidation of the two ministries and the creation of an alcohol and drug commission. More significant rationalization occurred in 1994 with consolidation of the separate entities into 17 regional health authorities, themselves further consolidated in 2003 to nine authorities.

A much deeper form of centralization occurred in 2008, with the introduction of Alberta Health Services as the single provincial delivery entity, taking over from the nine regions and the three central bodies (for cancer, mental health, and drugs and alcohol). AHS also assumed responsibility from several municipalities for direct delivery of emergency medical services. Some municipalities and private contractors continued in their previous roles, but now funded through AHS.

The mid-1990s creation of regional health authorities was a strategy pursued in several provinces (Hurley, Lomas, and Bhatia 1994) and, indeed, internationally (Philippon and Braithwaite 2008). This strategy offered the promise of improved allocative efficiency, as regions could now make local tradeoffs between hospital care and preventive strategies that might lead to longer-term gains. However, in Alberta as in the rest of the country, the strategy was more a potential than a delivered reality (Casebeer 2004; Hinings et al. 2003; Tomblin 2007).

The stimulus for the initial 1994 rationalization in Alberta was to contribute to deficit reduction via health system reform (Church and Smith 2008), and it could be interpreted as marking a shift from a dominant medical professionalism paradigm in health-sector administration to one of administrative efficiency (Reay and Hinings 2005). However, the change has also been described as being more about governance than service delivery reform (Philippon and Wasylyshyn 1996), a characterization also true of other provincial regionalization efforts (Lewis and Kouri 2004).

Health service regionalization in Canada was often accompanied by formula funding, offering the prospect of an economically or epidemiologically rational basis of resource allocation. Although a regional funding formula was introduced in Alberta that, prima facie, should have led to equitable distribution of resources (Smith and Church 2008), significant differences continue. For example, Duckett, Kramer, and Sarnecki (2012, 325) have shown that in 2008, "Edmonton residents were admitted to hospital at approximately 6% greater rate than residents of Calgary (on an age-gender standardized basis). The difference in bed utilization was even greater: Edmontonians consumed 25% more bed-days than Calgarians."

The creation of AHS in 2008 was a significant change to typical provincial health administrative structures. In some senses it may be seen as a continuation of the trend to consolidate administration: formally, AHS was created as a regional health authority under Alberta legislation. However, AHS's positioning as a single provincial provider is unique among the larger provinces. The reasons behind the creation of AHS are poorly documented, and speculation abounds as to the motivation for the change. Whatever the reasons for the new structure, it created the potential for significant savings in health spending.

Prior to the creation of AHS there was almost no intra-provincial benchmarking of system performance. The different regional health authorities used different definitions for key variables (e.g., measures of dependency), and inconsistent cost allocation and counting practices inhibited cost comparisons. The lack of benchmarking and intra-provincial information sharing led to significant differences in efficiency. Figure 12.12, for example, shows the payments for residential aged care in the 176 nursing homes in Alberta. It can be seen that there was a fourfold variation in the payment per resident-day. Creation of AHS highlighted the issue of intra-provincial equity in payments, with the AHS's response being to phase in a consistent payment approach over a five-year period.

Figure 12.12 Payments to nursing homes in Alberta per weighted resident-day, 2009

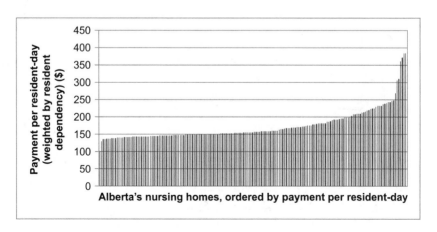

In AHS's second year (the 2009 budget year), significant spending reductions—around 10% on an operating basis—were required to bring spending into line with the provincial government allocation. The AHS Board approved a deficit budget for the organization for that year as part of a two-year strategy to achieve the government target, which included acute bed reductions in both Edmonton and Calgary.

Another strategy pursued by AHS was to reduce administrative costs. Consistent with the general pattern of higher expenditure in Alberta, administrative costs per head were lower in Alberta in the mid 1990s than in Canada as a whole, then diverged over the next decade so that by 2000 Alberta's costs were around 25% greater than the Canadian average (see Figure 12.13). The creation of AHS led to significant reductions in senior management across the province (Duckett 2011), but this also led to a one-off increase in administrative costs due to payment of severances. Albeit a single data point, the effects of the new, leaner structure were seen in the 2011 data: Alberta's cost was marginally below the Canadian average. It is unclear at this stage whether this advantage can be sustained.

Possibly the most significant change with the creation of AHS was a move realigning the government's strategy of delivery organization in two ways: (1) reducing the impact of intra-provincial rivalry, and (2) accepting government funding mandates rather than bypassing them with overspending and political action. There has always been significant

Figure 12.13 Health administrative expenses per capita, Alberta and Canada, 1995–2011

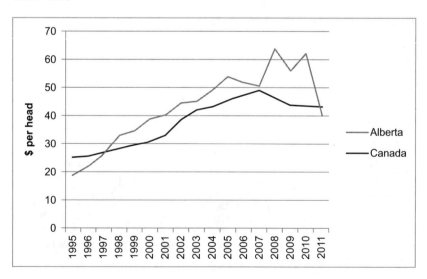

rivalry between Calgary and Edmonton, ranging from hockey to health care. Possibly because of the effects of Alberta's political culture, discussed below, government largesse in one city is often expected to be mirrored in the other.

Prior to the formation of AHS, there was no coordinated provincial planning or coordination; rather, the respective regional health authorities were engaged in a cost-increasing medical arms race. Creation of AHS mitigated the intra-provincial rivalry and provided an environment for sharing expertise, intra-provincial learning, and improved intra-provincial equity (Duckett 2011). Economies of scale in procurement were delivered through improved purchasing power, larger order sizes, and provincial standardization of stock-keeping units, yielding approximately $150–$200 million per annum in savings in procurement costs (Duckett 2010). Other benefits of the integrated structure allowed workforce planning linking frontline concerns and province-wide issues to be conducted for the first time (Bloom, Duckett, and Robertson 2012; Duckett, Bloom, and Robertson 2012), and the development of a provincial approach to addressing long waits in hospital emergency departments (Duckett and Nijssen-Jordan 2012).

What was not achieved at first was equal progress in spreading good clinical and governance practices across the province. This was perhaps a result of prioritizing the need to make significant spending reductions in AHS's second year (2009, see below), the delay in establishing a provincial framework for physician governance (new medical bylaws had to be created), and the delay in establishing organizational mechanisms for clinician engagement (eventually achieved with the Alberta Clinical Council and clinical networks).

The creation of AHS changed the dynamic of relationships among the new single provincial health service delivery organization, the health minister, and the ministry. Whereas in the past the minister and the ministry might have been required to adjudicate between regional entities competing for political access, influence, and resources, AHS was charged with internalizing priority choices among geographic areas and clinical services. Unification into a single delivery organization can eliminate conflict among minister, ministry, and health service only if the objective functions of all three are perfectly aligned. As mentioned above, Alberta has a tradition of populist politics, and the more populism is in the ascendancy (versus the economic rationalist strain in the Progressive Conservative Party), the more likely there is to be conflict between technocratically rational and politically rational decisions. A single delivery organization may, perversely, increase the potential for political decision-making by creating a single conduit for ministerial management.

The single provincial delivery organization also created an environment for confusion of roles. In an ideal world, the minister and ministry would "do strategy" and AHS would implement. But Alberta Health and Wellness (the ministry) had become essentially a policy-free zone as the politically powerful previous delivery entities pursued their own disparate agendas. So AHS developed its own strategy capacity and formulated its own policies, in part to ensure intra-provincial equity. To the extent that these policies needed ministerial approval, they were often delayed or not released publicly. Different ministers had different conceptions of their role, covering the full spectrum from arm's length to micromanagement, the latter leading to further confusion of roles and eventually resignation of almost half the AHS Board over ministerial interference relating to continued employment of the chief executive officer (Health Quality Council of Alberta 2012).

2009 was AHS's *annus horribilis*: the new organization was presented with a government budget that provided only enough funds to employ staff for about 10 to 11 months. AHS needed to implement about a 10% reduction in its spending rate in the absence of an established internal financial reporting system and no usable metrics (because of inconsistent definitions adopted for data collection by the previous regional health authorities), even while responding to the H1N1 virus. AHS's cost-containment decisions (e.g., tightening up on new recruitment) and proposed hospital bed closures attracted an avalanche of criticism, including high-profile campaigns by unions and other stakeholders designed to protect jobs and reverse the cuts. AHS planned to achieve the expenditure reductions over a two-year period, and it adopted a deficit budget for 2009. However, the borrowing necessary for this would appear on the provincial balance sheet, and increases in provincial borrowing were a subject of broader political contention (including within the provincial Progressive Conservative Party caucus and cabinet). Without such borrowing or some alternative means of financial support, AHS would not have been able to meet its payroll obligations in early 2010, which would have resulted in even worse publicity.

Opinion polling showed health to be a major political issue, a situation that continued up to the 2012 provincial election. An Environics poll conducted in 2007 showed health care as the second most important issue for the Alberta government to address. By 2011 health care was the dominant concern, mentioned by 36% of respondents, with the environment second at 14% (Environics Research Group 2011).

The most contentious strategies adopted by AHS—acute bed reductions in Edmonton and Calgary—were reversed following a revised budget for 2009 (approved in the lead-up to the 2010 government budget). The government also announced a new financial arrangement in the 2010 budget that was unique in providing for multi-year funding: a five-year term that guaranteed funding increases of 6% in each of the first three years and 4.5% in the remaining two years. The government also agreed to meet the planned 2009 deficit of AHS. These guaranteed funding increases represented a significant savings against previous spending patterns; they were based on estimates of the effect of inflation (2% per annum) and population growth and aging (2.5% per annum), with higher funding in the first three years to cushion the transition.

For its part, AHS agreed to fund technological change internally through improved efficiency and not to approach the provincial government for additional funding during the funding period, except in the case of significant unforeseen external and uncontrollable factors. However, AHS did not take responsibility for commissioning (and funding) all the capital works in the planning pipeline or subsequently announced by government. The 2013 budget overturned this agreement and provided for lower growth, requiring tighter spending control.

The new arrangement's effect was tested almost immediately as AHS negotiated a new collective agreement with nurses (through their union, the United Nurses of Alberta). The previous collective agreement had been negotiated on behalf of all the regions (and the province-wide entities) by a separate, jointly owned entity, the Health Boards Association of Alberta. Those negotiations were conducted without clear accountability (or even ownership) of the outcomes and resulted in a three-year cost of $620 million funded by government in addition to budget. In contrast, AHS represented an integrated and accountable management side in the negotiations, accepting that it would need to meet the full cost of the negotiated outcome from within the five-year funding envelope. Consequently AHS was able to take a tougher negotiating stance, with the result that the three-year cost of the new agreement was $120 million.

Internal structural change has been a recurring feature of AHS during its short existence, with almost annual changes in structure and CEO (four CEOS or acting CEOs between 2008 and 2013). The most significant change occurred in June 2013, when the AHS Board was dismissed, with the proximate cause being the board's refusing a ministerial request not to pay senior staff their earned bonuses. The board was replaced by an administrator. This muddied the distinction between government and AHS as an independent, arm's-length organization.

Privatization

Privatization has two distinct meanings: expansion of private funding of health care (more user payments or more private insurance) and expansion of private delivery. These are independent constructs, although an expansion of private funding would facilitate an expansion of private delivery. Alberta has flirted with expanding private funding, but this has not been a hallmark of its health system (Alberta, Premier's Advisory Council on Health 2001; Gregoire 2006).

Privatization of delivery is advocated by right-wing think tanks and business interests as a panacea that guarantees improved efficiency. It is a favoured cost-saving strategy in several provinces, including Alberta, where a private-delivery strategy was announced amid significant controversy in 2000 (Cairney 2000; Church and Smith 2006; Gray 2000). Although there are many examples of private delivery in Alberta, in terms of both freestanding delivery entities and outsourcing (e.g., cleaning, laboratory services), there is little evidence that these strategies have been cost-saving.

One of the earliest privatization implementations in Alberta was the complete privatization of cataract surgery in Calgary, with a parallel strategy, albeit at a smaller level of private delivery, being pursued in Edmonton (for a history of the development of private cataract provision in Calgary, see Armstrong 2000). The contracting process with Calgary providers was unique; it resembled the caucus race in *Alice's Adventures in Wonderland*, where everyone is a winner and everyone gets a prize. Dranove, Capps, and Dafny describe the process thus: "Facilities submit bids to AHS at regular intervals, and an evaluation committee takes all bids and averages or blends them to determine the price. ... this process does nothing to encourage either truthful bidding or low bidding. There is an implied risk that AHS might allocate more procedures to the lowest bidder(s), but in fact this has never occurred. The process might even encourage providers to inflate their bids to boost the average price" (2009, 22).

Dranove, Capps, and Dafny (2009) go on to recommend that the tendering process for cataracts in Calgary be put on a more regular basis. AHS did this in 2009–10, with the outcome that some previous providers were not offered contracts and the contract price dropped significantly. AHS committed to allocating the same budget to ophthalmology services, simultaneously expanding provision by 20% because of the reduced unit price. This suggests that AHS's previous contract processes were not designed to achieve the best outcome for the public. The providers who missed out on contracts conducted a public campaign to overturn the results of the 2009 public tender process. Following a high-profile intervention by the then minister for health, the losing tenderers were also awarded contracts at the new lower price, reintroducing caucus-race elements to the tender process.

Another high-profile engagement with the private sector was in orthopedics, when a contract with a private group to provide orthopedic services in Calgary was negotiated in 2004. The contract was negotiated after a long history of lobbying for public-sector contracts (Cairney 1998; Gibson and Clements 2012), with an initial contract for services costing $2.82 million in 2004–05 and rising to a peak of $8.3 million in 2008–09. The contract was time limited and the service was initially provided from leased premises. However, the owners of the service planned a move to a purpose-built facility and were eventually bankrupted. During the bankruptcy process there was significant public reporting, much of it suggesting that the private service was more efficient than the public. Internal AHS documentation released following freedom-of-information requests shows this not to have been the case: joint procedures were about 7% more expensive in the private facility compared to public provision, and foot and ankle procedures about 32% more expensive (Gibson and Clements 2012).

Cataracts and orthopedic surgery have been the most high-profile privatizations in Alberta, but they represent a very small proportion of total annual health spending—less than 0.4% (Ruseski 2009). Other privatization and outsourcing endeavours have been pursued, with one *cause célèbre* being payroll outsourcing. The former Calgary Regional Health Authority outsourced payroll processing, as well as some other aspects of the human resource management function, to Telus Sourcing Solutions for a very long contract period. In 2009, unions representing staff paid through this payroll system initiated legal action against Telus for poor performance (CBC News 2009). AHS subsequently negotiated to insource the Calgary payroll function.

Since the contracting out of surgery has been more prevalent in Calgary than Edmonton (e.g., $25 million in Calgary in 2008 versus $4.8 million in Edmonton), this has contributed to the popular but misleading perception that privatization in total is greater in Calgary (Church and Smith 2006). In fact the reverse is true, driven primarily by the former Capital [Edmonton] Health Region's outsourcing of laboratory services to private-sector provider Dynalife. Both the former Calgary and Capital Health Regions also outsourced other services such as linen services. Private provider K-Bro was recently awarded a new 10-year contract for linen supply in Edmonton that entailed "certain price concessions as compared to the existing services agreement" (CNW Newswire 2012). The details of the new contract are not in the public domain, but the fact that price concessions were announced for a new contract suggests that the former contract may have been overpriced.

The success of privatization and outsourcing as cost-containment strategies relies on good contract negotiations by the purchaser, in Alberta's case the former health regions and now AHS. What evidence that exists in the public domain shows that the former health regions did not negotiate contracts that were more efficient than public provision, and so privatization was not an effective cost-containment strategy. This raises the question as to why it was pursued; the answer lies possibly in the nature of provincial politics (see below).

Strategic repositioning to primary care

A third strategy pursued in Alberta is strategic repositioning. As shown above, Alberta has implicitly followed a hospital-led health-care development strategy, heavy on capital and leading to higher spending on hospital care. A 2010 strategy (Alberta and AHS 2010) provides, at least on paper, for a more balanced approach, identifying five goal areas: improve access and reduce wait times; provide more options for continuing care; strengthen primary health care; "be healthy, stay healthy"; and build one health system. It is unclear at this stage whether the ambitious goals set by the plan will be achieved; reports to date show mixed results. One very promising sign is that then-Premier Alison Redford made expansion of primary care a centrepiece of her health policy, committing to establishing 140 family-care clinics across the province in the three years from 2011.

Barriers to cost containment in Alberta

Alberta's track record on containing health-care costs is a sorry one. And Alberta's poor financial constraint has implications for all of Canada as, for example, its collective agreement outcomes become precedents for other provinces. It could be argued that Alberta's poor health system performance is determined by exogenous economic factors. This logic argues that Alberta is a higher-cost province, with higher median family incomes than the Canadian average, translating into higher factor prices and hence higher health costs. However, even adjusting for differential inflation results in Alberta being a higher-cost jurisdiction. There are probably two main factors that contribute to this overall poor performance: provincial wealth and politics.

Provincial wealth

Wealthier countries tend to spend more on health as a proportion of GDP (Anderson and Hussey 2001; Reinhardt et al. 2002). Several Canadian studies have examined interprovincial differences in health expenditure, adopting similar methods and yielding similar results to the international studies (Di Matteo 2009; Di Matteo and Di Matteo 1998; Landon et al. 2006). It is therefore not surprising that, as a relatively wealthy province, Alberta tends to spend more on health care on a per capita basis.

Health service stakeholders can be very persuasive when arguing for increased funding for their specialty, institution, or region. It is easy to manufacture crises and to enlist compliant media, inspired by the promise of new technology, in arguments for more funding. Until the creation of AHS there were no provincial structures to engage clinicians in orderly prioritization processes. As well, there was no clear budget constraint: the budget for health care increased dramatically year on year, with no real sense of opportunity costs either within or outside the health sector. In this environment, a key part of the management task became lobbying government for additional funding rather than managing expectations within an established budget. Whereas in other environments the health-care arms race between big-city rivals Edmonton and Calgary would be managed through application and affirmation of regional resource allocation formulae or other strategies, the political environment of Alberta was not conducive to that.

Any system reform involving redistribution or reprioritization creates winners and losers, and vociferous losers can increase the political cost of system reform. In the context of burgeoning oil and gas revenue, it would be very hard for politicians to withstand requests for service expansion when there was any money at all in the provincial coffers. The marginal political cost of rejecting spending requests was high and the monetary cost was often seen as easily affordable.

The *Canada Health Act* enshrines a privileged position for physician organizations: there is a legislated requirement for physician fees to be set by negotiation, with arbitration mandated if negotiation fails. The founding bargain of medicare had as its objective "to find a way of combining publicly supported universal coverage with the true essentials of professional freedom" (Taylor 1978). In reality, this meant that "organised medicine was able to improve the economic position of its members even while it preserved the contractual system of remuneration and private practice, protected the role of physicians at the centre of the healthcare system, and prevented major changes to primary healthcare" (Marchildon and Schrijvers 2011, 222).

In principle, this special place for physicians applies equally to Alberta as to any other province. A corollary of provincial wealth is the ability of the province, its media, its voters, and its politicians to see additional spending on health care as an easy solution to any perceived (or manufactured) "health crisis." So Alberta's wealth provides an important differentiating context, in allowing the province to respond more easily to rent-seeking by physicians than other provinces, resulting in "sweetheart deals" (Fierlbeck 2001) to avoid adverse publicity.

Although regionalization in Alberta involved a shift from a dominant medical-professionalism paradigm in health-sector administration to a business-efficiency one, this transition was able to be only partially accomplished: the "previously dominant logic of medical professionalism has been subdued rather than eliminated" (Reay and Hinings 2005). The medical profession, both through its organized arm, the Alberta Medical Association, and through ginger groups and individual mavericks, continues to challenge what it sees as undue constraint of budgets or as illegitimate priority setting.

Provincial politics

Two important characteristics of Alberta's provincial politics have implications for health-sector spending patterns: one-party dominance and rural gerrymandering. Prolonged periods of one-party dominance are associated with clientelism (Trantidis 2011), in which symbiotic exchange relationships develop that thwart meritocratic resource allocation processes (Hicken 2011). Calgary journalist Rick Bell recently described the situation in Alberta more colourfully: "A Tory loss would trigger Conservatives of convenience to head for the nearest lifeboat, since the PCs have about as much conviction as an empty bag of potato chips and are nothing without power. Not to break any hearts, but many Tory supporters do the supporting because they have an acute sense of smell—for the gravy at the trough" (Bell 2012).

Between 1992 and 2006, the Ralph Klein (Progressive Conservative) administration suffered several high-profile scandals about inappropriate distribution of government favours and investments (Bell and Jansen 2007; Vivone 2009). There is no evidence that the privatization and outsourcing that have occurred in health care in Alberta have been efficiency increasing. Church and Smith (2006) have documented some of the political links associated with privatization of services in Calgary. In terms of more recent examples, the board of Dynalife, the laboratory contractor in Edmonton, has several Progressive Conservative luminaries among its membership.

Another consequence of one-party dominance and lack of political competition could also be stifling of innovation; without a strong need to compete for votes, a dominant party may see less need to develop innovative policies that might "bend the cost curve." Alberta has a long-standing tradition of rural gerrymandering (Long 1969) that has contributed to the continuation of one-party dominance (Neitsch 2011). The rules for the most recent provincial redistribution (2010) allowed for the smallest constituency to be half the size of the average, which advantages rural constituencies—the mean population per constituency in rural Alberta is 39,737, compared to 42,618 in Calgary.

Clientelism plays out differently in the two large population centres as compared to rural settings. For Edmonton and Calgary, the regional health authority, clinical leaders, and (especially in Edmonton) municipal leadership saw advocacy for additional (both capital and operating) health spending as part of routine business. Leaders in each city scrutinized the largesse delivered to the other. As part of the exchange, political issues and poor publicity were managed. In rural Alberta, the health system was often seen as part of local wealth creation, with local employment prioritized over system efficiency and more contemporary service delivery modes and local procurement used to support local providers. Although there are clear links between employment and health, the motivation for these local decisions was more likely to be the result of clientelism than pursuit of a public health goal.

The petty corruption of clientelism is supplemented by the prevalence of pork-barrel politics. The direction of reform of mental health services internationally is clear: towards service integration and deinstitutionalization. The proportion of beds in mental hospitals to the total number of mental health beds has been used as a performance measure for mental health care, with a lower ratio being better (Jacob et al. 2007). Jacob and colleagues summarize good practice: "Large custodial mental hospitals need to be replaced by community-care facilities, backed by general hospital psychiatric beds and home care support" (2007, 1069–70). But in Alberta this is not the policy that has been pursued. A very large mental hospital in a rural centre (Ponoka) was rebuilt while the local member of the legislature was health minister, to the detriment of good access for residents of the major population centre of the region (Red Deer).

As noted above, the management role in regional health authorities became about advocacy and managing potentially poor publicity. Criticism of the government was reportedly managed through creation of a culture of intimidation. Although many people interviewed by the Health Quality Council of Alberta for a recent review reported no direct experience with intimidation,

> [o]n the other hand many interviewees identified, through their own personal experiences or experiences of others, disturbing situations where leaders (most often physicians or administrative leaders) had attempted to "muzzle" or intimidate physicians to prevent or cut short their advocacy. In some cases, this was attributed to leaders being "directed" from external sources, such as politicians or the government, to stop the advocacy. Interviewees described numerous situations in which physicians or prominent senior leaders had experienced severe negative repercussions while advocating for patients or system improvements. In some cases the intimidation was "subtle and nuanced and was career destructive," and in others the intimidation was "direct and focused." These experiences caused significant stress for some of the individuals involved and, in some instances, were life-altering, resulting in career changes or a move out of the province. These situations were seen to have sent a clear message that "if you speak up, this is what can happen to you," and were seen as having a "chilling effect" on others. Other individuals used strong language when describing their experience; one said "it was like I had rabies." (Health Quality Council of Alberta 2012, 31)

Clientelism is a culture in which meritocratic resource allocation processes take second place to exchange relationships. In such environments, normal democratic processes of advocacy (by both health stakeholders and external advocates) can become risky. Advocacy outside the dominant channels threatens the client relationship. Idiosyncratic resource allocation obscures the nature of any penalties for such behaviour but sends a clear message reinforcing the clientelist bargain.

One-party dominance also allows control of voice opportunities for public participation. Consultation processes can be stage-managed to provide a veneer of consultation without substance (Lesch 2009). Church and Smith (2008) also note that the major regional restructuring of health services in the province also involved a shift to boards appointed by the minister to effect change locally. Appointed boards helped to ensure that the new board members "could be trusted to move forward without question on implementing the new structures" (Church and Smith 2008, 232). Clientelism, through its impact on privatization and outsourcing decisions and because of its impact on strategic planning decisions, especially in rural areas, contributes to system inefficiency and militates against cost-reducing service rationalization.

Conclusion

The cost curve in Alberta is growing, and faster than the Canadian average. Alberta's relative wealth has meant that a high-cost health system has been affordable, and this wealth has been a contributing factor in making the province an expensive one in terms of health provision. Conservative political dominance might normally be expected to lead to antipathy towards government intervention or to a stronger government presence in any sector of the economy, but not in Alberta politics. This is because one-party dominance is associated with clientelism, and the iconic status of health care in Canada allows appropriation of health-care funding to meet clientelist obligations. One-party dominance, coupled with the reinforcing effect of populist politics, means that health care in Alberta becomes an instrument of reciprocity to a greater extent than in other provinces. Government MLAs, and their constituencies, expect not only access to decision-making but also some return for political support. Unprofitable investments—unprofitable when their return is measured in terms of gain in political capital rather than health gain—have become endemic in Alberta's health-care decision-making.

Politics and wealth intersect in Alberta. Think Alberta, think oil. This creates a peculiar dynamic that has an impact on health-care priority settings and delivery. There are many communities in Alberta that have not shared in the oil wealth through employment (or wealth-creating) opportunities. For a conservative government, which would normally be expected to eschew public enterprise and investment and employment creation, how can this wealth legitimately be shared? The answer lies in part in investment in the health sector. Capital funding of hospitals engages citizen support for medicare; it is seen as a legitimate way of distributing oil wealth, in the naive belief that it delivers health benefits to the community while at the same time being consistent with a conservative government ideology.

In Alberta, political dynamics trump the economic drivers, including cost containment. The politics of the province will probably conspire to keep health care in the province relatively expensive into the medium term, making it unlikely that the provincial cost curve could be bent significantly even if there were the political will to do so.

References

Alberta. Premier's Advisory Council on Health. 2001. *A Framework for Reform: Report of the Premier's Advisory Council on Health* [Mazankowski Report]. Edmonton: Premier's Advisory Council on Health.

Alberta and AHS (Alberta Health Services). 2010. *Becoming the Best: Alberta's 5-Year Health Action Plan, 2010–2015*. Edmonton: Alberta Health and Wellness Communications.

Anderson, G., and P. S. Hussey. 2001. "Comparing Health System Performance in OECD Countries." *Health Affairs* 20, no. 3: 219–32. http://dx.doi.org/10.1377/hlthaff.20.3.219.

Armstrong, W. 2000. *The Consumer Experience with Cataract Surgery and Private Clinics in Alberta: Canada's Canary in the Mine Shaft.* [Edmonton]: Alberta Chapter, Consumers Association of Canada.

Ashby, N. J., A. Bueno, and F. McMahon. 2012. *Economic Freedom of North America 2011.* Vancouver: Fraser Institute.

Bell, E., and H. Jansen. 2007. "Sustaining a Dynasty in Alberta: The 2004 Provincial Election." *Canadian Political Science Review* 1, no. 2: 27–49.

Bell, R. 2012. "Grit Future Hitched to Raj." *Toronto Sun*, 17 June. http://www.torontosun.com/2012/06/17/grit-future-hitched-to-raj. Accessed 21 April 2014.

Bloom, J., S. Duckett, and A. Robertson. 2012. "Development of an Interactive Model for Planning the Care Workforce for Alberta: Case Study." *Human Resources for Health* 10, no. 1: 22.

Cairney, R. 1998. "New Private Facility Woos Public Dollars in Calgary." *Canadian Medical Association Journal* 159, no. 5: 551–52.

———. 2000. "Will It Be Third Time Lucky for Ralph Klein?" *Canadian Medical Association Journal* 162, no. 3: 409.

Casebeer, A. 2004. "Regionalizing Canadian Healthcare: The Good—the Bad—the Ugly." *Healthcare Papers* 5, no. 1: 88–93. http://dx.doi.org/10.12927/hcpap..16845.

CBC News. 2009. "Health Workers File Lawsuit over Telus Payroll System." 21 May. http://www.cbc.ca/news/canada/calgary/health-workers-file-lawsuit-over-telus-payroll-system-1.861022. Accessed 21 April 2014.

Church, J., and N. Smith. 2006. "Health Reform and Privatization in Alberta." *Canadian Public Administration* 49, no. 4: 486–505. http://dx.doi.org/10.1111/j.1754-7121.2006.tb01995.x.

———. 2008. "Health Reform in Alberta: The Introduction of Health Regions." *Canadian Public Administration* 51, no. 2: 217–38. http://dx.doi.org/10.1111/j.1754-7121.2008.00016.x.

CNW Newswire. 2012. "K-Bro Announces New Alberta Health Services Contract." 7 May. http://www.newswire.ca/en/story/968943/k-bro-announces-new-alberta-health-services-contract. Accessed 18 June 2012.

Coleman, M. P., D. Forman, H. Bryant, J. Butler, B. Rachet, C. Maringe, U. Nur, E. Tracey, M. Coory, J. Hatcher, et al. 2011. "Cancer Survival in Australia, Canada, Denmark, Norway, Sweden, and the UK, 1995–2007 (the International Cancer Benchmarking Partnership): An Analysis of Population-Based Cancer Registry Data." *Lancet* 377, no. 9760: 127–38. http://dx.doi.org/10.1016/S0140-6736(10)62231-3.

Denis, C. 1995. "'Government Can Do Whatever It Wants': Moral Regulation in Ralph Klein's Alberta." *Canadian Review of Sociology and Anthropology/Revue canadienne de sociologie et d'anthropologie* 32, no. 3: 365–83. http://dx.doi.org/10.1111/j.1755-618X.1995.tb00777.x.

Di Matteo, L. 2009. "Policy Choice or Economic Fundamentals: What Drives the Public-Private Health Expenditure Balance in Canada?" *Health Economics, Policy, and Law* 4, no. 1: 29–53. http://dx.doi.org/10.1017/S1744133108004611.

Di Matteo, L., and R. Di Matteo. 1998. "Evidence on the Determinants of Canadian Provincial Government Health Expenditures, 1965–1991." *Journal of Health Economics* 17, no. 2: 211–28. http://dx.doi.org/10.1016/S0167-6296(97)00020-9.

Dranove, D., C. Capps, and L. Dafny. 2009. *A Competitive Process for Procuring Health Services: A Review of Principles with an Application to Cataract Services*. Calgary: School of Public Policy, University of Calgary.

Duckett, S. 2010. "Second Wave Reform in Alberta." *Healthcare Management Forum* 23, no. 4: 156–58. http://dx.doi.org/10.1016/j.hcmf.2010.08.006.

———. 2011. "Getting the Foundations Right: Alberta's Approach to Health-Care Reform." *Health Policy* 6, no. 3: 22–26.

Duckett, S., J. Bloom, and A. Robertson. 2012. "Planning to Meet the Care Need Challenge in Alberta, Canada." *International Journal of Health Planning and Management* 27, no. 3: e186–96. http://dx.doi.org/10.1002/hpm.2112.

Duckett, S., G. Kramer, and L. Sarnecki. 2012. "Alberta's Health Spending Challenge: A Policy-Oriented Analysis of Inter- and Intra-Provincial Differences in Health Expenditure." In *Boom and Bust Again: Policy Challenges for Commodity Based Economy*, edited by D. Ryan, 301–34. Edmonton: University of Alberta Press.

Duckett, S., and C. Nijssen-Jordan. 2012. "Using Quality Improvement Methods at the System Level to Improve Hospital Emergency Department Treatment Times." *Quality Management in Health Care* 21, no. 1: 29–33. http://dx.doi.org/10.1097/QMH.0b013e31824180f6.

Environics Research Group. 2011. *Public Opinion in Alberta: Summary of Survey Findings*.

Fierlbeck, K. 2001. "Cost Containment in Health Care: The Federalism Context." In *Federalism, Democracy and Health Policy in Canada*, edited by D. Adams, 131–78. Kingston, ON: McGill-Queen's University Press.

Gibson, D., and J. Clements. 2012. *Delivery Matters: The High Costs of For-Profit Health Services in Alberta*. Edmonton: Parkland Institute, University of Alberta.

Gray, C. 2000. "Alberta Is Back at It, Goading the Feds." *Canadian Medical Association Journal* 162, no. 3: 411.

Gregoire, L. 2006. "Alberta's Hybrid Public–Private 'Third Way.'" *Canadian Medical Association Journal* 174, no. 8: 1076–77. http://dx.doi.org/10.1503/cmaj.060330.

Health Quality Council of Alberta. 2012. *Review of the Quality of Care and Safety of Patients Requiring Access to Emergency Department Care and Cancer Surgery and the Role and Process of Physician Advocacy*. Calgary: Health Quality Council of Alberta.

Hicken, A. 2011. "Clientelism." *Annual Review of Political Science* 14, no. 1: 289–310. http://dx.doi.org/10.1146/annurev.polisci.031908.220508.

Hinings, C. R., A. Casebeer, T. Reay, K. Golden-Biddle, A. Pablo, and R. Greenwood. 2003. "Regionalizing Healthcare in Alberta: Legislated Change, Uncertainty and Loose Coupling." *British Journal of Management* 14 (Suppl. 1): S15–30.

Hurley, J., J. Lomas, and V. Bhatia. 1994. "When Tinkering Is Not Enough: Provincial Reform to Manage Health Care Resources." *Canadian Public Administration* 37, no. 3: 490–514. http://dx.doi.org/10.1111/j.1754-7121.1994.tb00874.x.

Jacob, K., P. Sharan, I. Mirza, M. Garrido-Cumbrera, S. Seedat, J. Mari, V. Sreenivas, and S. Saxena. 2007. "Mental Health Systems in Countries: Where Are We Now?" *Lancet* 370, no. 9592: 1061–77. http://dx.doi.org/10.1016/S0140-6736(07)61241-0.

Lampard, R. 2009. "The Hoadley Commission (1932–34) and Health Insurance in Alberta." *Canadian Bulletin of Medical History* 26, no. 2: 429–52.

Landon, S., M. L. McMillan, V. Muralidharan, and M. Parsons. 2006. "Does Health-Care Spending Crowd Out Other Provincial Government Expenditures?" *Canadian Public Policy* 32, no. 2: 121–41. http://dx.doi.org/10.2307/4128724.

Lesch, M. S. 2009. *The Politics of Loss Imposition: Health Care Reform in Ontario and Alberta.* Vancouver: University of British Columbia.

Lewis, S., and D. Kouri. 2004. "Regionalization: Making Sense of the Canadian Experience." *Healthcare Papers* 5, no. 1: 12–31. http://dx.doi.org/10.12927/hcpap.2004.16847.

Long, J. A. 1969. "Maldistribution in Western Provincial Legislatures: The Case of Alberta." *Canadian Journal of Political Science* 2, no. 3: 345–55. http://dx.doi.org/10.1017/S0008423900025105.

Marchildon, G. P., and K. Schrijvers. 2011. "Physician Resistance and the Forging of Public Healthcare: A Comparative Analysis of the Doctors' Strikes in Canada and Belgium in the 1960s." *Medical History* 55, no. 2: 203–22. http://dx.doi.org/10.1017/S0025727300005767.

Neitsch, A. T. 2011. "Political Monopoly: A Study of the Progressive Conservative Association in Rural Alberta, 1971–1996." PhD diss., University of Ottawa.

Philippon, D. J., and J. Braithwaite. 2008. "Health System Organization and Governance in Canada and Australia: A Comparison of Historical Developments, Recent Policy Changes and Future Implications." *Health Policy* 4, no. 1: e168–86.

Philippon, D. J., and S. A. Wasylyshyn. 1996. "Health-Care Reform in Alberta." *Canadian Public Administration* 39, no. 1: 70–84. http://dx.doi.org/10.1111/j.1754-7121.1996.tb00118.x.

Reay, T., and C. R. Hinings. 2005. "The Recomposition of an Organizational Field: Health Care in Alberta." *Organization Studies* 26, no. 3: 351–84. http://dx.doi.org/10.1177/0170840605050872.

Reinhardt, U. E., P. S. Hussey, and G. F. Anderson. 2002. "Cross-National Comparisons of Health Systems Using OECD Data, 1999." *Health Affairs* 21, no. 3: 169–81. http://dx.doi.org/10.1377/hlthaff.21.3.169.

Ruseski, J. E. 2009. "Competition in Canadian Health Care Service Provision: Good, Bad, or Indifferent?" School of Public Policy Research Papers. Calgary: University of Calgary.

Smith, N., and J. Church. 2008. "Shifting the Lens: The Introduction of Population-Based Funding in Alberta." *Healthcare Management Forum* 21, no. 2: 36–42. http://dx.doi.org/10.1016/S0840-4704(10)60544-3.

Taylor, M. G. 1978. *Health Insurance and Canadian Public Policy: The Seven Decisions That Created the Canadian Health Insurance System.* Montreal: Institute of Public Administration of Canada and McGill-Queen's University Press.

Tomblin, S. G. 2007. "Effecting Change and Transformation through Regionalization: Theory versus Practice." *Canadian Public Administration* 50, no. 1: 1–20. http://dx.doi.org/10.1111/j.1754-7121.2007.tb02000.x.

Trantidis, A. 2011. "The Micro-foundations of One-Party Hegemony: Development and Clientelism." Queen Elizabeth House Working Papers. Oxford: University of Oxford.

Vivone, R. 2009. *Ralph Could Have Been a Superstar: Tales of the Klein Era.* Kingston, ON: Patricia Publishing.

Wesley, J. J. 2011. *Code Politics: Campaigns and Cultures on the Canadian Prairies.* Vancouver: University of British Columbia Press.

thirteen
Saskatchewan and Manitoba: Managing Down

GREGORY P. MARCHILDON

Introduction

This chapter addresses the nature of the health-care cost curves in Saskatchewan and Manitoba and associated policy interventions by both provincial governments. The rationale for including both provinces in a single chapter—aside from their geographic juxtaposition—is the similarity of their respective demographics, health outcomes, and regional health authority (RHA) structures. Another striking similarity is that both provinces have proportionally the largest resident Aboriginal populations among all provinces. Many First Nations and Métis residents live in remote northern communities or poorer urban neighbourhoods that are often marked by unhealthy living conditions and higher rates of suicide and violence, circumstances that create greater-than-average demands on health services. As has often been noted, there is a large gap in health status and outcomes between the majority of Aboriginal residents and the majority populations in both provinces (Lemstra and Neudorf 2008; Martens et al. 2002, 2010).

At the same time, provincial governments (as opposed to the federal government) are responsible for ensuring that all residents, including "registered Indians" as defined under the federal *Indian Act*, have access to all medically necessary hospital and medical care services. Even with the federal government covering other health costs and benefits for eligible First Nations residents—including medical transportation and prescription drugs, as well as public health services and some long-term care and home care on the reserves—provincial responsibility for expensive hospital and medical services means that Saskatchewan and Manitoba, holding everything else constant, would be expected to have higher per capita health costs than most other provinces.

As will be seen, both provincial governments, working with and through their RHAs, have adopted very similar strategies to bend the cost curve. In terms of structure and policy action, these two prairie governments stand in marked contrast to their neighbours Alberta and Ontario. As described by Stephen Duckett and others, the Alberta government has created and pursued different structures and strategies since it created Alberta Health Services to replace the existing RHA structure in 2008 (Donaldson 2010; Duckett 2010, 2011). Ontario too has pursed a very different strategy of regionalization, initially rejecting the idea of creating RHAs and subsequently establishing Local Health Integration Networks (LHINs), which, unlike RHAs in Saskatchewan and Manitoba, are restricted to "purchasing" rather than providing services.

This chapter is divided into three sections. The first addresses government health spending and demographic trends to identify areas that face unique cost pressures in Saskatchewan and Manitoba. The second section examines the question of fiscal sustainability by putting provincial government health expenditures in the context of provincial revenues and expenditures, demographic pressures, and above-average human resource costs. The final section explores the key policy interventions that both provincial governments are relying on to bend down the health-spending cost curve.

Health spending trends in Saskatchewan and Manitoba

Figure 13.1 illustrates long-term trends in real health spending by the Saskatchewan and Manitoba governments. Although there is nothing overtly unique about the trajectory of either provincial government, two

Figure 13.1 Saskatchewan and Manitoba government real health expenditures per capita, 1975–2012 (1997 dollars)

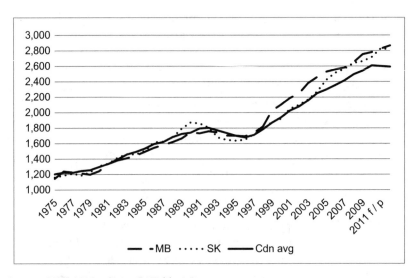

Source: CIHI 2012a, Series B, Table 4.7.

Figure 13.2 Provincial government nominal health expenditures per capita, standardized for age and sex, 2006–2009

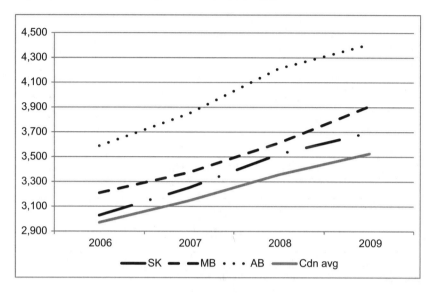

Source: Derived from CIHI 2011a, 40, Table 6.

matters are worth noting. The first is the sharp fiscal course correction made by the Saskatchewan in the early 1990s to reduce interest payments on an enormous accumulated public debt. Health spending cuts accompanied health reforms that included hospital consolidation and the introduction of health region and health reforms (Adams 2001; James 1999). As illustrated by a comparison to the Canadian average, this cost-cutting effort in Saskatchewan was simply an extreme version of what occurred in other provinces, including Manitoba. The second issue is the extent to which both the Saskatchewan and Manitoba trends in spending were nearly identical to the national trend until the late 1990s (in Manitoba's case) and the mid 2000s (in Saskatchewan's case), when both provinces spent more on a per capita basis than the national average.

The impact of the demographic profile of the two provinces will be examined in the next section, but it is nonetheless useful at this stage to compare provincial government per capita health spending standardized for age, since it could be argued that demographic factors may be contributing to the higher spending in both provinces. However, when age is considered as a factor (see Figure 13.2), Saskatchewan and Manitoba continue to show expenditures above the Canadian average, although not to the extent of Alberta. After decades of in-migration, Alberta has a demographically

Table 13.1 Provincial government per capita health expenditures, 2010 (current dollars)

	Saskatchewan	Manitoba	Provincial/Territorial Average
Hospitals	1,466	2,120	1,477
Physicians	793	923	779
Other institutions	582	701	417
Other professionals	24	29	29
Prescription drugs	301	295	296
Capital	146	197	222
Public health	379	320	237
Administration	27	53	45
Other health spending	274	388	189
TOTAL	4,239	5,024	3,692

Note: Due to rounding, individual columns may not add up to total figures.
Source: CIHI 2012a, Series C and D, Tables C.4.3, D.4.7.3, and D4.8.3

younger population than either province, so, holding everything else constant, one would expect its non-adjusted health spending to be lower than its prairie neighbours. However, this has not been the case, and adjusting for age simply increases the spending gap between the provinces.

When comparing specific categories of per capita health spending in Saskatchewan and Manitoba to the Canadian average, as shown in Table 13.2, there are some distinct differences between the two provinces. Manitoba's per capita expenditures on hospitals are well above those in Saskatchewan, while the latter province's hospital spending is close to the provincial average. As will be discussed in the third section, this is an area of expenditure that the Manitoba government targeted in its 2012 streamlining plan for consolidating regional health authorities and tertiary care (Manitoba 2012).

When it comes to public health, Saskatchewan's spending stands well above that of Manitoba and the provincial average, while Saskatchewan's spending on administration is well below that of Manitoba, which in turn is close to the Canadian average. While more investigation of the components that make up "administration" is required, it may also be worth exploring in future research whether the outcome for Saskatchewan is a statistical anomaly or the product of real efficiencies.

Both provinces stand well above the provincial average in terms of spending on non-hospital institutions, the majority of which are long-term care facilities. This last result may be more an effect of higher-than-average public subsidy for long-term care than it is a reflection of any inefficiency or an aging demographic—all potential hypotheses worthy of testing against the empirical evidence in more detailed research in the future.

To understand these spending trends, they must be placed in the context of provincial government revenues and expenditures as well as demographic trends. In addition, both provinces face cost pressures in competing for scarce health professionals, particularly doctors and nurses, against the adjacent provinces of Alberta and Ontario. As a consequence, their respective remuneration rates tend to be higher than the Canadian average. This is particularly true in Saskatchewan, where health organizations and communities compete directly with their counterparts in Alberta for doctors, nurses, skilled diagnostic technicians, and health system managers.

Fiscal sustainability

The word *sustainability*, as it applies to publicly funded health care, is a much used and abused term in the political arena, with scholars defining fiscal sustainability in many different ways (Di Matteo 2010; Marchildon 2004). These conflicting definitions are largely a result of the fact that the quantum and growth of health spending depend on many factors, most of which are exogenous to health ministries. As Joe Ruggeri points out in Chapter 14, two of these exogenous factors are paramount: (1) the growth in government revenues, or perhaps more explicitly, as Ruggeri puts it, the "capacity of the existing revenue structure to finance it, given all other demands on public funds," and (2) the performance of the provincial economy itself.

These factors are in turn affected by several underlying cost drivers, including demographic shifts; a health-sector inflation that deviates significantly from the general rate of inflation; changes (positive or negative) in the health of the population, including lifestyle behaviours that alter the relative burden of disease; the impact of major technological changes that alter the cost of diagnosis and treatment; and any changes in the elasticity of health service consumption to income (CIHI 2011b). The last is a particularly interesting feature of health care. The empirical evidence demonstrates that health care is what economists would classify as a "superior" or "luxury" good; that is, as incomes grow, we allocate larger shares of income to health spending. We do so as individuals in terms of private health spending and we do so collectively through public-sector health

Table 13.2 Saskatchewan and Manitoba government health spending as percentage of provincial GDP and provincial government revenues, 2000 and 2008

	Saskatchewan		Manitoba	
	2000	2009	2000	2009
Provincial GDP	6.0	6.8	7.7	9.3
Provincial revenues	26.6	37.6	30.2	36.8

Source: Author's calculations, based on CIHI 2011a and Statistics Canada 2011b.

funding managed by our respective governments. In fact, Don Drummond recently used Robert W. Fogel's (2009) estimate of 1.6 for the long-term income elasticity of health services to income in the United States to make the point that there should be "nothing necessarily surprising or alarming about healthcare rising as a percentage of public and private budgets" (Drummond 2011, 15).[1] This is not to say that all government initiatives aimed at bending the cost curve are doomed, but rather to recognize that the most diligent provincial government efforts to contain costs may still produce rates of health spending that exceed growth in provincial gross domestic product (GDP) or income.

In this chapter, *fiscal sustainability* is treated more narrowly as the relationship between provincial government health expenditures and government revenues. However, even this extremely truncated approach must consider the structure of provincial revenues, including tax increases or decreases and federal transfers provided (at least ostensibly) for provincial spending on health care. Since factors such as the relative burden of disease, the impact of technological change, and the income elasticity of health are not likely to differ greatly between two provinces as similar as Saskatchewan and Manitoba, the cost drivers more likely to produce differences are their respective demographic profiles and their respective rates of health-provider remuneration.

Before looking at this, the ratio between provincial government spending on health relative to all other provincial government expenditures is presented in Figure 13.3. To ensure that health expenditures are expressed as a proportion of all government obligations, payments on the public debt

---

1 There is an ongoing debate among health economists about the income elasticity of health, with Getzen (2000), for example, demonstrating that smaller units of analysis actually exhibit lower income elasticity than more populous units of analysis. For a summary of this literature and an exploration of the issue, see Di Matteo (2003).

Figure 13.3 Provincial government health expenditures as percentage of total program spending, including debt repayment, 1991–2011 (current dollars)

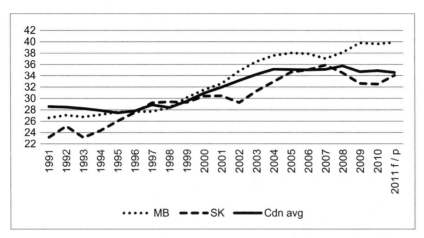

Source: CIHI 2012a, Series B, Table 4.5.

are included. As can be seen, the Manitoba government's expenditures as a share of total health spending grew rapidly after 2001 and now exceed the average of all provincial governments. In contrast, Saskatchewan remained near or under the national average for most years between 1990 and 2009.

Examining government health expenditures as a proportion of government revenues and provincial GDP reveals that provincial health expenditures play a larger part in Manitoba's economy than Saskatchewan's, largely as a consequence of Saskatchewan's resource boom, which has generated more rapid economic growth since the late 1990s. Despite this growth, Saskatchewan government health expenditure as a share of provincial revenues had exceeded that of Manitoba by 2009. This is likely because of more aggressive tax reductions in this period by successive provincial administrations in Saskatchewan, relative to the Manitoba government.

The majority of the funding for provincial health-care expenditures is raised directly by provincial governments. On a national basis, it is estimated that approximately 80% of provincial health spending is raised through own-source provincial taxation. The remaining 20% is made up of revenues collected by the Government of Canada and then transferred to the provinces through the Canada Health Transfer (CHT). The money is transferred on the condition that the provincial governments meet the five criteria—public administration, comprehensiveness, universality, portability, and accessibility—enumerated in the *Canada Health Act*. As a consequence of the new, pure per capita formula announced by the federal

Table 13.3 Dependency ratios in Saskatchewan and Manitoba compared to Canadian average, 2011 and 2031

Age Group	Dependency Ratio in 2011			Projected Dependency Ratio in 2031		
	SK	MB	Canada	SK	MB	Canada
0–14	27.7	23.9	23.7	30.6	26.4	26.7
65+	20.9	20.3	20.8	34.4	35.9	37.5
Total	48.6	44.2	44.5	65.0	62.3	64.2

Source: Statistics Canada 2011a.

government in December 2011, the CHT contribution to provincial health spending will decrease gradually over the next eight years (Marchildon and Mou 2013).

Federal funding is also provided through equalization. Historically, Saskatchewan and Manitoba have been equalization beneficiaries, but in recent years Saskatchewan in particular has not received equalization payments, and Manitoba has received proportionately less than it did in the past. Given the fact that the pure per capita CHT formula has fewer negative implications for Saskatchewan and Manitoba than for provinces with older populations, such as those in Atlantic Canada, and given the lessening importance of equalization for both provinces, federal transfer funding will not be examined further in this chapter.

An important demographic consideration when evaluating own-source taxation capacity is the age structure of the provincial population. Dependency ratios identify the proportion of a population too young or too old to be working (and therefore contributing taxes) and supported by public services paid for through the taxes of a working-age population. Indeed, many of those who argue the unsustainability of public funding of health care base their arguments on the demographic bubble caused by the baby-boom generation and the consequent increase in dependency ratios.

As of 2011, Saskatchewan's dependency ratio was substantially higher than the rate in Manitoba and the Canadian average. While Table 13.3 shows a substantial increase in dependency ratios for both provinces by 2031, the projected dependency ratio for Saskatchewan is forecast to be only slightly above the Canadian average, while that for Manitoba is expected to be considerably below the Canadian average. Judging by recent history, however, an aging population may represent less of a pressure on sustainability than other factors, in particular health-sector inflation—a factor that is more within the policy control of provincial governments (CIHI 2011b).

Figure 13.4 Average gross fee-for-service payment per physician earning minimum of $60,000, 2010–2011

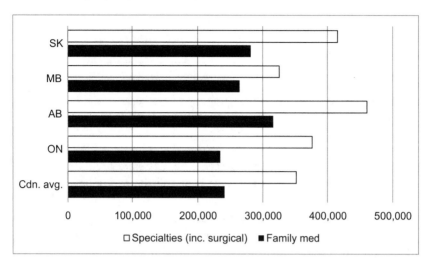

Source: Derived from CIHI 2012c, Table A5.1.

A CIHI (2011b) report on cost drivers in health care has highlighted the extent to which health-sector inflation above the rate of general inflation has been a cost driver in recent health spending in Canada. Between 1998 and 2008, the average annual growth (in nominal dollars) of all physician spending in Canada—almost all of which is financed by provincial governments—was 6.8%. Figure 13.4 compares Manitoba and Saskatchewan to the Canadian average and to Alberta and Ontario historically, the two provinces with the highest physician remuneration in Canada. Remuneration for family physicians in Manitoba and Saskatchewan is higher than the Canadian average and exceeded only by fee-for-service (FFS) remuneration in Alberta, which leads the rest of Canada by a considerable margin. While specialists in Manitoba, or at least those who receive FFS compensation, receive less than the national average, specialists in Saskatchewan receive the second highest compensation in Canada. Only Alberta specialists are paid more.

Nurses outnumber doctors by a factor of 5 to 1 in Canada, and almost all are paid from public sources (Marchildon 2013a). Using data disseminated by the Canadian Federation of Nurses' Unions, we can see that nurses in Saskatchewan are the highest paid in Canada, well above base and maximum salaries in Alberta. While Manitoba lags only slightly behind Alberta in terms of base salary, the maximum level is considerably lower than in

Table 13.4 Base and maximum annual salary by province, general-duty registered nurses*

	Saskatchewan**	Manitoba	Alberta**	Québec
Base	66,746	62,508	63,147	42,276
Maximum	86,644	73,692	82,881	62,966

* Figures are as of 2 July 2011, for contracts ending 31 March 2012.
** Collective agreements in Saskatchewan and Alberta have 2% added to the base rate for nurses with 20 or more years employment, to "recognize long-term services."
Source: CFNU 2011.

Alberta and Saskatchewan. To show the other extreme, Table 13.4 includes Québec, the province with the lowest base and the maximum salaries for nurses in Canada.

The majority of specialist physicians and registered nurses work in hospital settings. More efficient hospitals might compensate for more highly paid doctors and nurses, so it is worthwhile comparing hospital efficiency province by province. In the Canadian Hospital Report Project, CIHI now provides a comparative efficiency measure based on the cost per weighted case for 2007, 2008, and 2009. Using an average of the three years, hospital efficiency performance in Saskatchewan is considerably better than in Alberta, but not quite as good (by a perhaps insignificant margin) as hospital efficiency in Manitoba. Based on a productivity measure of inpatient work of nurses, Saskatchewan's nurses show higher productivity than those in Manitoba and Alberta. However, some caution should be used about drawing too firm a conclusion from these productivity and efficiency results. CIHI has only recently developed these indicators and the data are limited to three years' worth of observations (CIHI 2012d).

In the introductory chapter it was noted that all jurisdictions in Canada have experienced reductions in avoidable deaths through improvements in medical treatment and better disease prevention. Nonetheless, Saskatchewan and Manitoba have among the highest provincial rates of avoidable mortality in Canada, measured from either treatable causes or preventable causes. One possible explanation, especially for avoidable mortality for preventable causes, is the relative size of the Aboriginal populations in both provinces, and the fact that a significant number of First Nations and Métis people live on rural and remote reserves with limited local access to a broad range of health-care services.

More difficult to explain are the high mortality rates for preventable causes, given the significant spending by the federal government for

Table 13.5 Hospital efficiency by province, annual average, 2007–2009

	Saskatchewan	Manitoba	Alberta
Cost per weighted case	$5,280	$5,231	$5,821

Source: CIHI 2012b.

Table 13.6 Nurse productivity in hospitals by province, annual average, 2007–2009

	Saskatchewan	Manitoba	Alberta
Total worked hours per weighted case	51.0	61.7	58.2

Source: CIHI 2012a.

Table 13.7 Age-standardized avoidable mortality rates, 2006–2008 (pooled data)

	Avoidable Mortality from Treatable Causes	Avoidable Mortality from Preventable Causes
Saskatchewan	80	142
Manitoba	83	143
Canadian average	66	120
British Columbia	58	114
Ontario	67	110
New Brunswick	61	134
Newfoundland and Labrador	88	132

Source: CIHI 2012e.

on-reserve public health and illness prevention services. For this reason, Table 13.7 compares Saskatchewan and Manitoba results to two other provinces with rural and remote populations: New Brunswick and Newfoundland and Labrador. Only the latter province has a higher avoidable mortality rate, and this only for treatable causes. Table 13.7 includes British Columbia and Ontario simply because historically they have among the lowest rates of avoidable mortality in the country. The results for this aggregate indicator suggest that both provincial governments, perhaps acting in concert with the federal government, have considerable potential to extract greater value for money from future health spending.

Bending the cost curve: Recent interventions and reforms

This section examines the major policy changes enacted by the Saskatchewan and Manitoba governments in recent years to "bend the cost curve." Although this phrase is more a metaphor than a precise concept, it is nonetheless useful because it implicitly refers to longer-term change in expenditure patterns than what may be implied in shorter-term "cost-cutting" or "cost-containment" interventions. The most common approach used by governments in connection with their health spending is the notion of achieving greater value for money. The term *value for money* is a colloquial way of describing efficiency—the ability to obtain more output for the same set of inputs. However, value for money can also be consistent with the notion of bending the cost curve when it embraces health system reforms that lead to the sustainable use of fewer resources in the longer term.

These cross-cutting cost curve–bending reforms will be grouped into two categories, the first involving structural changes to the health system as a whole and the second involving process changes to improve the efficiency of health services delivery, including the substitution of providers to ensure care that is less costly but at least as appropriate as higher-cost care. A word of warning: this review selects what the author considers to be the most important reforms or interventions or those with the most future potential. Finally, it should be noted that most of these reforms and initiatives are of very recent vintage. As a consequence, there exist very few data and virtually no studies concerning the impact and effectiveness of these reforms.

Structural reforms

Bending the cost curve has always been one of the key reform objectives of provincial governments in creating regional health authorities (Marchildon 2006). One of the principal objectives of regionalization—first introduced in the midst of a contraction in government spending in the first half of the 1990s—was to attain long-term efficiencies and cost control through active management of a range of health services within a defined geographic area, an obvious contrast with the passive payment system previously administered by provincial governments (Axelsson et al. 2007). However, when the anticipated economies of scale and scope did not emerge from the new structures, the Saskatchewan and Manitoba governments further reduced the number of regional health authorities (RHAs). Neither government went to the extreme of the Alberta government in creating one single RHA for the province, but both provinces did go farther, and earlier, than Ontario in their regionalization efforts.

In 2002 Saskatchewan replaced its 33 health districts with 13 regional health authorities, and in 2012, the Manitoba government announced consolidation of its 11 regional health authorities into five larger RHAs (Manitoba 2012; McIntosh and Marchildon 2008). In both cases the provincial governments were motivated by a desire to increase the capacity of RHAs to achieve better value for money on behalf of the population they were serving. Although it is part of a growing trend in Canada, the evidence on the impact of regionalization is both limited and contradictory, and even more so for the current trend to greater centralization (Marchildon 2013a).

In the Manitoba case, the five larger RHAs have been tasked with finding cost savings everywhere possible and, especially in the case of the Winnipeg Regional Health Authority, to keep administrative costs below 3% of the operational budget. To back this up, the government has passed legislation that limits the amount of administrative spending in RHAs in order that more resources can be devoted to delivering health services. In addition, the government directed the Winnipeg health region to encourage greater specialization in order to reduce overlap and duplication among Winnipeg hospitals. The Government of Manitoba was explicit about its expectation that fewer RHAs should translate into a significant reduction in the number and cost of executive positions (Manitoba 2012).

In Saskatchewan, in contrast, there has been no further consolidation of RHAs since 2002. However, the government has attempted to achieve a similar outcome through another means, introducing its "Shared Services" initiative in 2012. Simply put, this is the government's effort to centralize back-office functions (e.g., payroll, laundry, information technology, procurement, and human resource training) without dismantling the RHAs. At the same time, the government made it clear to the RHAs that achieving progress on Shared Services would be essential to future survival of the existing RHA board and management structure (Marchildon 2013b).

Cross-cutting process reforms: Lean and provider substitution

Process reforms can be distinguished from structural reforms in that they attempt to change the ways in which health services are delivered and the relationships among those who deliver the services, rather than the underlying structures and institutions. Two main process reforms have been initiated by the Saskatchewan and Manitoba governments with a view to bending the cost curve. Saskatchewan has become a leader in Canada in the implementation of Lean process reforms, while Manitoba is ahead of most provinces in substituting some of the services of family physicians with those provided by allied professions, in particular nurses and physician assistants.

Lean is a workforce production methodology first developed by Toyota and eventually adopted by car manufacturers in North America. In recent years Lean methodologies have been adapted to health care, most prominently in the National Health Service (NHS) of the United Kingdom and by numerous health-care organizations in the United States (IHI 2005; Johnson et al. 2012; Papadopoulos 2011). Following the lead of the Institute for Healthcare Improvement and the Institute of Medicine in the United States, the Saskatchewan government introduced Lean processes to various health-care settings, with a focus on clinical environments (Fine et al., 2009; Saskatchewan 2012). Two of the earliest Lean initiatives targeted clinical process redesign for physician practices, work that was led by the Saskatchewan Health Quality Council, and work redesign reform that focused on hospital wards, known as "Releasing Time to Care" (Saskatchewan Health Quality Council 2012).

Negotiations for the 2012–14 collective agreement between the provincial government and the Saskatchewan Union of Nurses (SUN) was successfully concluded after SUN agreed to work with the health ministry and the RHAs on Lean initiatives. In a major effort to scale up the reform, the Saskatchewan ministry of health set several Lean targets. By 31 March 2013 it intended to implement Lean as part of all surgical service lines; establish Continuous Improvement (Lean) offices across the province; have a minimum of 240 health-care managers pursuing Lean certification and 500 staff engaging in "Rapid Process Improvement" workshops; and consolidate key back-office functions throughout the province through Shared Services initiatives (Saskatchewan 2012). Although the provincial health quality council is spearheading a major evaluation of Lean initiatives, there had been no systematic assessment of Lean's impact at the time of writing (Marchildon 2013b).

Although Lean has not had a similar impact in Manitoba, that province has also been implementing Lean process reforms. The government's main objective is to train more than 1,500 frontline professionals, including doctors, nurses, managers, and staff, in Lean Six Sigma methods to improve efficiency as well as quality and safety (Manitoba 2012). The government of Manitoba (and the government of Saskatchewan) has involved nurses in major Releasing Time to Care projects that are Lean-inspired.

Manitoba has gone much farther than Saskatchewan in implementing a substitution strategy. Although the provincial government justifies the reform on the basis on access and quality, the objective here is to substitute lower-cost providers for higher-cost physicians while still providing health services of equivalent quality or a set of services more appropriate to health needs. The Manitoba government is a leader among provinces in introducing physician assistants who support and extend the scope of practice of doctors, an important consideration in regions that face severe shortages of doctors. Although the position has long been a part of the armed forces in Canada, the first civilian physician assistant to use the title was in Manitoba. In 2008 the University of Manitoba became the first postsecondary institution to offer a civilian physician assistant program, and by 2010 Manitoba had 60 physician assistants (Jones and Hooker 2011).[2]

The other major initiative that falls into the category of provider substitution is nurse-based primary-care clinics. Although they have long been part of the health landscape of remote communities in northern Canada, the provincial government initiated nurse-based clinics in southern cities and urban towns. Known as "QuickCare clinics," these primary-care clinics are staffed by nurse practitioners and registered nurses who provide a range of diagnoses and treatment of minor medical problems. While intended to take pressure off family doctors in particular—given that they operate on a walk-in as well as an appointment basis and are open to the public for extended hours during the week, as well as on weekends—QuickCare clinics are likely intended to take the pressure off emergency departments as well (Manitoba 2012). The first QuickCare clinic opened in Winnipeg's North End in March 2012, while the second, in Selkirk, a bedroom community a little north of Winnipeg, opened a month later.

Conclusion

As shown above, the cost pressures faced by the Saskatchewan and Manitoba governments are very similar. Both provinces have proportionally large Aboriginal sub-populations with poor health status and higher-than-average health-care needs. While some of their needs are financed through federal programs and coverage, more expensive hospital and physician services are funded and administered by the two provincial governments. Age is less of a cost pressure, since the average age of the population in both provinces was below the Canadian average in 2011 and is forecast to remain below it until 2031. Nonetheless, neither provincial government spends as much per capita as Alberta, a result that becomes even more exaggerated when expenditures are adjusted for age.

---

2 This compares to 143 physician assistants in the Canadian Forces, 67 physician assistants in Ontario, many of whom were involved in pilot projects in that province, and almost none in the rest of the country.

Both provinces have high-cost structures for provider payment, as illustrated by physician and nurse remuneration that exceeds the national average. The situation in Saskatchewan is much more extreme than in Manitoba, likely because of the province's more intense competition with Alberta for scarce health professionals and the Saskatchewan government's greater fiscal capacity, due to resource royalty revenues. Provider remuneration is one area in which provincial governments have some policy control, given the periodic collective bargaining negotiations between provincial governments and health professionals. At the same time, some interprovincial collaboration is likely essential, given the knock-on effects of high wage and remuneration settlements in nearby provinces such as Alberta and Ontario and the prevalence of provider mobility throughout Canada (with the possible exception of Québec).

In reviewing interventions aimed at bending the cost curve, the structural reforms introduced by regionalization are the most long-standing. When first introduced, regional health authorities were expected to manage their respective areas in such a way as to find efficiencies among a broad range of services. To gain even more economies of scale and scope, both provincial governments reduced the number of RHAs. Saskatchewan consolidated down from 33 to 13 RHAs in 2002, while Manitoba moved from 11 to five RHAs in 2012. Still, neither province has gone as far as Alberta in creating a single RHA; they have pursued alternative strategies, including Saskatchewan's Shared Services initiative.

In terms of process reforms, Saskatchewan has been a leader in Canada in the introduction of Lean processes to improve both quality and efficiency. Manitoba has tended to rely more heavily on a substitution strategy, being the first jurisdiction in Canada to promote physician assistants. More recently, the Manitoba government facilitated the establishment of QuickCare clinics, which rely on nurse practitioners and registered nurses to provide a variety of basic treatment and diagnostic services. Both strategies have some potential to bend the cost curve, but it will take years of experimentation to determine the precise impact these reforms will have on bringing costs down without damaging access or quality.

References

Adams, D. 2001. "The White and the Black Horse Race: Saskatchewan Health Reform in the 1990s." In *Saskatchewan Politics: Into the Twenty-First Century*, edited by H. Leeson, 267–93. Regina: CPRC Press.

Axelsson, R., G. P. Marchildon, and J. R. Repullo-Labrador. 2007. "Effects of Decentralization on Managerial Dimensions of Health Systems." In *Decentralization in*

Health Care, edited by R. B. Saltman, V. Bankauskaite, and K. Vrangbæk, 141–66. New York: McGraw Hill and Open University Press.

CFNU (Canadian Federation of Nurses' Unions). 2011. *Overview of Key Nursing Contract Provisions*. Ottawa: CFNU.

CIHI (Canadian Institute for Health Information). 2011a. *National Health Expenditure Trends, 1975–2011*. Ottawa: CIHI.

————. 2011b. *Health Care Cost Drivers: The Facts*. Ottawa: CIHI.

————. 2012a. National Health Expenditure Database, 1975–2011. Ottawa: CIHI.

————. 2012b. *Canadian Hospital Reporting Project 2012: Financial Indicator Trending*. Ottawa: CIHI.

————. 2012c. National Physician Database, 2010–2011 Data Release. Ottawa: Canadian Institute for Health Information.

————. 2012d. *Canadian Hospital Reporting Project: Technical Notes for Financial Indicators*. Ottawa: CIHI.

————. 2012e. *Health Indicators 2012*. Ottawa: CIHI.

Di Matteo, L. 2003. "The Income Elasticity of Health Care Spending: A Comparison of Parametric and Nonparametric Approaches." *European Journal of Health Economics* 4, no. 1: 20–29. http://dx.doi.org/10.1007/s10198-002-0141-6.

————. 2010. "The Sustainability of Public Health Expenditures: Evidence from the Canadian Federation." *European Journal of Health Economics* 11, no. 6: 569–84. http://dx.doi.org/10.1007/s10198-009-0214-x.

Donaldson, C. 2010. "Fire, Aim … , Ready? Alberta's Big Bang Approach to Healthcare Disintegration." *Health Care Policy* 6, no. 1: 22–31.

Drummond, D. 2011. "Therapy or Surgery? A Prescription for Canada's Health System." Benefactors Lecture. Toronto: C. D. Howe Institute.

Duckett, S. 2010. "Second Wave Reform in Alberta." *Healthcare Management Forum* 23, no. 4: 156–58. http://dx.doi.org/10.1016/j.hcmf.2010.08.006.

————. 2011. "Getting the Foundations Right: Alberta's Approach to Health-Care Reform." *Health Policy* 6, no. 3: 22–26.

Fine, B. A., B. Golden, R. Hannan, and D. Morra. 2009. "Leading Lean: A Canadian Healthcare Leaders' Guide." *Healthcare Quarterly* 12, no. 3: 32–41. http://dx.doi.org/10.12927/hcq.2013.20877.

Fogel, R. W. 2009. "Forecasting the Cost of U.S. Healthcare in 2040." *Journal of Policy Modeling* 31, no. 4: 482–88. http://dx.doi.org/10.1016/j.jpolmod.2009.05.004.

Getzen, T. E. 2000. "Health Care Is an Individual Necessity and a National Luxury: Applying Multilevel Decision Models to the Analysis of Health Care Expenditures." *Journal of Health Economics* 19, no. 2: 259–70. http://dx.doi.org/10.1016/S0167-6296(99)00032-6.

IHI (Institute for Healthcare Improvement). 2005. *Going Lean in Health Care*. Cambridge, MA: ICI.

James, M. 1999. "Closing Rural Hospitals in Saskatchewan: On the Road to Wellness?" *Social Science and Medicine* 49, no. 8: 1021–34. http://dx.doi.org/10.1016/S0277-9536(99)00180-X.

Johnson, J. E., A. L. Smith, and K. A. Mastro. 2012. "From Toyota to the Bedside: Nurses Can Lead the Lean Way in Health Care Reform." *Nursing Administration Quarterly* 36, no. 3: 234–42. http://dx.doi.org/10.1097/NAQ.0b013e318258c3d5.

Jones, I. W., and R. S. Hooker. 2011. "Physician Assistants in Canada: An Update on Health Policy Initiatives." *Canadian Family Physician/Médecin de famille canadien* 57, no. 3: e83–88.

Lemstra, M., and C. Neudorf. 2008. *Health Disparity in Saskatoon: Analysis to Intervention*. Saskatoon: Saskatoon Health Region.

Manitoba. 2012. *Focused on What Matters Most: Manitoba's Plan to Protect Universal Health Care*. Winnipeg: Government of Manitoba.

Marchildon, G. P. 2004. "Introduction: The Many Worlds of Fiscal Sustainability." In *The Fiscal Sustainability of Health Care in Canada*, edited by G. P. Marchildon, 3–23. Toronto: University of Toronto Press.

———. 2006. "Regionalization and Health Services Restructuring in Saskatchewan." In *Health Services Restructuring in Canada: New Evidence and New Directions*, edited by C. M. Beach, R. P. Chaykowski, S. Shortt, F. St-Hilaire, and A. Sweetman, 33–57. Montreal: McGill-Queen's University Press for the John Deutsch Institute for the Study of Economic Policy.

———. 2013a. *Health Systems in Transition: Canada*. Toronto: University of Toronto Press.

———. 2013b. "Implementing Lean Health Reforms in Saskatchewan." *Health Reform Observer/Observatoire des réformes de santé* 1, no. 1. http://dx.doi.org/10.13.162/hro-ors.01.01.01

Marchildon, G. P., and H. Mou. 2013. "The Conservative 10-year Canada Health Transfer Plan: Another Fix for a Generation?" In *How Ottawa Spends, 2013–2014. The Harper Government: Mid-term Blues and Long-term Plans*, edited by C. Stoney and G. B. Doern, 47–63. Montreal: McGill-Queen's University Press.

Martens, P. J., J. Bartlett, E. Burland, H. Prior, C. Burchill, S. Huq, L. Romphf, J. Sanguins, S. Carter, and A. Bailly. 2010. *Profile of Metis Health Status and Healthcare Utilization in Manitoba: A Population-Based Study*. Winnipeg: Manitoba Centre for Health Policy.

Martens, P. J., R. Bond, L. Jebamani, C. Burchill, N. Roos, S. Derksen, M. Beaulieu, C. Steinbach, L. MacWilliam, R. Walld, et al. 2002. *The Health and Healthcare Use of Registered First Nations Peoples Living in Manitoba: A Population-Based Study*. Winnipeg: Manitoba Centre for Health Policy.

McIntosh, T., and G. P. Marchildon. 2008. "The Fyke in the Road: Health Reform in Saskatchewan from Romanow to Calvert and Beyond." In *Saskatchewan Politics: Crowding the Centre*, edited by H. Leeson, 337–53. Regina: CPRC Press.

Papadopoulos, T. 2011. "Continuous Improvement and Dynamic Actor Associations: A Study of Lean Thinking Implementation in the UK National Health Service." *Leadership in Health Services* 24, no. 3: 207–27. http://dx.doi.org/10.1108/17511871111151117.

Saskatchewan. 2012. *Ministry of Health Plan for 2012–13*. Regina: Government of Saskatchewan.

Saskatchewan Health Quality Council. 2012. *Accelerating Excellence in Saskatchewan*. Series of articles for *Healthcare Quarterly*. Saskatoon: Saskatchewan Health Quality Council.

Statistics Canada. 2011a. *Population Projections for Canada, Provinces and Territories, 2009 to 2036*. Cat. no. 91–520-X. Ottawa: Statistics Canada.

———. 2011b. *Provincial and Territorial Economic Accounts*. Cat. no. 13–018-XWE. Ottawa: Statistics Canada.

fourteen
Atlantic Canada: The Impact of Aging on the Cost Curve

JOE RUGGERI[1]

Introduction

The sustainability of the current system of public financing of health care in Canada is the subject of a long-standing and increasingly polarized debate among policymakers, media pundits, and scholars.[2] This paper focuses on the four Atlantic provinces, where the foundations of fiscal stability have been shaken by recent federal and provincial income tax reductions, deteriorating economic conditions, and mounting pressures on health-care spending caused by acceleration in the rate of population aging. The aging effect may be stronger in Atlantic Canada because of its projected faster rate of population aging. Individually these provinces account for a small share of the Canadian population, but they have common features that facilitate aggregation for the purpose of analysis.

The question of fiscal sustainability is addressed by analyzing trends in health-care spending from 1998 to 2009 and identifying the major cost drivers and their relative contribution. It shows that for Atlantic Canada, as for the rest of Canada, the effect of non-demographic factors—extra health-spending inflation, increasing utilization, and technological changes—on the growth of inflation-adjusted health-care spending was higher than the combined effect of population growth and aging. The chapter then projects key economic and fiscal indicators to 2031 for two scenarios, with details on the methodology in the appendix. The results show that, for all provinces and territories combined, the effect of demographic factors on health-care spending over the period from 2011 to 2031 will be lower than that from 1998 to 2009, with the aging effect more than offset by a lower rate of population growth. However, the opposite result is found for Atlantic Canada. A stronger aging effect is compounded by a projected higher rate of population growth. Finally, the chapter discusses by health expenditure category the

1 I am thankful to James Ayles, Livio Di Matteo, Mike Joyce, Greg Marchildon, and Shaun MacNeill for providing relevant information and helpful comments.
2 A comprehensive review of studies on ways to reform the Canadian health-care system is found in Prada and Brown (2012).

main policy instruments introduced recently by the four Atlantic provinces to curb health-expenditure growth. The concluding section summarizes the results and points out that the issue of health-care sustainability in Atlantic Canada has both spending and revenue dimensions. In particular, it indicates that the current structure of federal transfers for health care is biased against provinces with above-average rates of population aging.

Spending pressures in health care: The past 20 years[3]

A key pressure on health spending in Atlantic Canada is rooted in demographics. The long-term sustainability of Canada's publicly financed health-care system depends on the growth of public spending on health care, the capacity of the existing revenue structure to finance it, and the performance of the economy, all of which in turn are affected by demography. A summary indicator of population aging is the median age of the population. Values of this indicator for 2011 and 2031 are shown in Table 14.1, which demonstrates population aging in Canada and each of the four Atlantic provinces, with Atlantic Canada aging at a faster rate than the country as a whole. Table 14.2 shows that, for both Canada and Atlantic Canada, the share of the population 65 years and over will increase substantially, but the rate of increase will be higher in Atlantic Canada. As well, as Table 14.3 shows, Atlantic Canada historically has serious difficulties attracting and retaining immigrants. Although there has been a noticeable upward trend during the past decade, even the highest population share of net immigration into Atlantic Canada (2009–10) still amounts to only 40% of the national average.

Table 14.1 Median age of population, Canada and Atlantic provinces, 2011 and 2031

	2011	2031	Change
Canada	39.9	42.8	2.9
Newfoundland and Labrador	43.8	49.2	5.4
Prince Edward Island	42.1	45.1	3.0
Nova Scotia	43.0	45.9	2.9
New Brunswick	43.0	47.3	4.3
Atlantic Canada	43.3	46.9	3.6

Source: Author's calculations, based on Statistics Canada 2011a, Projection M-1, Tables 11–1 to 11–5.

3 The data used in this section are found in reports and databases published by the Canadian Institute for Health Information (CIHI).

Table 14.2 Population shares of selected age groups, Canada and Atlantic provinces, 2011 and 2031

| | Age Group | | | |
	0–4	5–19	20–64	65+
Canada				
2011	5.6	17.2	62.8	14.4
2031	5.2	16.8	55.2	22.8
Change	−0.4	−0.4	−7.6	8.4
Atlantic Canada				
2011	4.7	16.2	62.8	16.3
2031	4.2	14.7	53.0	28.1
Change	−0.5	−1.5	−9.8	11.8
Difference				
2011	0.9	1.0	0.0	−1.9
2031	1.0	2.1	2.2	−5.3

Source: Author's calculations, based on Statistics Canada 2011a, Projection M-1, Tables 11–1 to 11–5.

Table 14.3 Immigration and interprovincial migration, Canada and Atlantic provinces, selected years

| | % of Population | | |
	Net Immigration	Net Interprovincial Migration	Total Migration
Canada			
2001–02	0.70	—	0.70
2006–07	0.69	—	0.69
2009–10	0.75	—	0.75
Atlantic Canada			
2001–02	0.06	−0.23	−0.17
2006–07	0.18	−0.50	−0.32
2009–10	0.30	0.06	0.36

Source: Statistics Canada 2011b, Tables 1.2–1 to 1.2–5.

The major forces driving demographic change—natural increase (or decrease), immigration, and interprovincial migration—together will produce over the next 20 years a population in Atlantic Canada that will grow at a lower rate than the national average and age at a faster rate than the national average. These differences will have important implications for economic growth, health-care spending, and fiscal sustainability in Atlantic Canada.

For the period from 1998 to 2009, provincial/territorial health expenditures (in current dollars) increased at an average annual rate of 7.0% in Atlantic Canada and 7.4% for the country as a whole. Following the approach used by CIHI (2011c), I identify three categories of cost drivers: general inflation, demographic changes, and other factors. The first cost driver is measured by the trend in the implicit price deflator for current government expenditures. I applied the same rate to Canada and to the Atlantic region, with any differences between the two captured by the "other" category. Demographic factors include growth of the population and changes in its age structure. The effect of population aging was measured by comparing the growth rates of two hypothetical levels of health spending in 2009. The first was derived by multiplying the per capita health expenditures by selected age group in 1998 by the actual population in 2009. In the second, the same procedure was repeated by using the 2009 level of the population with its 1998 age distribution. The effect of all other factors was calculated as a residual, a catch-all category that includes excess inflation in the health-care sector, increases in utilization, and technological change. For the Atlantic region it also includes excess growth of its implicit price deflator over the national growth. The results are shown in Table 14.4.

For the country as a whole, general inflation accounted for 40% of the increase in health-care spending by provincial and territorial governments, while demographic factors added 26%, split almost evenly between population growth and population aging. The remaining cost drivers had an impact nearly one-third higher than that of demographic factors. Inflation-adjusted spending increased at an average annual rate of 4.4%, with population aging accounting for slightly less than 1 percentage point of this growth, or 21%.

Health-care spending by provincial governments in Atlantic Canada increased at a slightly lower rate. As discussed above, the aging effect was stronger in Atlantic Canada, reflecting its faster rate of population aging, but the overall effect was 43% lower because its population level fell slightly while that of Canada increased by 1% per year. The contribution of "other" cost drivers was 20% higher in Atlantic Canada, partly because of its higher rate of inflation of government current expenditures (0.33 percentage point). The contribution of the "other" category, net of this extra general inflation, was very similar for both Canada (2.47%) and Atlantic Canada (2.63%). From 1998 to 2009, provincial government spending on health care in Atlantic Canada, adjusted for the national level of inflation, grew by 4.1% per year. Population aging contributed 1.2 percentage points, or 29%, to this growth.

Table 14.4 Cost drivers of health care by provincial/territorial governments, 1998–2009

	Canada		Atlantic Canada	
	% Points	%	% Points	%
Total growth (average annual rate)	7.37		7.02	
Contribution by				
General inflation*	2.95	40.0	2.95	42.0
Population growth	1.02	13.8	−0.09	−1.3
Population aging	0.93	12.6	1.20	17.1
Subtotal: Demographic factors	1.95	26.4	1.11	15.8
Other	2.47	33.6	2.96	42.2
Growth of inflation-adjusted spending	4.42		4.07	
Growth of real GDP	2.38		2.43	

* Implicit price deflator for current government expenditures in Canada.
Source: Author's calculations, based on: CIHI 2011a; Statistics Canada 2011c, Tables 3 and 5.

The growth of inflation-adjusted health-care spending by provincial/territorial governments exceeded the growth rate of real GDP, implying that the ratio of health expenditures to GDP increased over time. The magnitude of this increase was slightly higher for the country as a whole (1.9 percentage points) than for the four Atlantic provinces combined (1.7 percentage points). Also, in 2009 the share of provincial government revenues in Atlantic Canada claimed by health-care expenditures was 5.1 percentage points lower than the national average.[4]

The next 20 years

Two forecasting scenarios are presented. In the first scenario, real provincial/territorial health-care spending is assumed to increase at a rate determined by known cost drivers: (a) the effect of demographic factors over the period from 2011 to 2031, and (b) continuation of the growth rate of non-demographic factors that occurred from 1998 to 2009. The population-growth effect in this first scenario is based on Statistics Canada's

---

4 Author's calculations.

Table 14.5 Projected contribution of demographic factors to growth of real provincial/territorial health-care spending, 2009–2031

| | Contribution (% Points) | |
	Canada	Atlantic Canada
Population growth	1.01	0.37
Population aging	0.97	1.41
Total	1.98	1.78

Source: Author's calculations, based on CIHI 2011b and Statistics Canada 2011a.

medium population projection (M1), and the population aging effect was calculated in the same manner as for the 1998–2009 period, by using per capita provincial/territorial health-care spending in 2009. Table 14.5 shows that for Canada as a whole, demographic factors will make the same contribution to health spending as they did during the 1998–2009 period, because a slight reduction in the contribution of population growth is offset by a small increase in the contribution of population aging.

Different conditions materialize in Atlantic Canada, as both demographic factors will have stronger effects. Population growth is projected to become positive and the population aging effect will rise substantially. As a result, the contribution of demographic factors to provincial government health-care spending will increase from 1.11 percentage points in 1998–2009 to 1.78 percentage points in 2011–31. It should be noted that population growth and population aging have different effects on health-care spending. For a given age distribution, an increase in the population puts pressure on health-care spending by raising the demand for health services and leaving per capita spending unchanged. In contrast, population aging alone affects health-care spending by raising the average per capita expenditure.

Health-care sustainability indicators for the first scenario are shown in Table 14.6, assuming that the contribution of non-demographic factors to real health expenditures by provincial and territorial governments will continue at the same level as during the period from 1998 to 2009. For Atlantic Canada, the differential increase in the implicit deflator for government current expenditures is assumed to vanish. As explained in the Appendix, it is assumed that real GDP will increase at an average annual rate of 2.1% in Canada and 1.7% in Atlantic Canada, and that provincial/territorial government revenues will rise in line with real GDP, minus the reduction in federal transfers resulting from the change in 2014–15 to a pure per capita transfer. This scenario addresses the following

Table 14.6 Scenario 1: ratio of real health-care spending by provincial/territorial governments to GDP and government revenues, 2011 and 2031

	2011	2031	Change	Average Annual % Change
Health expenditures (no inflation, C$ million)				
Canada	130,344	311,358	181,014	4.45
Atlantic Canada	9,942	23,567	13,625	4.41
	Ratio to GDP			
Canada	7.9	12.4	4.5	
Atlantic Canada	9.7	16.3	6.6	
	Ratio to Revenues			
Canada	43.3	68.3	25.0	
Atlantic Canada	39.8	67.3	27.5	

Sources: Author's calculations, based on Statistics Canada 2011c; Canada, Department of Finance 2011; provincial and territorial government figures for 2012; and appendix to this chapter.

question: If the experience of 1998–2009 with non-demographic cost drivers is repeated over the next 20 years, what share of GDP and provincial government revenues will be claimed by health-care spending in 2031? The answer to this question is shown in Table 14.6.

In this scenario, inflation-adjusted health expenditures expand at similar average annual growth rates for both Canada and Atlantic Canada. This rate of growth would be more than double that of real GDP and real government revenues. As a result, the ratio of health spending to GDP and revenues rises substantially over the next 20 years. For the country as a whole, the GDP ratio would increase by 4.5 points (57%), reaching 12.4% in 2031, and the revenue ratio would increase by 25 percentage points. By 2031, health spending would claim more than two-thirds of the combined revenues of all provinces and territories. A similar pattern would materialize in Atlantic Canada. The real GDP ratio would rise at a faster rate than for Canada (6.6 percentage points, or 68%), because of the slower projected growth of real GDP, and would reach 16% in 2031. A larger increase would also occur in the revenue ratio, which would rise by 28 percentage points and reach 67% in 2031.

Such large increases in the revenue share of health spending would leave limited resources for financing other provincial government programs. In Atlantic Canada, to maintain the same fiscal balance as in 2011, real expenditures for non-health programs would have to decline by an

Table 14.7 Scenario 2: growth of real health-care spending by provincial/territorial governments, ratio to GDP and government revenues constant at 2011 value

	Average Annual % Change, 2011–2031
Health expenditures (no inflation, C$ million)	
Canada	2.10
Atlantic Canada	1.70
Demographic Factors	
Canada	1.98
Atlantic Canada	1.78

Sources: Author's calculations, based on Statistics Canada 2011c; Canada, Department of Finance 2011; provincial and territorial government figures for 2012; and appendix to this chapter.

average of 1.36% per year. By 2031, real spending for these programs would be 24% lower than it was in 2011.

In the second scenario, it is assumed that the ratio of real provincial expenditures on health care to real GDP remains constant at its 2011 level, meaning that real health-care spending will grow at the same rate as real GDP, namely, 2.1% per year for all Canadian provinces and 1.7% a year for Atlantic Canada. This case addresses the following question: what portion of the cost drivers can be financed if the ratio of health-care expenditure to GDP is not allowed to increase from its 2011 level? The answer to this question is shown in Table 14.7. For the country as a whole, a growth rate of real provincial/territorial health-care spending of 2.1% per year will be capable of covering the cost pressures from demographic factors. However, only 5% of the cost pressures from non-demographic factors experienced during 1998–2009 can be financed by this constrained growth of health spending. In Atlantic Canada, a constant ratio to real GDP will not be sufficient even to pay for the cost arising from demographic pressures. Although the spending pressures from demographic factors will be lower in Atlantic Canada—primarily because of substantially lower population growth—population aging will have a much higher effect on labour supply, employment, and real GDP in the Atlantic region.[5]

---

5 There is an additional issue. Starting in 2017–18, the growth rate of the Canada Health Transfer will track a three-year moving average of the growth of nominal GDP. If inflation runs at an

The governments of the Atlantic provinces have three painful fiscal options for addressing the spending pressures from accelerated rates of population aging: (1) they can raise taxes as spending pressures mount, (2) they can shift higher taxes to future generations by borrowing, or (3) they can cut spending for other programs. Under any of these three options, maintaining current standards of health-care services requires a reduction in private consumption (for current or future generations) or a reduction in the consumption of public services. The painful effects of the above fiscal measures could be mitigated through measures that will reduce the cost of providing a certain health-care service, thus "bending the cost curve." The extent to which this supplemental policy option is being implemented by provincial governments in Atlantic Canada is discussed in the rest of this chapter.

Bending the cost curve in health care

The overwhelming share of government spending on health care in Atlantic Canada (see Table 14.8) is used for direct health services, with the lion's share going to acute care, which is delivered by hospitals (nearly half of the total) and other institutions (15%). In evaluating efforts at bending the cost curve, it is important to distinguish between changes in the level of spending and changes in rates of growth. For example, a one-time reduction in administrative costs will shift the curve downwards but will not affect the long-term growth rate. Also, controlling health-care costs by reducing the quality of services or shifting the cost to patients does not really bend the cost curve but rather shifts the burden from the public to the private sector. Moreover, part of the costs shifted to individuals will be borne by governments through personal income tax credits for medical expenses.

Policymakers in Atlantic Canada have started to address health-care spending issues by using both general and targeted measures. The general measures represent initial responses that followed the path of least resistance, focusing on internal adjustments that did not affect service delivery. These general measures included wage freezes for civil servants, restructuring of departmental organization, and moratoriums on hiring. With administration accounting for a minute share of total health-care spending, it soon became clear that structural adjustments were needed. Some targeted measures have been introduced, while others are under consideration. Since making structural changes to the delivery of health care requires courageous

---

average of 2% per year, the new formula will cut the growth rate of real federal transfers almost in half (from 4% to 2.1%). Compared to the current formula, the new formula will by 2031 lead to a reduction in the real value of the transfer of nearly C$1 billion to the Atlantic provinces.

Table 14.8 Atlantic Canada provincial government spending on health care by use of funds, 2011

Function	% of Health-Care Spending, 2011	Average Annual % Change		
		1975–2011	1990–2011	2005–2011
Hospitals	46.0	6.83	4.37	6.46
Other institutions	14.7	10.40	7.16	8.00
Physicians	18.4	7.96	6.16	6.54
Other professionals	0.4	3.96	−1.02	7.13
Drugs	6.8	11.50	6.41	6.98
Capital	3.5	4.83	4.09	5.29
Public health	3.7	7.90	6.53	8.37
Administration	1.9	7.52	7.10	7.61
Other	4.6	12.03	8.01	8.27
Total	100.0	7.60	5.35	6.87
Inflation*		4.30	2.41	2.86
Inflation-adjusted		3.30	2.94	4.01

* Implicit price deflator for current government expenditures in Canada.
Source: Author's calculations, based on CIHI 2011b.

and painful political decisions, provincial governments first try to gain some political cover by seeking recommendations from separate bodies. One example is the establishment of the Office of Health Systems Renewal in New Brunswick in 2012; its purpose is "identification and implementation of health innovation and best practices most promising to health renewal in New Brunswick." Another targeted measure is the gradual introduction of electronic health records. Although this initiative will actually add to cost pressures in the short term, it has the potential to enhance the effectiveness of health-care delivery over the long run. Provincial governments have also begun to take specific steps to curb the growth of health-care spending.

Prevention

There are two categories of policies under disease prevention. The first is confined to government policies directed at reducing the incidence of illness through the programs of ministries of health. The second category includes all other government policies that may affect a person's health status, directly or indirectly, but that are aimed at non-health objectives.

Although prevention may be thought of as a pre-care activity, in the operations of health departments and in the National Health Expenditure (NHEX) database, it is categorized as public health. This includes traditional programs directed at communicable disease control (immunization), environmental health (air and water quality), food safety, and health emergency preparedness, as well as more recent programs focusing on healthy living. All four Atlantic provinces have introduced these newer prevention programs; their focus is primarily on expectant mothers, early childhood, school-age children, and youth.

There are three major obstacles to the formulation and implementation of effective long-term prevention programs. First, the determinants of healthy living that are under the control of individuals remain an individual choice. Thus, although healthy living may generate large externalities, the extent to which it is amenable to policy influences remains an open question. Second, prevention cannot be compartmentalized, because the determinants and effects of health status are widespread and transcend the mandates of single departments. This is particularly true for children. Healthy children not only impose lower health costs on society but also perform better in school and, later, become more productive workers (see Ruggeri 2006), thereby also boosting government revenues. Thus prevention policies become instruments of human capital development. Third, public policy is often framed within a short-term horizon, while the benefits of prevention tend to materialize over the long run.

Without ignoring the permanent need to search for efficiencies in public service delivery, prevention is an area where spending cuts would likely be self-defeating and where cost savings from cutting public health programs would be minimal. In Atlantic Canada, public health accounts for less than 4% of total provincial government health-care spending. Moreover, in this region, spending on public health as a percentage of total health-care spending is less than half the national average.[6]

Physicians

In 2011, payments to physicians accounted for 18.4% of health-care spending by provincial governments in Atlantic Canada (18.8%, if other professionals are included). Total expenditures on physicians' services (E) can be

---

6 Author's calculations, based on CIHI 2011b.

expressed as the product of the total number of services provided (S) and the average cost of each service (AC):

(1) $E = S \times AC$

If all payments were under a fee-for-service (FFS) arrangement, AC would measure the average fee charged per unit of service. Expression (1) can be rewritten as:

(2) $E = P\,(D/P)(S/D) \times AC,$

where P = population, D = number of doctors, and S = number of services provided.

The growth of expenditures can be approximated by the sum of the growth rates of four components in (2), with different potential for government policy. Population growth is exogenous. The number of doctors serving a given population depends partly on private decisions (enrolment in medical school, location choice after graduation) and partly on government policy. The number of service units performed on average by each physician is partly endogenous, originating with an individual who perceives the need to consult a physician. It also depends on the size and age distribution of the population and on the factors that affect population health. The physician, however, determines the number of follow-up services and referrals to specialists.

Government policy is confined largely to determination of the health services it will pay for in terms of the coverage basket. The average cost per unit of service depends on negotiated arrangements between the government and the physicians' bargaining unit. Although there are a variety of payment arrangements—the traditional fee for service and alternative approaches such as capitation, salary, contract, or block funding—each type of arrangement is the result of negotiations between two monopolists: the government and the medical association.

With respect to fee-for-service (FFS) payments, a report on cost drivers by CIHI (2011c) concluded that, from 1998 to 2008, "increases in fee schedules contributed more than half (3.6%) of the growth" of total FFS payments, adding that "physician remuneration grew faster than the average weekly wage of other health and social services workers during the past decade" (p. 20). The main policy tool used by provincial governments in Atlantic Canada to affect physician expenditure has been a shift to alternative payments for physicians. As shown in Table 14.9, from 1999–2000 to 2009–10, the share of alternative payments in total clinical payments increased in all four provinces. The highest increases in percentage points were recorded in Prince Edward Island and Nova Scotia; by 2009–10 the share of alternative

Table 14.9 Spending on alternative payments as percentage of total clinical payments

Province	Share (%)		
	1999–2000	2009–10	Change
Newfoundland and Labrador	27.3	31.7	4.4
Prince Edward Island	22.4	41.2	18.8
Nova Scotia	27.2	45.3	18.1
New Brunswick	16.4	31.3	14.9

Source: CIHI 2011d, Tables A.1.1 and A.1.3.

payments in those two provinces exceeded 40%. There is no conclusive evidence, however, that this change in the type of payments had a significant effect on the growth of spending on physicians' services.

Provincial governments have also tried to introduce ad hoc short-term cost-containing measures through negotiations. For example, the New Brunswick government was able to secure a two-year freeze on fee levels for physicians. The Prince Edward Island government has taken a more general approach by planning to hold the annual growth rate of health care at 3.5%. However, given the interprovincial competition for physicians and the difficulty of attracting and retaining physicians in rural areas, the potential for restraint in payments to physicians to make a major contribution to bending the health-care cost curve remains very limited.

Hospitals

The overwhelming majority of Canadian hospitals are operated by not-for-profit entities—private or publicly controlled organizations such as community boards of trustees or regional health authorities—that often manage a variety of facilities. Provincial governments provide most of the funding for these entities, which is negotiated annually between the boards or regional authorities and the government. In Newfoundland and Labrador, Prince Edward Island, and Nova Scotia, the final amount is set by ministerial discretion. In New Brunswick, funding is determined by a line-by-line approach, that is, negotiations on specific services, the sum of which in the end determines the total amount of government support.

Hospitals represent the largest share of total provincial government health-care spending. In Atlantic Canada this share in 2011 was 46%, two and a half times the share of spending on physicians. It will not be possible to meaningfully bend the cost curve in health-care spending without curbing the growth of spending on hospitals. So far, the measures introduced by provincial governments—the merging of various administrative units

(Nova Scotia), interprovincial co-operation (Prince Edward Island), more in-depth scrutiny of specific expenditures (New Brunswick)—are capable of generating relatively small savings. Moreover, these may be short-term savings only, with little impact on the long-term growth rate.

Other institutions

The category "other institutions" refers to various types of long-term care facilities where the chronically ill or disabled live more or less permanently. It includes homes for the aged (nursing homes) and residential facilities for people with physical or psychological disabilities or alcohol and drug problems, and children with emotional problems. This category accounted for nearly 15% of health spending by provincial governments in Atlantic Canada. Moreover, it has been the fastest-growing area of health budgets over the past 20 years. The major spending pressures in this category come from the long-term care facilities for the aged. The care of aging parents is still largely a family responsibility. However, provincial governments have decided as a matter of policy to provide financial assistance to families that do not have sufficient financial means. Provincial governments set the daily rates in nursing homes and cover the difference between those rates and what clients can afford, based on a means test.

The major cost-containment initiative by provincial governments in Atlantic Canada is the expansion of home care, an initiative that tries to keep seniors in their homes as long as possible, thus avoiding pressures to build additional facilities. Home-care services are largely non-medical in nature, so the overall cost of care is lower than in a nursing home or even in assisted living facilities. Thus, even if the health-care costs did not change, the overall cost to government would be reduced. Moreover, eliminating the shock of leaving one's home and being separated from family members and friends, as well as providing an opportunity to continue in familiar routines, may contribute to better health, thus lessening the cost pressures arising from population aging. Recognizing the benefits of home care for both the client's well-being and the public purse, all four provincial governments in Atlantic Canada have committed additional funds in their more recent budgets.

Drugs

All Atlantic provinces offer financial assistance for drug costs incurred by low-income seniors, residents of nursing homes, clients of departments of social services or social development, and individuals with selected medical conditions such as multiple sclerosis and cystic fibrosis. The coverage of these programs differs somewhat among provinces. In addition, the governments of Nova Scotia and Newfoundland and Labrador also offer a public drug program for the uninsured. The differences in coverage, particularly the different treatment of the uninsured, are reflected in per capita drug expenditures by the provincial governments. New Brunswick and Prince Edward Island spend almost identical per capita amounts, which are substantially lower than those of the other two Atlantic provinces. Overall, spending on drugs per person by provincial governments in Atlantic Canada is lower than the national average. Only in Nova Scotia does it exceed the national average.[7]

The main policy tool used so far to reduce spending on drugs is reducing the price of generic drugs from 45% to 35% of brand-name prices. This shifts the cost curve down in the short run but does not change its slope, thus having little effect on the growth rate of spending. Still, the level of spending over both the medium and long term will be lower than in the absence of the policy change.

Conclusions

Provincial governments in Atlantic Canada are aware of the fiscal pressures arising from the health-care sector and have started taking action, but public policy has been largely confined to restraint in administrative costs, short-term restraint on fees for physicians, and reductions in the price of generic drugs. The effect of these measures on the growth of health-care spending is quite modest. Whether provincial governments will be able to introduce bold structural changes is not yet known. Seeking efficiencies in the delivery of public services is an obligation of elected officials regardless of the fiscal situation, and an imperative under unsustainable fiscal conditions. Basing health policies on the belief that efficiencies in the delivery of services can secure sustainability of the publicly funded health-care system ignores fiscal realities and the complex factors that determine spending and cost pressures in health care.

The sustainability of Atlantic Canada's health-care systems has both cost and revenue dimensions, and provincial governments do not have the capacity to exercise full control over either of them. The demand for services is complex and affected by genetic factors, individual lifestyle choices, decisions by firms that affect the health status of people, working conditions and social developments, and government policies that affect the rate of unemployment and the level of poverty (a major determinant of population health) and allow persistence of negative health externalities. On the cost side, they are constrained by powerful interest groups and voters' reactions to drastic structural reforms. On the revenue side, they are constrained by the structure of federal transfers, which are largely controlled by the federal government.

---

7 Source: CIHI 2011b, Table D.4.

The existing formula for federal health transfers is biased against the Atlantic provinces because it fails to take into account the faster rate of population aging in the Atlantic region. The adjustments in 2014 (equal per capita payments) and 2017 (lower growth rate of transfers) will further aggravate the situation by cutting almost by half the growth in real federal transfers. Ruggeri and Zou (2004) suggest that this bias could be eliminated by introducing a special federal transfer related to a provincial rate of population aging in excess of the national average. The Senate Special Committee on Aging (Senate of Canada 2008) also recognized this issue and presented a variety of options, including the one proposed by Ruggeri and Zou.

The sustainability of publicly funded health systems in Atlantic Canada cannot be secured by relying exclusively on efficiency gains in the delivery of health-care services; it requires a coordinated and multifaceted approach that involves all stakeholders. In particular, individuals must take concrete steps towards healthier lifestyles; all levels of government must promote economic development policies aimed at reducing unemployment and the incidence of poverty; workplaces must be made safer and working conditions less stressful; provincial governments must be more aggressive in pursuing structural changes; and the federal government must honour its long-standing commitment to share the cost of financing health-care spending, taking into consideration interprovincial differences in spending pressures arising from population aging.

References

Canada. Department of Finance. 2011. *Economic and Fiscal Update*. Ottawa: Department of Finance.

CIHI (Canadian Institute for Health Information). 2011a. *National Health Expenditure Trends, 1975 to 2011, Report*. Ottawa: CIHI.

———. 2011b. *National Health Expenditures Database, 1975–2011*. Ottawa: CIHI.

———. 2011c. *Health Care Cost Drivers: The Facts*. Ottawa: CIHI.

———. 2011d. *National Physician Database*. Ottawa: CIHI.

Prada, G., and T. Brown. 2012. *The Canadian Health Care Debate: A Survey and Assessment of Key Studies*. Toronto: Conference Board of Canada.

Ruggeri, G. C., ed. 2006. "The Environment and the Health of Children." Fredericton: Policy Studies Centre, University of New Brunswick.

Ruggeri, J., and Y. Zou. 2004. *Population Aging and Per Capita Cash Payments under the Canada Health Transfer*. Ottawa: Caledon Institute of Social Policy.

Senate of Canada. Special Committee on Aging. 2008. *Issues and Options for an Aging Population: Second Interim Report*.

Statistics Canada. 2011a. *Population Projections for Canada, Provinces and Territories, 2009 to 2036*. Cat. no. 91–520-X. Ottawa: Statistics Canada.

———. 2011b. *Annual Demographic Estimates: Canada, Provinces and Territories*. Cat. no. 91–215-X. Ottawa: Statistics Canada.

———. 2011c. *Provincial and Territorial Economic Accounts*. Cat. no. 13–018-XWE. Ottawa: Statistics Canada.

Appendix

This appendix discusses the methodology used in my calculations with respect to cost drivers in health care, economic growth, and provincial/territorial government revenues. I followed the general approach used by the Canadian Institute for Health Information (CIHI 2011c), which identifies three major categories of cost drivers: general inflation, demographic factors, and non-demographic factors. For general inflation, I used the same index employed by CIHI, namely the implicit price deflator for government current expenditures. The two major demographic factors affecting health-care spending are population growth and population aging. For a given level of per capita health-care spending and a given age distribution of the population, the contribution of the former equals the average annual growth rate of the population.

The contribution of population aging was calculated as follows. For the period from 1998 to 2009 (the period for which detailed data on health spending by age group are available), I started with per capita provincial/territorial health-care spending by age group and the share of each age group of the population for Canada and Atlantic Canada. Next I estimated the population by age group in 2009, assuming the 1998 age distribution. Then I calculated total provincial/territorial health-care spending as the sum of the age-specific spending, derived as the product of 1998 age-specific per capita spending, and estimated the 2009 population with the 1998 age distribution. I repeated the above exercise using the actual age distribution of the 2009 population.

The difference in the average annual growth rates between the two scenarios yields the contribution of population aging to the growth of health spending. I performed the same calculations for the period 2009 to 2031 by using as a starting point the age distribution of the population in 2009 and the age-specific health-care spending for the same year. I applied the population growth and population aging effects to the analysis of projected trends from 2011 to 2031, using Statistics Canada's (2011) medium population projection M1.

The growth of real GDP can be measured as the growth of employment plus the growth of labour productivity (output per person employed).

Employment growth is determined by the interactions between the demand for and supply of labour. The demand for labour depends on both domestic and international developments, specifically demand by domestic and foreign consumers (individuals, businesses, and governments). The supply of labour depends upon the size of the working-age population (15 years and over), its age composition, and age-specific labour force participation rates. The bulk of the working-age population is in the age group between 20 and 64 years. This is also the age group with the highest participation rate. Statistics Canada's population projections indicate that, for the country as a whole, over the period from 2011 to 2031 this age group will grow at an average annual rate of 0.42%—less than half the growth of the entire population. There are limited opportunities for increasing this group's participation rates, which are already high. Participation rates are also unlikely to rise for those in the age group 15–19, as efforts are being made to reduce dropout rates and to increase participation in postsecondary education programs. The only boost to the participation rate will come from people over 65, especially those in the 65–75 age group. I have taken into consideration this potential effect and have assumed that, on average over the next 20 years, employment in Canada will increase by 0.6% per year.

Projections of labour productivity growth do not lend themselves to such a direct analysis; therefore I relied on existing projections from other sources. According to the fall 2011 Department of Finance economic and fiscal update, the private-sector forecast consensus assumes labour productivity growth of 1.1% per year from 2011 to 2016. I assumed a moderate acceleration of this growth in response to tightening labour market conditions and used a rate of 1.5% for the entire 20-year period. Thus, for the country as a whole I have assumed an average annual growth rate of real GDP of 2.1%.

The effect of population aging on the labour supply is much stronger in Atlantic Canada because the population in the 20–64 age group is projected to decline at an average annual rate of 0.44% from 2011 to 2031. I still assume positive employment growth over the entire period but at one-third the rate assumed for Canada, for the following reasons. First, there is still some slack in the labour supply, given the above-national-average unemployment rates. Second, participation rates are lower than the national average. Third, there is greater potential for increased labour supply from people 65 and over, because this age group will represent a larger share of the total population compared to the country as a whole. Assuming the same growth of labour productivity as for Canada yields an average growth rate of real GDP in Atlantic Canada of 1.7%.

For all provinces and territories combined, government revenues increased at about 80% of the rate of growth of GDP from 1998 to 2009, partly as a result of provincial tax cuts implemented in this period. Total revenues, however, increased at 94% of the growth of GDP. Similar results are found for Atlantic Canada, where during the same period total revenues increased by 91% of the growth of GDP. Since provincial and territorial governments will not have the fiscal capacity for further tax reductions in the time frame of my analysis, I assume that real government revenues will increase at the same rate as real GDP in both Canada and Atlantic Canada. From the value so derived for 2031, I subtracted $15 billion for the country as a whole and $1 billion from Atlantic Canada, which represents my estimates of revenue reduction from the new health-care financing formula.

PART IV

What Can Canada Learn from the International Evidence?

fifteen

The United States

GERARD ANDERSON

Introduction

It is not necessary to cite many numbers about the level of health-care spending in the United States, as they all tell the same story. Compared to all other countries in the world, the US is number one in nearly every category of health spending (Commonwealth Fund). As shown in Table 15.1, it spent considerably more than Canada and other OECD countries in 2009. The trends are even more troubling: if US health-care spending growth continues at its current pace, by 2030 all of the improvement in productivity in the US health-care economy will be going to pay for higher health-care bills (Chernew, Hirth, and Cutler 2009).

Instead of dwelling on the numbers showing the higher level of spending in the United States, this chapter discusses why the US has been so ineffective in controlling health-care spending, in spite of innumerable efforts. More specifically, the chapter argues why there is a lack of a political constituency for cost containment in the US. The discussion then turns to why the US is so expensive, discusses the more significant US cost-containment initiatives, presents what the US is likely to try in the future,

Table 15.1 Health spending in Canada, the United States, and other OECD countries, 2009

Indicator	Canada	United States	OECD Median
Per capita health spending ($)	4,363	7,960	3,180
% of GDP spent on health care	11.4	17.4	9.5
Public health spending per capita ($)	3,081	3,795	2,400
Private health spending per capita ($)	646	3,189	193
Hospital spending per discharge ($)	13,483	18,142	6,222

Source: OECD 2012.

makes some additional suggestions for controlling health spending, and offers some suggestions for Canada.

Why the US has failed to control health spending

Let's begin with a stakeholder analysis. Corporations, unions, individuals, health insurers, providers, and government should be concerned about the level of health-care spending, and all of them argue that cost containment is necessary for the United States. Therefore the more important question is, in spite of their statements, whether any of these stakeholders really want to control health-care spending.

US corporations should have a strong self-interest in cost containment, since private industry pays most of the health insurance premiums in the US. In addition, private industry pays taxes that support the public insurance programs, Medicare and Medicaid. A reason why these companies are not more aggressive in controlling health spending is that they profit from health care. If you examine the 25 largest corporations in the US (ranked by total revenues), only seven do not have a major portion of their revenues coming from the health-care industry (CNN 2012). These corporations are oil companies such as Exxon, auto companies such as Ford, and financial companies established by the US government (Fannie Mae and Ginnie Mae). Four of the largest 25 companies receive nearly all their revenues from health care (McKesson, CVS Caremark, Cardinal Health, and United HealthCare Group), while the others receive a significant portion of their total revenues from health-care services. For example, in 2011, General Electric had total revenues of $143 billion, with $18 billion coming from health care (General Electric 2012). If you broaden the list to include the entire Fortune 500, most of the companies have a significant health-care presence. This is not really surprising when you realize that health care represents 18% of the GDP and is one of the few industries in the US that is growing rapidly. In addition, many of the companies without a major presence in health care are philosophically opposed to the government's regulating any industry, so any policies that involve government regulation are generally opposed.

Unions should also have a strong interest in controlling health spending because, as most economists argue, corporations do not really pay for health insurance. In reality, it is the worker who pays the health insurance premium by accepting lower wages (Emanuel and Fuchs 2008). However, if you look at the unions with the largest enrolment, many are in the education and health-care sectors (US Bureau of Labor Statistics 2012). While these union members want lower health insurance premiums, they also want to maintain their jobs.

Individuals should also want to control health spending, because they are ultimately the ones that pay for health care. However, it is difficult for most individuals to understand how much it costs to provide health care. Moreover, because most Americans have health insurance, they are sheltered from paying directly for health services. There is a limited political constituency for rationing, queuing, or even taking costs into consideration when making a medical decision in the United States. Once insurance is paying the bill, the patient is less interested in how much it costs.

Health insurers should be a logical constituency for controlling health spending. However, there are several reasons why they have not been strong advocates for controlling spending. First, they receive an administrative fee for administering claims. Second, many of them want to insure hospitals, doctors, pharmaceutical companies, and other industries that provide health-care services. A health insurer known to deal aggressively with health-care providers is unlikely to be able to attract their business. Third, in many parts of the country, one private insurer is the dominant health insurer in that state, so there is little competition among private insurers.

Health-care providers are concerned about health-care spending, and many have taken action to reduce the level of spending. Some of those initiatives will be discussed later in this chapter, but the bottom line is that providers want to maximize their revenues. In most countries, government is the primary impetus for controlling health-care spending, because the government accounts for the majority of health funding. The United States is the only major OECD country where the public sector does not fund most health care. And it is an outlier in several other respects. First, the public health insurance programs, Medicare and Medicaid, were established as part of a political compromise in 1965 designed to minimize the ability of the government to control health spending. Cost containment was not the focus of the original design of the programs; in fact, hospitals were guaranteed to have their costs paid and physicians could have great latitude in setting their own prices. In addition, the Medicare and Medicaid programs are not permitted by law to interfere with the practice of medicine.

Second, compared to the private insurers, the government has been relatively aggressive in controlling health-care prices. The Medicare program pays 30% less on average than the private insurers, and the Medicaid program even less. The concern for public insurers such as Medicare and Medicaid is that lower prices could reduce access for their beneficiaries. Providers might not accept public patients if the rates are set too low compared to the private sector; indeed, this has already been an issue in some states.

Third, there is little consensus among politicians on the best approach to controlling health spending. One approach, advocated primarily by the Democrats, is to use regulation to control spending and to rely on providers to make the decisions about what is cost-effective medical care. A contrasting approach, favoured primarily by Republicans, is to allow the market to control spending and to give more information to individuals so they can make more informed decisions. The lack of a policy consensus on this fundamental issue explains why so little government policy has been implemented.

Finally, the lobbying process means that various interests exert considerable influence in protecting certain industries. For example, many large drug companies have their headquarters in the state of New Jersey, so it is not surprising that attempts to control drug prices are opposed by even liberal members of the New Jersey political establishment.

Prior attempts at cost containment

In spite of the lack of a political constituency for cost containment, the United States has attempted a whole series of initiatives going back as far as the 1920s. For example, the American Medical Association established a committee in 1926 designed to investigate and solve the problems associated with a rising level of medical-care spending. During the Second World War the US government made a tax policy decision that fostered the growth of private health insurance and set the country on a different course than most other OECD countries. The main implication of this tax decision was that the US relied on competition among private health insurers to control spending, while most other OECD countries (such as Canada) relied on government rate-setting and supply-side controls.

This raises an important policy question: have private insurers been able to control health-care spending in the United States? Most of the evidence suggests that they have not been successful. The first piece of evidence comes from reasonably long-term spending data. Over the 1970 to 2008 period, the annual rate of increase in per capita health-care spending in the private sector averaged 9.3% per year, compared to 8.3% in the Medicare program. Second, data from the Medicare Prospective Payment Assessment Commission (MedPAC) show that the private sector is paying 30% more to providers than Medicare for equivalent services. While some have argued that the Medicare program pays too little and private insurers have to pay more because of the cost shift, there is little domestic or international evidence to support the claim that hospitals, physicians, and pharmaceutical companies are underpaid in the United States.

Third, private insurers in the US have much higher administrative costs than public insurers. The typical public insurer has an administrative cost of 2–3%, while the administrative costs of private insurers routinely exceed 20%. Finally, one of the bargaining points with the hospitals and physicians in establishing the Medicare and Medicaid programs was a prohibition against the federal government's negotiating directly with providers. As part of this political deal, hospitals were paid their own costs and physicians were permitted to set their own rates.

Most cost-containment efforts have been government initiated. Federal initiatives include

- certificates of public need;
- President Nixon's wage and price controls;
- all-payer state rate setting;
- President Carter's hospital cost–containment legislation;
- the Medicare prospective payment system, or diagnosis-related groups (DRGs);
- the Medicare resource-based relative value scale (RBRVS); and
- the sustainable growth rate (SGR) system.

The "certificate of public need" was the US government's attempt at supply-side controls by limiting the amount of hospital beds and equipment; it is generally recognized to have been unsuccessful in controlling the number of beds or new technology. Most of the other attempts focused on prices paid to hospitals and doctors; some never passed or lasted only a short time (e.g., wage and price controls, cost containment).

The DRG system has been used since 1983 to control the rate of growth of hospital spending in the Medicare program. It is difficult to assess the impact of a large program such as the DRGs, since there is no reasonable control group, but most of the evidence suggests that it succeeded in controlling Medicare spending without having an adverse impact on access to or quality of care (Mayes and Berenson 2006). RBRVS has been used since 1989 to control physician spending in the Medicare program by establishing a fee schedule; it has also been successful in controlling Medicare spending, and most physicians still participate (Hsaio, Dunn, and Verrilli 1993). The SGR system was an attempt at a global budget for physician spending in the Medicare program; the idea was that if physician volume increased faster than projected, the payment rates would be reduced. However, the system was never allowed to go into effect.

The main private-sector cost-containment initiative was managed care. The most successful expansion of managed care occurred in the early to mid 1990s, when managed-care plans were able to contract with a limited number of providers and negotiate price reductions. However, the public did not like having restrictions placed on which providers they could use, and managed-care plans were forced to expand their panels of providers and thereby reduce their bargaining power with providers. Health insurance premiums increased at a much slower rate in the first half of the 1990s, as managed care was able to control providers. However, premiums went back up in the latter half of the 1990s, when the managed-care companies could no longer restrict the number of providers.

There were several initiatives to control spending in both the public and private sectors after 2000, but the next large initiative was the *Affordable Care Act*, also known as "Obamacare." Despite its title, the main purpose of the Act was to expand health insurance coverage rather than control health spending. Before the legislation was even debated, President Obama and Congress made deals with providers on the level of cost containment that each provider group would be expected to contribute. The rationale for negotiating those deals in advance was the experience of President Clinton's health-care reform initiative in the 1990s, when health-care providers were kept out of the political process. They were generally opposed to the legislation because they feared it would reduce their revenues.

Learning from this experience, President Obama and his team told the providers how much they needed in cost savings and recruited them to help develop the legislation. Because of this approach, the providers were more willing to support the legislation. The pharmaceutical industry, for example, had been fearful that the government would impose price controls within the Medicare program. Instead it negotiated a price reduction for drugs for certain Medicare beneficiaries and escaped any direct negotiation with Medicare over prices. President Obama and Congress got the savings they needed and the pharmaceutical industry got a policy it could accept.

The Congressional Budget Office projected that the *Affordable Care Act* would save $220 billion over the 2012 to 2021 period. However, some of those "savings" are price reductions to providers, while others are actually tax increases to the public. In Congressional Budget Office calculations, anything that lowers spending or increases revenues to the federal government is counted as savings.

Perhaps the most controversial provision in the *Affordable Care Act* is the creation of the Independent Payment Advisory Board (IPAB). As envisioned in the law, a 15-member board will propose ways to control rates of increase in Medicare spending. However, the board is prohibited from altering Medicare benefit design and will control spending primarily by limiting provider rates. The range of providers is limited, however, because some providers have already negotiated deals until 2019, and they will supposedly have immunity from further cuts until after that date. The projected $15 billion in savings will come mostly from physicians and home health-care services. However, it should also be noted that the IPAB will not address spending in the private sector. None of its members have been announced and it is unclear when the board will be established.

The initiative that has received the most attention is the Center for Medicare and Medicaid Innovation (CMMI). It provides $10 billion over 10 years to establish pilot programs that will work with public programs to lower health spending. The basic idea is that hospitals and physicians know how to reduce health-care spending and that it is the current set of rules and regulations and the current payment system that keep them from achieving those savings. The expectation is that reducing those rules and changing the financial incentives will encourage providers to devise alternatives that will lower spending and improve outcomes.

Affordable care organizations (ACOs) are the most visible initiative from the CMMI to date (Center for Medicare and Medicaid Services 2012). Their goal is to help patients, especially the chronically ill, get the right care at the right time while avoiding unnecessary duplication of services and preventing medical errors. When an ACO succeeds in both delivering high-quality care and spending health-care dollars more wisely, it will share in the savings it achieves for the Medicare program. Medicare offers several different ACO programs, depending on how much financial risk the provider is willing to accept. The Medicare Shared Savings Program helps Medicare fee-for-service providers become ACOs by allowing them to share in the savings if utilization in their community is lower than what Medicare projects; in that case the provider would get a bonus from Medicare. However, there are no penalties if the provider does not control utilization. The Advance Payment initiative is for plans that are willing to accept financial risk if they do not control utilization. The trade-off is that more potential savings are possible if they are able to control utilization, but there are financial penalties if they cannot. The Pioneer ACO Model is a program designed for health plans that have already implemented some form of coordinated care and have demonstrated success. Pioneer ACOs have the greatest possibilities of financial reward, but also the greatest financial risk. The projected savings for ACOs are quite small—in the $5 million to $1 billion range over the next several years.

Other initiatives in the *Affordable Care Act* that are not part of the CMMI include the Patient-Centered Outcomes Research Institute (PCORI), electronic medical records, a "Cadillac tax" on very expensive private health insurance benefits, some administrative savings, and savings from reduced fraud and abuse. None of these savings are expected to be substantial in the 2012 to 2021 period.

Moving forward

US policymakers and health services researchers are always coming up with new initiatives to control health-care spending. Some of the most discussed initiatives include introducing malpractice reform, creating comparative effectiveness entities, reducing regional practice variations, improving end-of-life care, increasing consumer cost-sharing, and changing the Medicare program from a defined benefit to a defined contributions program. A recent Institute of Medicine report found that the United States could save $750 billion a year if it made several changes to the health-care system, including eliminating unnecessary services ($210 billion), reducing excess administrative costs ($190 billion), eliminating inefficiently delivered services ($130 billion), lowering health-care prices ($105 billion), reducing fraud ($75 billion), and eliminating missed prevention opportunities ($55 billion) (Institute of Medicine 2011). These are mostly guidelines intended to inspire policymakers to take concrete action and to show them where the largest savings are possible. Most of these proposals have been discussed for years, but actually putting any of the options into practice has proven to be difficult.

Malpractice reform is the perennial favourite of physicians, who argue that malpractice premiums are too high and that malpractice suits lead to defensive medicine. When the Congressional Budget Office tried to determine how much in savings would be generated by changing the malpractice laws, it found they were not very large; there is in fact limited empirical evidence of substantial savings with malpractice reform (Elmendorf 2009). Second, malpractice premiums represent a small portion of total health spending. Trying to identify "defensive medicine" has also proven to be elusive.

Another approach is to look at geographic areas with high rates of utilization. Analysis of Medicare data by researchers at Dartmouth College found a two-to-one differential in medical-care spending across geographic areas. Additional research has shown that most of the variation occurs in services where there is considerable disagreement over the best clinical approach to addressing a medical problem. The Dartmouth researchers also noticed an association between geographic areas with the most physicians per capita and the most utilization per capita—hence the term *supplier-induced demand*. Their policy proposal therefore is to change the geographic distribution of physicians or, more recently, to change the economic incentives by encouraging the creation of ACOs. The problem with trying to alter the geographic distribution of physicians is that prior attempts to induce physicians to locate in medically underserved areas have generally been unsuccessful.

Medicare beneficiaries in their last six months of life spend approximately 30% of the Medicare budget (Hogan et al. 2001). Because the American public is opposed to rationing—or any other approach that will lead to limiting access to services that might prolong life—efforts have focused on benefits that will provide better care to Medicare beneficiaries through the hospice program, thereby saving money when a person with a terminal illness is given palliative care rather than intensive acute care. The challenge is that the hospice program has not saved Medicare substantial money.

Another approach has been to increase the level of cost sharing. The RAND health insurance experiment conducted in the 1970 and 1980s showed that people with higher levels of cost sharing used fewer medical-care services and that quality of care was not seriously adversely affected. This caused public and private insurers to advocate an increase in the level of cost sharing that continues today. The challenge is that most of the health-care dollars are spent by a small portion of the population, and you cannot expect those individuals to continue to pay high out-of-pocket amounts every year. Effectively this means that most of the expensive users of health care reach their out-of-pocket maximum reasonably quickly and the effect of cost sharing is minimized. Many of the most contentious labour–management negotiations in recent years have been over increasing the level of cost sharing.

The policy idea that has received the most attention recently is the defined contribution proposal by Congressman Paul Ryan, chair of the House of Representatives Budget Committee and the Republican vice-presidential candidate in the 2012 election. The proposal would transform the Medicare program from a defined benefit to a defined contribution program. Under the current defined benefit system, the Medicare beneficiary is entitled to unlimited Medicare-covered services. Under the defined contribution proposal, the idea is to take the current value of the Medicare benefit and index it forward at the rate of increase in overall inflation, as measured by the consumer price index (CPI). This would become the amount the Medicare beneficiary would receive from the federal government; the beneficiary would then purchase health insurance from private insurers. The problem with this proposal is that unless private insurers are somehow able to control spending—something that so far they have been unable to do—the Medicare beneficiary will be left paying a larger and larger proportion of the premium. The Congressional Budget Office estimated that under the Ryan plan, in 2030 Medicare would pay only 32% of the total amount the beneficiary would spend on health care.

Long-term projections of health spending

Long-term projections for health care spending in the United States are dire. Projections by Medicare actuaries and Congressional Budget Office economists suggest that by 2030 the US will be spending 25% of the gross domestic product on health care, and that it will reach 45% by 2080 (Congressional Budget Office 2007). By the time health spending reaches 30% to 35% of gross domestic product, all productivity improvements in the US economy will be going to increased health-care spending (Chernew, Hirth, and Cutler 2009). However, if the country decided to control health spending it could look in two areas: prices and people with multiple chronic conditions.

Promising areas for future control of US health spending

Prices are substantially higher in the United States than in other industrialized countries, yet little is being done to bring them in line with other countries. One paper argues "It's the Prices, Stupid" as the explanation for the higher level of spending in the US (Anderson et al. 2003). It is more difficult to show this for hospital and physician services and easiest to compare prices of brand-name drugs, because the products are identical. Price differentials vary from drug to drug and from country to country, but on average the US pays almost twice as much for brand-name drugs as other OECD countries. While it is more difficult to compare prices for other medical services, the data suggest that the fees for physician services and for hospital discharges are substantially higher in the United States, and that most of the difference is not attributable to case-mix differences, length of stay in the hospital, or other factors that would suggest quantity or service-intensity differences.

The challenge has always been to find a way to lower prices in the US. The Medicare program is already paying 30% less than private insurers for hospital and physician services, and in most states, Medicaid programs pay even less than Medicare. If the public sector lowered rates even further and the private insurers did not match the lower prices, providers might not accept Medicare and Medicaid patients, thereby reducing access to needed care for publicly insured patients. The challenge, therefore, is to get the private sector to pay lower prices if the US is to pay international rates for medical services.

There is wide geographic variation in the amount that the private sector pays in comparison to Medicare. The Medicare program's objective is to pay the costs for an efficient hospital plus a small operating surplus, adjusting rates for cost-of-living differences. However, if you look at private-sector payment rates in comparison to Medicare rates, wide discrepancies are encountered across geographic areas. This is because the rates are based on price negotiation and reflect the relative bargaining power of the insurers and providers. Overall it does not appear that the private insurers have an approach that leads to lower prices, since they pay higher prices than the public sector.

If the private sector cannot control prices, then all-payer rate setting may be necessary. Perhaps the best examples of all-payer rate setting in a multi-insurer environment are Germany and Japan, which have been using the method for many years. It is also a concept that the state of Maryland has been using since the early 1970s. Another approach is to prohibit private insurers from paying more than Medicare rates. From a political perspective, both approaches are difficult to implement, since most stakeholders have an aversion to rate regulation, and providers will not want to have their rates reduced.

People with multiple chronic diseases are responsible for 60% of all health-care spending in the United States, and 70% of spending in the Medicare program is for beneficiaries with five or more chronic conditions (Anderson 2010). In the US, as in other industrialized nations, the challenge is that the health-care system remains oriented towards acute care. The research infrastructure, educational system, payment and delivery system, and quality metrics were all designed to treat acute illnesses. The problem is that the burden of disease has changed and most people now seek medical care to treat a chronic condition. Changing this orientation will require fundamental changes in how research is conducted, clinicians are educated, providers are paid, care is delivered, and quality measured.

The problem begins with the lack of an evidence base for treating people with chronic conditions, as such people are often excluded from randomized clinical trials. Combining the best practices for treating individual conditions has been shown to be an effective approach for persons with multiple chronic conditions (Boyd et al. 2005). The problem created by having an acute-care orientation extends to medical school and during residency, when most teaching focuses on a particular organ or part of the body instead of the whole person. The United States has moved away from the advice of William Welch, one of the founders of the Johns Hopkins medical school, who wrote: "It is much more important to know what sort of patient has a disease than what sort of disease a patient has" (Johns Hopkins 2000). The financing and delivery system are still oriented to acute illness; the financing system, for example, typically pays only for services that lead to an improvement in health. However, for people with chronic conditions such as Alzheimer's, the emphasis should be not on improvement but on maintenance. Financing also involves problems in the payment system, since often payments are for specific services and cannot be coordinated with care across multiple providers. Quality metrics also focus on treatment of specific diseases and not the whole person.

Conclusion

The United States remains number one in health spending—a distinction that it has held for the past 40 years. It is not for lack of trying or good ideas that the US is unable to control health spending. While there have been constant calls for cost containment and many initiatives, there does not appear to be an economic or a political constituency for cost containment, or a political agreement on the best approach to controlling spending. As a result, most initiatives have had limited success.

Canada has an opportunity to take some ideas from the US and actually implement them. The ideas are often good; it's just that the US tends to be less successful in implementing them. Two distinct advantages that Canada has are an all-payer system and universal coverage. In the US, each insurer has its own unique relationship with each provider. This obviously adds to administrative costs, but much more important is that it does not allow any one insurer to negotiate effectively with the providers. As noted earlier, a main reason why the United States is so expensive is that the US pays providers much higher prices, and the providers prefer this relationship. The current financing system gives providers more negotiating power than in other industrialized countries. As Uwe Reinhardt said in his presentation at the "Bending the Cost Curve in Health Care" conference, Canada should embrace its all-payer system and use it to its full advantage.

Two ideas that Canada should consider are accountable care organizations (ACOs) and a focus on people with multiple chronic conditions. Accountable care organizations are designed to encourage hospitals, physicians, and other clinicians to work together to improve the health of the population. Canada should consider adapting ACOs to its own circumstances, as the fee-for-service payment system does not provide the same sorts of incentives. Second, most health spending in Canada is for treating people with multiple chronic conditions, but the current system remains focused on acute illness. Canada would be well advised to review some of the US programs that focus on people with multiple chronic conditions.

References

Anderson, G. 2010. "Chronic Care: Making the Case for Ongoing Care." Robert Wood Johnson Foundation. Accessed 23 April 2014. http://www.rwjf.org/en/research-publications/find-rwjf-research/2010/01/chronic-care.html.

Anderson, G. F., U. E. Reinhardt, P. S. Hussey, and V. Petrosyan. 2003. "It's the Prices, Stupid: Why the United States Is So Different from Other Countries." *Health Affairs* 22, no. 3: 89–105. http://dx.doi.org/10.1377/hlthaff.22.3.89.

Boyd, C., J. Darer, C. Boult, L. Fried, L. Boult, and A. Wu. 2005. "Clinical Practice Guidelines and Quality of Care for Older Patients with Multiple Comorbid Diseases: Implications for Pay for Performance." *Journal of the American Medical Association* 294, no. 6: 716–24. http://dx.doi.org/10.1001/jama.294.6.716.

Center for Medicare and Medicaid Services. "Accountable Care Organizations." Accessed 26 August 2012. http://www.cms.gov/Medicare/Medicare-Fee-for-Service-payment/ACO/index.html?redirect=/ACO/.

Chernew, M. E., R. A. Hirth, and D. M. Cutler. 2009. "Increased Spending on Health Care: Long-Term Implications for the Nation." *Health Affairs* 28, no. 5: 1253–55. http://dx.doi.org/10.1377/hlthaff.28.5.1253.

CNN (Cable News Network). 2012. "Fortune 500: Our Annual Ranking of America's Largest Corporations." Accessed 26 August 2012. http://money.cnn.com/magazines/fortune/fortune500/2012/full_list/.

Commonwealth Fund. "Multinational Comparisons of Health Systems Data, 2011." http://www.commonwealthfund.org/Publications/Chartbooks/2011/Dec/Multinational-Comparisons-of-Health-Data-2011.aspx. Accessed 26 August 2012.

Congressional Budget Office. 2007. *The Long-Term Outlook for Health Care Spending.* Washington, DC: Congress of the United States Congressional Budget Office.

Elmendorf, D. 2009. Letter to Senator Orrin G. Hatch, October 9. Accessed 26 August 2012. http://www.cbo.gov/sites/default/files/cbofiles/ftpdocs/106xx/doc10641/10-09-tort_reform.pdf.

Emanuel, E., and V. Fuchs. 2008. "Who Really Pays for Health Care: The Myth of 'Shared Responsibility.'" *Journal of the American Medical Association* 299, no. 9: 1057–59. http://dx.doi.org/10.1001/jama.299.9.1057.

General Electric Company. 2012. *GE Works: 2011 Annual Report.* Accessed 26 August 2012. http://www.ge.com/ar2011/pdf/GE_AR11_EntireReport.pdf.

Hogan, C., J. Lunney, J. Gabel, and J. Lynn. 2001. "Medicare Beneficiaries' Costs of Care in the Last Year of Life." *Health Affairs* (Millwood) 20, no. 4: 188–95. http://dx.doi.org/10.1377/hlthaff.20.4.188.

Hsiao, W. C., D. L. Dunn, and D. K. Verrilli. 1993. "Assessing the Implementation of Physician-Payment Reform." *New England Journal of Medicine* 328, no. 13: 928–33. http://dx.doi.org/10.1056/NEJM199304013281306.

Institute of Medicine. 2011. *The Healthcare Imperative: Lowering Costs and Improving Outcomes –Workshop Series Summary*. Washington, DC: Institute of Medicine.

Johns Hopkins Health System and Johns Hopkins University. 2000. *William H. Welch: Pioneer of Twentieth-Century Medicine*. Online exhibit. Accessed 26 August 2012. http://www.medicalarchives.jhmi.edu/welch/welcome.htm.

Mayes, R., and R. Berenson. 2006. *Medicare Prospective Payment and the Shaping of U.S. Health Care*. Baltimore, MD: Johns Hopkins University Press.

OECD (Organisation for Economic Co-operation and Development). 2012. OECD Health Data 2012. Accessed 26 August 2012. http://www.oecd.org/health/health-systems/oecdhealthdata2012.htm.

United States Bureau of Labor Statistics. 2012. "Table 3: Union Affiliation of Employed Wage and Salary Workers by Occupation and Industry." *Economic News Release*. Accessed 26 August 2012. http://www.bls.gov/news.release/union2.t03.htm.

sixteen

Australia

STEPHEN DUCKETT

Context

The Commonwealth of Australia is a federation with six states and two territories (collectively called "the states"), and a federal government based in the national capital, Canberra. With 22.5 million people (2011 census), it is one of the world's least densely populated countries, though heavily urbanized. Most of the population is centred on the eastern seaboard, with a pocket around Perth in the southwest of the continent. For three of the states, more than 70% of their population lives in the capital city, while about two-thirds of New South Wales residents live in the capital.

Like the platypus, Australia's health system is a curious hybrid: of public and private financing and provision, with federal and state roles in governance and provision. There is an ideological divide between the main political parties—Labor at the centre or centre left, Liberals on the centre right—in terms of their attitudes to key health policies at the federal level (Duckett 2008). Australia was governed nationally by a conservative government, a Liberal–Country Party coalition, from 1949 to 1972. Health policies in this period emphasized subsidies for private insurance, with residual schemes for pensioners. Public hospitals, established by state governments, also provided residual schemes to enable pensioners to access inpatient and outpatient care without direct charge (Kewley 1973). There was a major policy shift with the election of a Labor national government in 1972, which had a mandate to introduce a national universal health insurance scheme.

Australia was thus a relative latecomer to universality in health care. Its national scheme, Medibank, was introduced in 1975, over significant opposition from the medical profession and private insurance interests (Duckett 1979, 1980, 1984; Scotton and Macdonald 1993). This first implementation proved fragile; it was slowly dismantled by the Liberal government elected a couple of months after the last state joined the scheme. Universality was restored in 1984 with re-election of a Labor government, accompanied by a name change for the scheme from Medibank to Medicare. Despite the introduction of universal coverage (for both hospitals and medical care), private insurance organizations maintained their revenue by marketing insurance against the costs of treatment in private hospitals and of "ancillary" services, particularly dental care and allied health care.

After decades of opposition to universal health insurance (Wooldridge 1991), the Liberal Party (then out of power), recognized the political popularity of Medicare and reversed its stance before the 1996 election. The differences between the two main parties now focus mainly on the extent to which private financing and provision should be encouraged.

Australia's constitution gives the national parliament power to make laws about "the provision of ... pharmaceutical, sickness and hospital benefits, medical and dental services (but not so as to authorize any form of civil conscription)." The Australian High Court originally determined that the civil conscription limitation was quite restrictive, and it overturned limits on the way medical practitioners could write prescriptions for medications. More recently, the Court has taken a narrower view of what is proscribed (Mendelson 1999). Nevertheless, the civil conscription limitation has been seen as one barrier to the Commonwealth government's regulation of medical practitioners' fees.

Commonwealth power is thus quite extensive, and it is supplemented in practice by the power to make grants to the states on matters over which it otherwise has no power. The states cannot levy excise taxes, nor do they impose income taxes. However, all net revenue from the federal goods and services excise tax is allocated to the states according to a complex equalization formula (Williams 2012). Accounting for about one-quarter of all state revenue, this transfer has no conditions attached. Commonwealth grants, with strings attached, account for a further one-quarter of state revenue.

The Commonwealth government in Australia, through this combination of constitutional power and funding, has a much greater presence in health policy than its Canadian counterpart. The federal government is responsible for funding physician services (registration of health professionals is also a national function), aged care, regulation (and subsidy) of health insurance, and pharmaceutical benefits. States maintain responsibility for public hospitals, which are primarily owned by state governments and managed by state-appointed boards. A few publicly funded hospitals are operated by Roman Catholic organizations. Public hospitals account for about two-thirds of hospitals in Australia.

Although Australia's Medicare is based on Canada's medicare system, its design was heavily influenced by the peculiarities of the Australian federation and service provision. Historically, public hospitals have been creatures of the states, which had little interest in medical services outside hospitals (Scotton and Macdonald 1993). Australia also has a dense network of so-called private hospitals, run by for-profit chains, Roman Catholic religious orders and other not-for-profit groups, and smaller independent entities. Although the system parameters have evolved marginally over time, the 1970s elements are still there:

- Public hospitals are provided by state entities (although a few Catholic hospitals function as public hospitals), with the Commonwealth government providing grants towards the costs of their operation. Although around 50% of costs were initially covered, the proportion covered federally is now around 30% to 35%. All Australian residents are entitled to hospital services without charge from public hospitals.
- Medical services (outside public hospitals) are provided mostly by private practitioners, who can set their own fees. The Commonwealth government sets a fee schedule and provides rebates. Medical practitioners can choose to bill the government directly and accept the rebate as full settlement of the account. This practice varies in direct relation to market power, by both geography and specialty (Essue et al. 2011; Young and Dobson 2003).
- Insurance against the cost of private hospital treatment is available on a regulated modified community-rated basis by private insurers (and one currently publicly owned), with premiums increasing by 2% per year above age 30, based on the age from which coverage has been continuously maintained. In the 1990s the Liberal government introduced a 30–40% subsidy against the cost of insurance and other tax incentives for middle- to high-income earners to take out health insurance.
- Because of a combination of mandatory copayments (e.g., for pharmaceuticals), limited public coverage and provision of allied health services and dental care, and market-based copayments for medical services, Australians meet a higher proportion of healthcare costs out of their own pocket than is the case in most other developed countries (Duckett and Kempton 2012).

The effect of these system features is that there is no centralized control for health system reform. States are the "system managers" for hospitals, the Commonwealth is the principal funder of primary medical care, and the private sector (hospitals, insurers, medical profession) plays a major role in provision.

Until the most recent round of system reforms, the Commonwealth was not directly exposed financially to increases in costs of public hospital care, and hence it had no financial incentive to use the levers it controlled to reduce demand for hospital care. Cost-shifting between the states and the Commonwealth (and vice versa) is endemic, with each party blaming the other for system shortcomings. Despite this complexity, Australia performs well on international health expenditure comparisons, sitting almost exactly on the trend line of health share of GDP against national wealth and marginally below prediction on some measures. Life expectancy in Australia and potential years of life lost are also better than the OECD average. The main exception is the health status of Australia's indigenous peoples (Aborigines and Torres Strait Islanders), who suffer considerably worse health status on every measure than other Australians.

Trends

There are three distinct periods in terms of change in gross domestic product (GDP) and patterns of health expenditure growth in Australia over the period 1989–90 to 2009–10 (see Figure 16.1). From 1989–90 to 1991–92, Australia's GDP contracted as part of a global recession, but wage-dominated health spending is "sticky downwards" and continued to

Figure 16.1 GDP and health expenditure, Australia, 1989–1990 to 2009–2010 (2009–2010 Australian dollars)

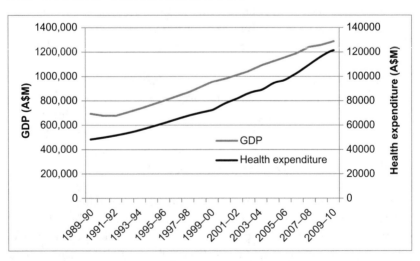

Source: Australian Institute of Health and Welfare 2012.

Figure 16.2 Health expenditure as share of GDP and per capita health spending, Australia, 1989–1990 to 2009–2010

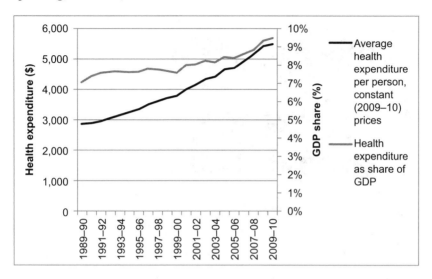

Source: Australian Institute of Health and Welfare 2012.

increase. For the next decade, growth in health spending paralleled GDP growth: both increased 40% over 1991–92 to 1999–2000 (constant prices).

The new millennium saw a change, with health spending rising faster than GDP in every year. From 1999–2000 to 2009–10, health spending grew 68% in constant dollars compared to a 35% growth in GDP. In several years in this decade, real health spending growth was more than two or three times growth in GDP: in 1999–2000 to 2000–01 (7.1% versus 2.1%), 2003–04 to 2004–05 (6.3% versus 3.0%), and 2007–08 to 2008–09 (7.1% versus 1.4%). Figure 16.2 shows this pattern in terms of share of GDP spent on health care and per capita health spending. Per capita health spending shows an upward trend over the whole period, albeit with faster growth in the latter decade (32% growth in 1989–90 to 1999–2000, 46% growth in 1999–2000 to 2009–10). As can be expected from the patterns seen in Figure 16.2, health expenditure share of GDP increased only marginally over the first decade, from 7.4% to 7.8% in 1997–98 and back to 7.6% in 1999–2000. The second decade showed a very different pattern, with GDP share increasing from 7.6% in 1999–2000 to 8.6% in 2006–07 (the last full year of the Liberal Howard government) to 9.4% in 2009–10.

Growth in total health expenditure has not been primarily price-driven. Australian health inflation over the past two decades averaged around

Figure 16.3 Composition of health expenditures by source of funds, Australia, 1995–1996 to 2009–2010

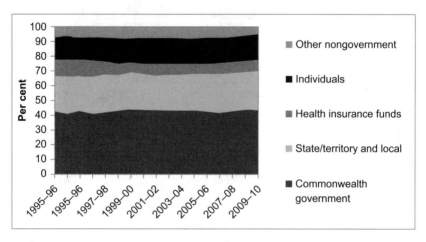

Source: Australian Institute of Health and Welfare 2012.

2.8% per annum, compared to general inflation at 2.6%. The past two decades saw some changes in sources of funding (see Figure 16.3, for which the time period is shorter because of earlier changes in data definitions). The most dramatic change over the period was the declining share of total health expenditure met by health insurance funds. In 1999–2000 private insurance met 11.3% of total expenditure. Following the Howard government's introduction of a private insurance subsidy in 1997, the share met from the privately paid component of health insurance premiums declined to around 7% in 2000–01, increasing to 7.6% by 2009–10. Out-of-pocket costs have increased significantly over the past two decades: from 15.6% in 1995–96 to 16.3% in 1997–98 and to 18.1% by 2001–02, subsequently easing to around 17.5%. Australia's reliance on out-of-pocket costs is high relative to most OECD countries (Duckett and Kempton 2012; Jan, Essue, and Leeder 2012), and this exposure of consumers to health costs may have helped to restrain health inflation, albeit with negative equity consequences. The health insurance changes accounted for the major shift in total private share, which declined from just over one-third of spending in 1995–96 to 30% in 2009–10.

Besides cost pressures, the state government's share is affected by the relative generosity of Commonwealth transfer payments, so the state share shows volatility over the period, increasing from 23.1% in 1995–96 to 25.3% in 1997–98 before declining to 23.8% in 2004–05. Since then the state share has shown a steady increase, reaching 26.3% of total spending in 2009–10. The Commonwealth share was relatively stable over the period, fluctuating slightly from a minimum of 41.2% in 1996–97 to a maximum of 44.3% in 2000–01. Coupled with the phenomenon of health spending outstripping GDP growth over the past decade, this has resulted in considerable interest by different stakeholders in cost-containment strategies.

Of course, cost containment can be antithetical to good policy in cases where the benefits of additional expenditure exceed the costs. The high proportion of health expenditure met by government tends to lead to policy discussions focusing on cost containment rather than economic efficiency (balancing benefits and costs). However, as shown below, some aspects of cost containment in Australia have been through pursuit of measures designed to ensure that additional expenditures are economically justified.

Bending the cost curve: Commonwealth government strategies

Commonwealth cost-control strategies have been influenced by the political environment and the main areas of spending. The Hawke-Keating Labor government was in office from 1983 to 1996 and the Howard Liberal–National coalition from 1996 to 2007; Labor was re-elected in 2007 and held office until 2013, with two prime ministers (Rudd to 2010, Gillard thereafter). Although the key political achievement of the Hawke-Keating government was the reintroduction of Medicare, expenditure growth was remarkably constrained in that period, possibly because of careful attention to system design as part of Medicare's reintroduction and a continuing fear of being characterized as allowing uncontrolled spending. In contrast, the Howard years show more rapid cost escalation, with little attempt to introduce cost-containment strategies. The Rudd–Gillard years also show high cost growth, primarily associated with new programs rather than with uncapping inflation.

Medical services

Spending on medical services has outpaced inflation. Australia has not been successful in controlling total spending on medical services, and spending has grown faster than inflation every year for the past two decades. However, service growth, not inflation per se, has been the principal issue. Medical services per capita increased from 7.2 in 1984–85 to 14.1 in 2010–11. Some (but not all) of this growth may be a statistical artifact,

Table 16.1 Targets of medical services cost control

	Demand Side	Supply Side
Price	• Use of price signals on consumers	• Control of rebates to medical practitioners • Control of total outlays
Volume	• Control of new items on fee schedule • Primary-care reform	• Control of number of medical practitioners

as some Medicare items were split over time, so two items might be billed where one was billed previously.

The spending growth is also partly accounted for by demographic factors: growth and aging of the population. However, the principal causes of utilization growth are not demographic but rather changes in patterns of practice: utilization is increasing dramatically for each age group, so total utilization would be increasing even without a change in demographic composition.

The Commonwealth government has pursued a mixture of supply- and demand-side strategies, involving both price and volume instruments (see Table 16.1).

Price signals

The use of consumer price signals in a universal health system is somewhat problematic and involves a trade-off between equity and expenditure control (Evans 1997; Evans et al. 1994). In contrast to Canada, the medical fee schedule in Australia can be set unilaterally by the federal government and thus used to control outlays. However, again unlike Canada, medical practitioners are not constrained in what they can bill patients: if government payments become out of line with practitioner expectations or aspirations, they can respond by increasing fees—what in Canada is known as extra billing. In specialties or locations where there is a relative shortage of medical practitioners, they are the price setters, and fee increases will not be offset by reductions in demand. In such circumstances, rather than controlling total costs, price signals become a way of shifting costs from government to consumers, an example of "shear," in Evans's categorization (Evans 1990).

Figure 16.4 shows the growth in Commonwealth government medical rebate spending and consumer out-of-pocket spending for each five-year period of the past two decades. Commonwealth government spending

Figure 16.4 Average annual growth (real terms) in Commonwealth government spending on medical services and consumer contributions, Australia, five-year periods, 1989–1990 to 2009–2010

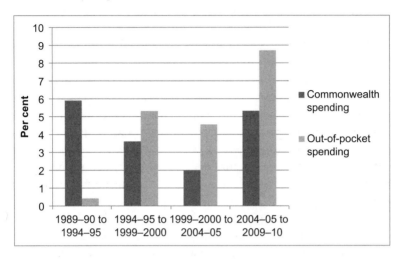

Source: Australian Institute of Health and Welfare 2012.

oscillated between 87% and 89% of combined Commonwealth and personal spending over this period. The first five-year period saw the highest growth in Commonwealth spending and almost negligible growth in out-of-pocket, suggesting that medical practitioners were satisfied with the level of government remuneration over that period. The pattern changed thereafter, with tightening of government spending growth and increased patient contributions.

In general practitioner direct Medicare ("bulk") billing, medical practitioners send their bills directly to Medicare Australia (the administering agency) and the consumer faces no out-of-pocket expenses. This practice peaked in 1997–98 at 83.8%, shortly after the change in government from Labor to Liberal. The Liberal Party had a history of opposition to Medicare and direct billing; with its absence of any copayment or other financial incentive on consumers, direct billing was not consistent with the conservative philosophy of the government. The decline in direct billing continued, down to 70.5% in 2003–04, and lower on a quarterly basis (Elliot 2003). Average copayments increased by about A$1 (from $6.86 to $7.95) between 1991–92 and 1995–96 but increased A$5 between 1995–96 and 2002–03 (Hopkins and Speed 2005). These increases in out-of-pocket payments were politically unpopular; they evinced a government response that involved incentives on general practitioners to direct-bill particular target groups, a change from the previous universality principles of Medicare (Jones, Savage, and Hall 2004; Swerissen 2004). Even after these changes, 6.3% of the population reported delaying seeing a general practitioner because of costs (Australian Bureau of Statistics 2010).

The Commonwealth government also attempted to reduce the salience of out-of-pockets by allowing medical practices to lodge claims on the patient's behalf (which speeds up the refund process). Widespread availability of credit card transactions also means that the immediate impact of out-of-pocket costs is deferred. The policy changes were fully implemented by the last five-year period, during which there were substantial increases in both government spending and out-of-pockets. In the absence of a counterfactual—how much would out-of-pocket payments have changed in the absence of the government policies?—it is difficult to make a definitive conclusion about the success of these policies in terms of impact on cost containment. The targeted incentives to direct-bill might have further strengthened the market power of doctors in relevant geographic areas, insulating them from the demand-constraining effects of out-of-pocket costs.

Control of total outlays

A handful of major companies are responsible for a significant proportion of pathology (laboratory) services in Australia. A unique approach to controlling total government outlays for pathology services has been in place since 1996. The most recent variant of these arrangements is the 2011 five-year Pathology Funding Agreement, which provides for adjusting rebates during the year if there is greater than expected growth in pathology tests. The aim of the adjustments is to ensure that the increase in total pathology outlays falls within agreed bands, as shown in Table 16.2.

In the event that total growth in outlays fall outside these bands, the Agreement mandates negotiations between the parties (government and providers) to identify proposed rectifying action, such as adjustments to

Table 16.2 Agreed growth-rate caps and floors (per cent) for pathology services, Australia, 2011–2016

	2011–12	2012–13	2013–14	2014–15	2015–16
Growth-rate floor	4.375	4.4	4.45	4.45	4.7
Growth-rate cap	4.875	4.9	4.95	4.95	5.2

rebates. If agreement can't be reached, there is provision for mediation or for termination of the Agreement. Commonwealth government budget documents claim the moderated growth rate will save A\$550 million over the life of the five-year agreement compared to what might otherwise have occurred (Australia 2011). Much of this reflects success in the government's ensuring a dividend to taxpayers from significant productivity improvements in the pathology sector due to technological advances, automation, and economies of scale.

Control of new items on the fee schedule

Australia has been a world leader in introducing cost-effectiveness requirements as part of the decision-making process for public funding of pharmaceuticals and medical services, including new diagnostic technologies. Since 1998, proposals for new items to be added to the Medicare schedule are considered by an independent committee known as the Medical Services Advisory Committee. This committee uses cost-effectiveness criteria to determine its recommendations, based on open processes with a full account of deliberations published on its website. Although it has not gone without criticism (Petherick et al. 2007), a recent review of health technology assessment essentially endorsed the current approach, albeit with minor suggested improvements. Although the Committee's approach includes assessment of new technologies against a nominated comparator (typically current practice), its processes have not been successful in identifying superseded or redundant technologies, or those that produce little value for money, in a way that would facilitate their removal from the fee schedule (Elshaug, Moss, et al. 2009; Elshaug, Watt, et al. 2009).

Primary-care reform

In common with other developed countries, Australia's population is aging, bringing new challenges to the health system. The principal method of paying for physicians in Australia, as in Canada, is still fee-for-service, a model based on the implicit assumption that health care involves a series of independent visits (or services) that should be subject to separate payments. Government and the medical profession have recognized the importance of introducing other modes of payment for general practitioners to encourage different practice patterns. However, the outcome has been a proliferation of new, largely item-based additions to the fee schedule with no overarching strategic vision or end point for the future of general practice (Beilby 2007).

Moreover, and despite the changes, it appears that longer general-practice consultations—necessary for a more preventive approach to patient management—are declining (Taylor et al. 2010). There has been an increase in shorter consultations, the reasons for which are contested but are possibly related to increased use of nurses employed by physician practices whose services now attract rebates (Britt, Fahridin, and Miller 2010).

After more than a decade of experience, the strategy of grafting incentives for different practice approaches onto the existing fee-for-service system seems to be largely ineffective. More fundamental strategies will thus be required, but such changes face an uphill battle, given the attachment to fee-for-service of the main medical profession lobby group, the Australian Medical Association. Recent attempts by the government to introduce relatively modest capitation arrangements for diabetes care were considerably watered down in response to opposition by the Association.

Control of numbers of medical practitioners

Although there is debate in the academic literature about the extent of supplier-induced demand for health care (McGuire 2000), Australian health policymakers are convinced that additional medical practitioners lead to additional government health spending. The additional spending is not only for rebates paid for consultations but also for downstream impacts through referrals, diagnostic tests, and prescriptions for medication. Further, an increase in medical supply, at least in the ranges observed to date in Australia, does not appear to create competitive pressures to lower fees (Richardson, Peacock, and Mortimer 2006).

Medical workforce policies have involved a trade-off between the costs of additional workforce supply and the benefits of improved access. During the mid 1990s, the emphasis was on restricting workforce supply, including reductions in intakes to medical schools. Graduation from medical school was also delinked from automatic rights to Medicare rebates by requiring new graduates to complete specialist training (including training through the Royal Australian College of General Practitioners). There was no parallel scheme to ensure that access concerns were being met by expanding the use of substitute practitioners such as nurse practitioners. This meant that access issues would inevitably increase, which they did, creating pressure to increase medical school intakes.

Medical school intakes (and graduation rates) were held constant for much of the 1990s, producing around 1,300 medical graduates per annum. The past decade has seen an explosion of intakes, with graduations increasing sharply from 2005 to a projected level of around 3,000 per annum (Joyce 2012).

Because of the long lead times involved in specialist training, it will be five to ten years before we can judge whether the medical school expansion policy, introduced to improve access, has changed the market power of the medical profession to constrain out-of-pocket costs. Regardless of the impact on out-of-pockets, the increase in medical practitioners will lead to a substantial increase in government and total spending on medical services.

Hospitals and health insurance

The Commonwealth government cannot directly influence total spending on public hospitals. Total current public hospital spending is determined by state governments; the Commonwealth contribution is related to neither state spending nor actual utilization of public hospitals.[1] The effect of the funding formulae was to make states responsible for the full marginal costs of any changes in hospital utilization and spending.

The Commonwealth contribution to public hospitals was defined in a series of five-year agreements with the states as the basis for Commonwealth grants and conditions on the grants (Deeble 2002; Duckett 2002, 2004; Paterson 2002; Pearse 1994; Reid 2002). Negotiations were usually fractious affairs characterized by brinkmanship; the states would argue that system deficiencies were the result of Commonwealth underfunding during the course of the prior agreement and would demand improved funding in the upcoming agreement. The funding formulae in the agreements were essentially population driven, with the arguments being about base quantum and indexation arrangements.

The Commonwealth's only option for controlling its hospital spending was through these regular negotiations. However, state rhetoric was generally effective in persuading the media and the public that some of the problems of their systems were due to lack of Commonwealth funding, which in turn constrained Commonwealth parsimony.

Private health insurance incentives

The most dramatic attempt to change the nature of these negotiations, as well as health policy discourse in Australia, was the move by the Howard Liberal government to introduce tax subsidies for private health

---

1 Changes that came into effect on 1 July 2014 provide that the Commonwealth government will pay 45% of the costs of growth in public hospital services, funded at an independently determined "national efficient price." The 2014 Commonwealth Budget foreshadowed ending this arrangement from 2017.

insurance in the late 1990s. Although total health insurance coverage had been declining from the early 1980s, almost the entire decline was among people covered for the costs of private treatment in a public hospital, a product that was increasingly irrelevant with the introduction of universal compulsory insurance through Medicare. Insurance for private hospital care had been remarkably stable over this period (Duckett and Willcox 2011).

Nevertheless, the government argued that the decline in health insurance was one of the reasons for increased demand for public hospital services. Rather than increasing grants to the states, it would support public hospital care indirectly by supporting private hospital care, claiming that in doing so the government would be shown to be "the best friend Medicare ever had" (Elliot 2006). A series of carrots and sticks was introduced to increase health insurance uptake:

- Tax penalties on high-income earners who did not have insurance were based on the rationale that such people were "unfairly" taking public hospital beds from poorer people. Because the threshold for the tax surcharge was not indexed, this penalty over time affected an increasing proportion of taxpayers.
- A subsidy for the general population provided a 30% rebate against the cost of health insurance, including both hospital insurance and ancillaries such as dental care, with a higher rate of subsidy available for older people. Part of the Howard government "middle-class welfare" initiatives (Tingle 2012), the subsidy was partly funded by the government's taking a tough position in the contemporary health-care agreement negotiations, thus effectively shifting funding from the public sector to the private sector.
- A change was made in the basis of community rating for private health insurance to "lifetime community rating," whereby health insurers could charge increased premiums to people who first purchased health insurance after age 30. Policy implementation was accompanied by advertisements with the slogan "Run for cover," showing people with insurance being rushed past other people on public hospital waiting lists (Ellis and Savage 2008).

The new policies were implemented in swift succession in the first few years of the Howard government (1997–2000), so it is difficult to disentangle their individual impact (Frech, Hopkins and MacDonald 2003; Palangkaraya and Yong 2005, 2007), but the lifetime rating change probably had the most significant impact (Butler 2002; Ellis and Savage 2008).

Together the changes led to a 50% increase in the proportion of people insured, a shift that may only have been politically feasible given the prior introduction of the subsidies. However, there has been little discernible shift from public care to private care (Moorin, Brameld, and Holman 2006; Moorin and Holman 2006a, 2006b, 2006c, 2007; Sundararajan et al. 2004) and hence little evidence to suggest that the espoused intent of the policy—of reducing demand for public hospital care—has been accomplished. Moreover, the policy has not been cost-reducing.

The 2007 election saw the government change back to Labor, with a consequent change in priorities. Support for private health insurance was no longer the *sine qua non,* and direct Commonwealth support to address public hospital access issues was championed by the new prime minister. The Rudd government started with high aspirations and a greater emphasis on health policy than its predecessor (Dowding et al. 2010). Rudd's initial foray into health policy involved a substantial increase in grants to the states for public hospital services.

But Rudd's agenda was broader. Contrary to the advice of its National Health and Hospitals Reform Commission, his government proposed a majority Commonwealth funding role for public hospital services (Hall 2010). The policy did not achieve the unanimous support of the states. Following a change of leadership in 2010, Prime Minister Gillard proposed more modest but still fundamental reforms that left the "system manager" role for public hospitals with the states. Gillard's emphasis has been on public hospital renewal rather than private health insurance, reinforcing her image as a (moderate) reforming leader in the tradition of her Labor predecessors (Johnson 2011).

Despite the fact that premium increases are subject to a government approval process (Biggs 2009), health insurance premiums have been increasing at more than double the rate of the consumer price index (Biggs 2012), in part driven by utilization increases. The cost to government of the open-ended private health insurance rebate has thus been escalating rapidly, increasing 50% in the five years from 2004–05 to 2009–10. After several unsuccessful attempts by the Rudd government to pass legislation to rein in financial assistance or incentives for insurance, following the 2010 election the Gillard government was able to use a changed composition in the Senate to pass legislation to means test the rebate and index the tax penalty threshold for middle-to-high-income earners without health insurance. The subsidies and penalties, indexed annually, are shown in Table 16.3. Although the changes were vociferously opposed by the then Liberal opposition (who also promised to restore the status quo when fiscally responsible), the effect of the tax penalty was still to

Table 16.3 Private health insurance income tiers for determining rebates and tax penalties, 1 July 2013–30 June 2014

	No Change	Tier 1	Tier 2	Tier 3
Income level (A$)				
Singles	88,000 or less	88,001–102,000	102,001–136,000	136,001+
Families	176,000 or less	176,001–204,000	204,001–272,000	272,001+
Private health insurance rebate (%)				
Under 65 years	30	20	10	0
65–69	35	25	15	0
70+	40	30	20	0
Medicare levy surcharge: tax penalty for those without private health insurance (%)				
All ages	0.0	1.0	1.25	1.5

encourage taxpayers in tiers 2 and 3 (at least) to take out private health insurance, albeit now with a reduced subsidy.

Medications

Unlike Canada, Australia has had a national scheme to subsidize access to medications, the Pharmaceutical Benefits Scheme (PBS), since 1948. Expenditure on medications is increasing rapidly: Commonwealth government expenditure rose an average of 11% per annum (constant dollars) in the period 1999–2000 to 2004–05, moderating to 6% per annum in 2004–05 to 2009–10. Mandated consumer copayments increased at almost identical rates.

Using its power as a monopsony, the Commonwealth government employs an array of measures to control medication expenditure (see Table 16.4).

Patient copayments and brand substitution

Mandated patient copayments ("moiety") have been part of the PBS since 1960 and are structured separately for the general population and for concession-card holders (Sweeny 2009). The PBS provides some protection from the cumulative impact of these copayments through annual safety-net thresholds.

Since 1994 pharmacists have been allowed to dispense generically identical forms of a drug where the pharmaceutical is listed on the PBS under more than one brand name (unless specifically directed not to do so by

Table 16.4 Elements of medication cost control

	Demand Side	Supply Side
Price	• Require patient copayments • Encourage prescription of generic (non-brand-name) drugs	• Negotiate prices based on lowest in other countries • Negotiate "risk-sharing" arrangements with suppliers (as volume increases, price declines)
Volume	• Institute prior approval scheme	• Limit inclusion on approval list (including through use of cost-effectiveness analysis) • Provide education program to pharmacists and doctors

the prescribing medical practitioner on the prescription form). If generic equivalents are available, the PBS will pay only for the least costly product and the consumer meets any additional costs for a specific brand-name alternative in addition to the copayments described above. An additional moiety is also payable if other pharmaceuticals in the same therapeutic class are deemed to be equivalent and an exemption on clinical grounds has not been granted for that patient. This policy (known as "therapeutic group premiums") was introduced in 1998. It applies to certain medications used to treat cardiovascular disease and peptic ulcers, and has reduced government expenditure for those classes of medication (Ioannides-Demos, Ibrahim, and McNeil 2002).

The memorandum of understanding effective until 30 June 2014 introduced another tool to slow government expenditure on pharmaceuticals. Under strengthened mandatory price-disclosure arrangements, manufacturers will be required to disclose the actual price paid by pharmacists to obtain medicines; this information will then trigger further price reductions by government. Although the price paid in Australia for most drugs is lower than the average in the United States, comparison with other countries such as New Zealand and England is less favourable (Duckett et al. 2013).

Controls on prescribing certain medications

Controls on the prescribing of some drugs have been introduced by requiring special approval ("authority") to prescribe them, over and above medical registration. Obtaining authority requires contacting the administering agency of the PBS and may, for example, require the medical practitioner to certify that specific indications for use of the medication are present.

Perception of the authority scheme is mixed (Liaw et al. 2003; Lu et al. 2005) but it does provide a platform for tailoring access to new and expensive genetically targeted medication (Hall et al. 2005).

Cost-effectiveness criteria

Through legislation passed in 1987, Australia was one of the first countries in the world to introduce cost-effectiveness considerations in pharmaceutical policy. A retrospective study of the decision-making process showed that in the early 1990s new pharmaceuticals costing more than A$68,913 per life-year saved were generally not listed on the PBS, while those that cost less than A$36,450 were listed. No apparent decision rules have been found to apply to the intermediate zone (George, Harris, and Mitchell 2001). Although there does not appear to be a formal basis for these criteria, they are consistent with a more rigorous approach in Australia to identifying the perceived economic value of human life for policy purposes (Abelson 2003).

Price incentives for suppliers

Historically the Australian government has been able to use its monopsony power to achieve lower prices relative to those paid in international markets. However, its ability to do this appears to be weakening as other countries establish schemes similar to the PBS and monitor international pricing negotiations (Löfgren 1998; Duckett et al. 2013).

In addition to consumer price incentives, the PBS pricing from suppliers is also used to reduce expenditure. Some of these are mandatory (e.g., when a generic equivalent comes onto the market, a 12.5% reduction on the ex-manufacturer price is automatically imposed), and some negotiated as part of listing decisions. One of the most powerful supply-side strategies involves risk-sharing with suppliers, such as using price–volume contracts to reduce the price paid under the PBS as volume increases. As of June 2010 the Pharmaceutical Benefits Pricing Authority reported 90 risk-sharing arrangements in place or under development (Pharmaceutical Benefits Pricing Authority 2010).

A new round of PBS reforms introduced in 2007 and phased in over five years was also designed to reduce prices paid by government, by driving mandatory price reductions and changing the basis for the comparator in cost-effectiveness analyses. Although the government is claiming savings in the order of billions of dollars up to 2018 (Australia 2010), many of those savings have yet to be realized; thus it is probably premature to evaluate the full effect of these changes (de Boer 2009; Searles et al. 2007). Changes introduced in 2012 were designed to allow the government to harvest discounts to pharmacists on prices that it had previously negotiated with manufacturers; these have reduced prices but not to international benchmarks.

Quality use of medicines

Reducing utilization through education of patients and prescribers is relatively weak in Australia. Although such a policy could involve a mix of strategies, the emphasis has been on sporadic consumer and prescriber educational programs rather than systematic use of incentives on manufacturers or medical practitioners. Such campaigns encourage consumers to be more judicious in their use of medication or attempt to educate medical practitioners to reduce their prescribing. Education of prescribers has mostly been through the National Prescribing Service, which rates well in terms of process measures (e.g., quality of materials) but is able to show few cost savings from changes in prescriber behaviour (Beilby et al. 2006).

Bending the cost curve in hospital care: State government strategies

State government expenditure is more focused than the Commonwealth's. More than two-thirds of total state health spending is on public hospital services, and significant differences in performance are seen between the states (see Table 16.5). Overall costs of public hospital admissions are somewhat similar across Australia, with the least expensive state (Tasmania) having per capita costs 6% below the Australian average, and the most expensive state (South Australia) having costs 9% above the Australian average (the two territories are excluded from this analysis because of smaller populations and somewhat different age/gender/ indigenous composition). In part because different incentives at the state level lead to different practices in recording admissions, and in part because of different patterns of private hospital provision, decomposition of total costs shows a wider variation: costs per admission vary from 12% below the Australian average (in Victoria) to 14% above (in Tasmania). There is also a wide variation in admission rates, from 14% above the Australian average (in Victoria) to 17% below (in Tasmania).

Historically, states attempted to control costs through input controls, but these were seen as ineffective, as well as inconsistent with contemporary public-sector budget development practices (Spigelman 1967), and were abandoned in the 1970s to be replaced by "global budgeting." States

Table 16.5 Public hospital admissions and costs, Australia, 2010–2011

	New South Wales	Victoria	Queensland	Western Australia	South Australia	Tasmania	Australian Capital Terr.	Northern Terr.	Australia (average)
Cost of admitted patients per capita (A$)	1,119	1,157	1,129	1,146	1,261	1,088	1,369	1,762	1,153
Cost per admission (A$)	5,104	4,284	5,273	4,790	5,313	5,557	5,238	3,868	4,871
Admissions per 1,000 population	219	270	214	239	237	196	261	456	237

also tried to control expenditures by closing beds and/or hospitals, especially in rural areas. This approach was generally strongly opposed by local communities. Local attachment to these hospitals stemmed in part from their historical origins where they were developed by local subscription; the communities felt they still "owned" the hospitals (Horsburgh 1977).

The 1980s and 1990s also saw the introduction of new industrial relations practices in Australia, including enterprise bargaining, in which negotiations attempted to identify productivity improvements to offset wage increases (Bray et al. 2005; Willis, Young, and Stanton 2005). Although these practices led to some local success, they did not markedly shift the cost trajectory.

Centralization of governance

The late 1990s saw centralization of governance become a common theme as a means to bend the cost curve (Dwyer 2004). Victoria and South Australia were exceptions, but the other states abolished separate board-governance arrangements such as regional health authorities in favour of direct management lines from the state ministry or department to the bedside. Restructuring was generally preceded by a review that typically identified the need to improve primary care (and cited the increased prevalence of chronic disease), but such recognition was not translated into deeds. Another common theme of these reviews was opportunistic inclusion of a range of technical efficiency and effectiveness measures, from ideas in good currency or known productivity opportunities. For example, almost every one recommends a call centre, a Web-based method of sharing innovations, amalgamation of support services where relevant, and improvements in the effectiveness of information systems and use of information (Dwyer 2004).

Variants of the English "targets and terror" performance measurement and management approach (Propper et al. 2008) were pursued, along with improved benchmarking. Several strategies to enhance management of hospitals were pursued nationally and at the state level. New South Wales initiated a "clinical process redesign" program, and there was a similar strategy in South Australia. These were local-level service redesign initiatives that focused on patient flow to improve efficiency and waiting times (Ben-Tovim, Bassham, et al. 2008; Ben-Tovim, Dougherty, et al. 2008; McGrath et al. 2008; O'Connell et al. 2008; Phillips and Hughes 2008). The New South Wales variant was led centrally by the health ministry.

At the national level, the National Demonstration Hospitals Program, a collaborative knowledge exchange–oriented initiative, operated from 1995 to 2003. It reported positive changes in the four areas of its focus: managing elective surgery, integrated bed management, integrated acute care, and improved hospital-based options for older Australians.

Activity-based funding

The alternative, a quasi-market strategy, was followed in Victoria and South Australia. In Victoria, arm's-length health service boards were retained, albeit with single institutional boards being amalgamated into multi-service bodies. Introduced in 1993, activity-based funding (Duckett 1995) was accompanied by significant budget reductions of around 15% over three years (Lin and Duckett 1997), and there is evidence that public hospitals were operating at the efficiency frontier shortly after the introduction of the new policy (Yong and Harris 1999).

However, activity-based funding is a neutral instrument in terms of efficiency; the critical policy variable is the payment per (weighted) case, and this can be set lower or higher than the prior average. Although activity-based funding clearly drove efficiency improvements in Victoria in the years around its introduction, in subsequent years funding was somewhat more generous and efficiency (in terms of cost per case) slipped (Duckett 2008). Although different data sources give somewhat different results, after 15 years' experience with activity-based funding, cost per admission in Victoria is still well below the Australian average.

A downside of activity-based funding is the incentive to increase (recorded) admissions. This risk is mitigated in Victoria by admission caps, established as part of the budget process: hospitals are not funded for admissions above a predetermined threshold. Victoria has also established and funded a "hospital admission risk program" designed to reduce hospital admissions by improving continuity of care and community services (Bird et al. 2007; Smith et al. 2003). Despite these efforts, reported admission rates in Victoria remain above the Australian average.

Future policy initiatives

One of Prime Minister Rudd's early actions was to establish a sweeping independent review of the Australian health-care system. The review body, the National Health and Hospitals Reform Commission, reported in 2009, making 123 separate recommendations (NHHRC 2009). The Commission identified a policy lacuna: Australia had almost no effective national policy coordinating structures—there were only Commonwealth bodies and inter-jurisdictional bodies, the latter often stymied by politics. Two of the three elements of a cybernetic model of health system leadership and governance (Smith et al. 2012)—priority setting and performance monitoring—were non-existent at the national level. The Commission recommended that "the Commonwealth, state and territory governments would agree to establish national approaches to health workforce planning and education, professional registration, patient safety and quality (including service accreditation), e-health, performance reporting (including the provision of publicly available data on the performance of all aspects of the health system), prevention and health promotion, private hospital regulation, and health intervention and technology assessment" (NHHRC 2009, recommendation 88.9).

New national bodies have been created to address several of these functions, including the Australian National Preventive Health Agency and the National Health Performance Authority, and in the longer term these may have helped "bend the cost curve," but both have been slated for abolition or merger in the 2014 Commonwealth Budget. A key Commission recommendation was designed to expand the use of funding approaches that promote efficiency. Specifically it recommended "that incentives for improved outcomes and efficiency should be strengthened in health care funding arrangements," involving a mix of

- activity-based funding (e.g., fee for service or case-mix budgets), which should be the principal mode of funding for hospitals;
- payments for care of people over a course of treatment or time period, with a greater emphasis on this mode of funding for primary health care; and
- payments to reward good performance in outcomes and timeliness of care, with a greater emphasis on this mode of funding across all settings. (NHHRC 2009, recommendation 95)

There was widespread acceptance in the policy community that public hospital efficiency could be improved: a separate independent review had identified potential to improve efficiency by about 10% (Forbes et al. 2010; Productivity Commission 2010). Recognizing this, governments established the Independent Hospital Pricing Authority to set a "national efficient price" for public hospital services, and agreed to implement a national approach to activity-based funding in all states.

Although the Commonwealth government supported a move towards episodic (care over a time period) physician payments, this was opposed by elements of the medical profession. A three-year trial, known as the Diabetes Care Project, was initiated instead. There has been no discernible progress on systematic implementation of the third limb of the recommendation—rewarding good performance.

Conclusion

The Australian health-care system performs well on key comparative metrics: it sits in the above-average performance quadrant internationally on both spending as a share of GDP and life expectancy. In contrast, Canada sits in the poorly performing quadrant, with higher costs per capita than the OECD average and marginally worse life expectancy (Duckett 2012).

Unlike in Canada, excess health cost inflation has not been the principal driver of health's increasing share of GDP in Australia; service growth and changed patterns of practice have driven the increase in costs. Health-sector wages (total hourly rates of pay) have tracked overall wages closely. Much like in Canada, Australia's health system has multiple loci of power, and there exists neither a national integrated plan to achieve efficiencies nor established national bodies to provide leadership. Policy development has been incremental rather than according to a synoptic ideal (Braybrooke and Lindblom 1970; Lindblom 1965), with policy being shaped by individuals and networks of influence (Lewis 2005). National associations of private-sector stakeholders (especially the Australian Medical Association and the association of private health insurers) have been key players in setting the agenda and shaping policy in areas of their interest.

At the national level, Australia has had a consensus on the broad parameters of policy since the mid 1990s—predominantly tax-funded access to public hospitals, medical care, pharmaceuticals, and long-term care for the frail aged. As a consequence of agreement on these parameters, a largely consistent direction has underpinned health policies in Australia for the past 20 years, even though the preferred levers, methods, and emphases vary among governments; some policies are more effective than others, while a few are palpably wrong-headed.

However, although the rhetorical differences are sharper than in practice, there are clear differences between the national political parties on aspects of health policy—specifically the importance of subsidies for private health insurance—and on the role of government generally. Differences in emphases in health policy should be expected to continue into the future. The differences are not so marked at the state level: both left and right parties support technocratic cost-containment policies (specifically activity-based funding) and strategies to enhance access to public hospital care.

In general terms, Australia has followed the three broad phases of policy priorities common to most developed countries: the first addressing access (and here Australia was a relative latecomer), the second controlling costs, and a third phase variously described as enhancing management of the system (Evans 1995), improving incentives (Cutler 2002), or improving strategic design (Tuohy 2012). Australia has kept health inflation in line with inflation in the rest of the economy, but costs still rise because of demographic factors and changes in practice patterns (more services per patient). The Australian experience also shows that there's no magic bullet for achieving an efficiency nirvana—multiple strategies are pursued by multiple players across multiple sectors. Cost constraint has been achieved by an array of initiatives, including those that target price and volume, acting on demand and supply. This approach probably represents recognition of Australian pragmatism and an absence of ideological obsession with either demand- or supply-side strategies.

References

Abelson, P. 2003. "The Value of Life and Health for Public Policy." *Economic Record* 79: S2–13. http://dx.doi.org/10.1111/1475-4932.00087.

Australia. 2010. *The Impact of PBS Reform: Report to Parliament on the National Health Amendment (Pharmaceutical Benefits Scheme) Act 2007*. Canberra: Department of Health and Ageing.

Australia. 2011. *Budget 2011*. Part 2, "Expense Measures: Health and Ageing." http://www.budget.gov.au/2011-12/content/bp2/html/bp2_expense-12.htm.

Australian Bureau of Statistics. 2010. *Health Services Patient Experiences in Australia, 2009*. Cat. no. 4839.0.55.001. Canberra: Australian Bureau of Statistics.

Australian Institute of Health and Welfare (AIHW). 2012. *Health Expenditure Australia 2010–11*. Cat. no. HWE56. Canberra: AIHW.

Beilby, J. 2007. "Primary Care Reform Using a Layered Approach to the Medicare Benefits Scheme: Unpredictable and Unmeasured." *Medical Journal of Australia* 187, no. 2: 69–71.

Beilby, J., S. Wutzke, J. Bowman, J. M. Mackson, and L. M. Weekes. 2006. "Evaluation of a National Quality Use of Medicines Service in Australia: An Evolving Model." *Journal of Evaluation in Clinical Practice* 12, no. 2: 202–17. http://dx.doi.org/10.1111/j.1365-2753.2006.00620.x.

Ben-Tovim, D. I., J. E. Bassham, D. M. Bennett, M. L. Dougherty, M. A. Martin, S. J. O'Neill, J. L. Sincock, and M. G. Szwarcbord. 2008. "Redesigning Care at the Flinders Medical Centre: Clinical Process Redesign Using 'Lean Thinking.'" *Medical Journal of Australia* 188 (6 Suppl.): S27–31.

Ben-Tovim, D. I., M. L. Dougherty, T. J. O'Connell, and K. M. McGrath. 2008. "Patient Journeys: The Process of Clinical Redesign." *Medical Journal of Australia* 188, no. 6: 14–17.

Biggs, A. 2009. *Private Health Insurance Premium Increases: An Overview*. Canberra: Parliamentary Library.

———. 2012. *Private Health Insurance Premium Increases: An Overview and Update*. Canberra: Parliamentary Library.

Bird, S. R., W. Kurowski, G. K. Dickman, and I. Kronborg. 2007. "Integrated Care Facilitation for Older Patients with Complex Health Care Needs Reduces Hospital Demand." *Australian Health Review* 31, no. 3: 451–61. http://dx.doi.org/10.1071/AH070451.

Bray, M., P. Stanton, N. White, and E. Willis. 2005. "The Structure of Bargaining in Public Hospitals in Three Australian States." In *Workplace Reform in the Healthcare Industry: The Australian Experience*, edited by P. Stanton, E. Willis, and S. Young, 63–90. Basingstoke, UK: Palgrave Macmillan.

Braybrooke, D., and C. E. Lindblom. 1970. *A Strategy of Decision: Policy Evaluation as a Social Process.* New York: Free Press.

Britt, H. C., S. Fahridin, and G. C. Miller. 2010. "Ascendancy with a Capital A: The Practice Nurse and Short General Practice Consultations." *Medical Journal of Australia* 193, no. 2: 84–85.

Butler, J. R. G. 2002. "Policy Change and Private Health Insurance: Did the Cheapest Policy Do the Trick?" *Australian Health Review* 25, no. 6: 33–41. http://dx.doi.org/10.1071/AH020033.

Cutler, D. M. 2002. "Equality, Efficiency, and Market Fundamentals: The Dynamics of International Medical-Care Reform." *Journal of Economic Literature* 40, no. 3: 881–906. http://dx.doi.org/10.1257/jel.40.3.881.

de Boer, R. 2009. "PBS Reform: A Missed Opportunity?" *Australian Health Review* 33, no. 2: 176–85. http://dx.doi.org/10.1071/AH090176.

Deeble, J. S. 2002. "Funding the Essentials: The Australian Health Care Agreements." *Australian Health Review* 25, no. 6: 1–7. http://dx.doi.org/10.1071/AH020001c.

Dowding, K., A. Hindmoor, R. Iles, and P. John. 2010. "Policy Agendas in Australian Politics: The Governor-General's Speeches, 1945–2008." *Australian Journal of Political Science* 45, no. 4: 533–57. http://dx.doi.org/10.1080/10361146.2010.517174.

Duckett, S. J. 1979. "Chopping and Changing Medibank, Part 1: Implementation of a New Policy." *Australian Journal of Social Issues* 14: 230–43.

———. 1980. "Chopping and Changing Medibank, Part 2: An Interpretation of the Policy Making Process." *Australian Journal of Social Issues* 15: 79–91.

———. 1984. "Structural Interests and Australian Health Policy." *Social Science and Medicine* 18, no. 11: 959–66. http://dx.doi.org/10.1016/0277-9536(84)90266-1.

———. 1995. "Hospital Payment Arrangements to Encourage Efficiency: The Case of Victoria, Australia." *Health Policy* 34, no. 2: 113–34. http://dx.doi.org/10.1016/0168-8510(95)94014-Y.

———. 2002. "The 2003–2008 Australian Health Care Agreement: An Opportunity for Reform." *Australian Health Review* 25, no. 6: 24–26. http://dx.doi.org/10.1071/AH020024.

———. 2004. "The Australian Health Care Agreements, 2003–2008." *Australia and New Zealand Health Policy* 1, no. 1: 5.

———. 2008. "Casemix Development and Implementation in Australia." In *The Globalization of Managerial Innovation in Health Care*, edited by J. Kimberly, G. de Pouvourville, and T. d'Aunno, 231–53. Cambridge: Cambridge University Press.

———. 2012. *Where to from Here? Keeping Medicare Sustainable.* Montreal: McGill-Queen's University Press.

Duckett, S., P. Breadon, L. Ginnivan, and P. Venkataraman. 2013. *Australia's Bad Drug Deal: High Pharmaceutical Prices.* Carlton, VIC: Grattan Institute.

Duckett, S., and A. Kempton. 2012. "Canadians' Views about Health System Performance." *Health Policy* 7, no. 3: 88–104.

Duckett, S., and S. Willcox. 2011. *The Australian Health Care System.* Melbourne: Oxford University Press.

Dwyer, J. M. 2004. "Australian Health System Restructuring: What Problem Is Being Solved?" *Australia and New Zealand Health Policy* 1, no. 1: 6.

Elliot, A. 2003. *The Decline in Bulk Billing: Explanations and Implications.* Canberra: Parliamentary Library.

———. 2006. "'The Best Friend Medicare Ever Had'? Policy Narratives and Changes in Coalition Health Policy." *Health Sociology Review* 15, no. 2: 132–43. http://dx.doi.org/10.5172/hesr.2006.15.2.132.

Ellis, R., and E. Savage. 2008. "Run for Cover Now or Later? The Impact of Premiums, Threats and Deadlines on Private Health Insurance in Australia." *International Journal of Health Care Finance and Economics* 8, no. 4: 257–77. http://dx.doi.org/10.1007/s10754-008-9040-4.

Elshaug, A. G., J. R. Moss, P. Littlejohns, J. Karnon, T. L. Merlin, and J. E. Hiller. 2009. "Identifying Existing Health Care Services That Do Not Provide Value for Money." *Medical Journal of Australia* 190, no. 5: 269–73.

Elshaug, A. G., A. M. Watt, J. R. Moss, and J. E. Hiller. 2009. *Policy Perspectives on the Obsolescence of Health Technologies in Canada.* Ottawa: Canadian Agency for Drugs and Technologies in Health.

Essue, B., P. Kelly, M. Roberts, S. Leeder, and S. Jan. 2011. "We Can't Afford My Chronic Illness! The Out-of-Pocket Burden Associated with Managing Chronic Obstructive Pulmonary Disease in Western Sydney, Australia." *Journal of Health Services Research and Policy* 16, no. 4: 226–31. http://dx.doi.org/10.1258/jhsrp.2011.010159.

Evans, R. G. 1990. "Tension, Compression, and Shear: Directions, Stresses, and Outcomes of Health Care Cost Control." *Journal of Health Politics, Policy and Law* 15, no. 1: 101–28. http://dx.doi.org/10.1215/03616878-15-1-101.

———. 1995. "Healthy Populations or Healthy Institutions: The Dilemma of Health Care Management." *Journal of Health Administration Education* 13, no. 3: 453–72.

———. 1997. "Going for the Gold: The Redistributive Agenda behind Market-Based Health Care Reform." *Journal of Health Politics, Policy and Law* 22, no. 2: 427–65.

Evans, R. G., M. Barer, G. L. Stoddart, and V. Bhatia. 1994. *Who Are the Zombie Masters, and What Do They Want?* Toronto: Premier's Council on Health, Well-Being and Social Justice.

Forbes, M., P. Harslett, I. Mastoris, and L. Risse. 2010. "Measuring the Technical Efficiency of Public and Private Hospitals in Australia." Paper presented at Australian Conference of Economists, Sydney, 27–29 September.

Frech, H. E., III, S. Hopkins, and G. MacDonald. 2003. "The Australian Private Health Insurance Boom: Was It Subsidies or Liberalised Regulation?" *Economic Papers* 22, no. 1: 58–64. http://dx.doi.org/10.1111/j.1759-3441.2003.tb00336.x.

George, B., A. Harris, and A. Mitchell. 2001. "Cost-Effectiveness Analysis and the Consistency of Decision Making: Evidence from Pharmaceutical Reimbursement in Australia (1991 to 1996)." *PharmacoEconomics* 19, no. 11: 1103–9. http://dx.doi.org/10.2165/00019053-200119110-00004.

Hall, J. 2010. "Health-Care Reform in Australia: Advancing or Side-Stepping?" *Health Economics* 19, no. 11: 1259–63. http://dx.doi.org/10.1002/hec.1652.

Hall, W. D., R. Ward, W. S. Liauw, and J. A. Brien. 2005. "Tailoring Access to High Cost, Genetically Targeted Drugs." *Medical Journal of Australia* 182, no. 12: 607–8.

Hopkins, S., and N. Speed. 2005. "The Decline in 'Free' General Practitioner Care in Australia: Reasons and Repercussions." *Health Policy* 73, no. 3: 316–29. http://dx.doi.org/10.1016/j.healthpol.2004.12.003.

Horsburgh, M. 1977. "Some Issues in the Government Subsidy of Hospitals in New South Wales: 1858–1910." *Medical History* 21, no. 2: 166–81. http://dx.doi.org/10.1017/S0025727300037698.

Ioannides-Demos, L. L., J. E. Ibrahim, and J. J. McNeil. 2002. "Reference-Based Pricing Schemes: Effect on Pharmaceutical Expenditure, Resource Utilisation and Health Outcomes." *PharmacoEconomics* 20, no. 9: 577–91. http://dx.doi.org/10.2165/00019053-200220090-00002.

Jan, S., B. M. Essue, and S. R. Leeder. 2012. "Falling Through the Cracks: The Hidden Economic Burden of Chronic Illness and Disability on Australian Households." *Medical Journal of Australia* 196, no. 1: 29–31. http://dx.doi.org/10.5694/mja11.11105.

Johnson, C. 2011. "Gillard, Rudd and Labor Tradition." *Australian Journal of Politics and History* 57, no. 4: 562–79. http://dx.doi.org/10.1111/j.1467-8497.2011.01614.x.

Jones, G., E. Savage, and J. Hall. 2004. "Pricing of General Practice in Australia: Some Recent Proposals to Reform Medicare." *Journal of Health Services Research and Policy* 9 (Suppl. 2): 63–68. http://dx.doi.org/10.1258/1355819042349899.

Joyce, C. 2012. "The Medical Workforce in 2025: What's in the Numbers?" *Medical Journal of Australia* 1 (Suppl. 3): 6–9. http://dx.doi.org/10.5694/mjao11.11575.

Kewley, T. H. 1973. *Social Security in Australia, 1900–72.* Sydney: Sydney University Press.

Lewis, J. M. 2005. *Health Policy and Politics: Networks, Ideas and Power.* Melbourne: IP Communications.

Liaw, S. T., C. M. Pearce, P. Chondros, B. P. McGrath, L. Piggford, and K. Jones. 2003. "Doctors' Perceptions and Attitudes to Prescribing within the Authority Prescribing System." *Medical Journal of Australia* 178, no. 3: 203–6.

Lin, V., and S. J. Duckett. 1997. "Structural Interests and Organisational Dimensions of Health System Reform." In *Health Policy in Australia*, edited by H. Gardner, 64–80. Melbourne: Oxford University Press.

Lindblom, C. E. 1965. *The Intelligence of Democracy: Decision Making through Mutual Adjustment.* New York: Free Press.

Löfgren, H. 1998. "The Pharmaceuticals Benefit Scheme and the Shifting Paradigm of Welfare Policy." *Australian Health Review* 21, no. 2: 111–23. http://dx.doi.org/10.1071/AH980111.

Lu, C. Y., J. Ritchie, K. M. Williams, and R. O. Day. 2005. "Recent Developments in Targeting Access to High Cost Medicines in Australia." *Australia and New Zealand Health Policy* 2: 28.

McGrath, K. M., D. M. Bennett, D. I. Ben-Tovim, S. C. Boyages, N. J. Lyons, and T. J. O'Connell. 2008. "Implementing and Sustaining Transformational Change in Health Care: Lessons Learnt about Clinical Process Redesign." *Medical Journal of Australia* 188, no. 6: 32–35.

McGuire, T. G. 2000. "Physician Agency." In *Handbook of Health Economics*, Vol. 1A, edited by A. J. Culyer and J. P. Newhouse, 461–536. Amsterdam: Elsevier. http://dx.doi.org/10.1016/S1574-0064(00)80168-7.

Mendelson, D. 1999. "Devaluation of a Constitutional Guarantee: The History of Section 51(xxiiiA) of the Commonwealth Constitution." *Melbourne University Law Review* 23, no. 2: 308–44.

Moorin, R., K. J. Brameld, and C. D. Holman. 2006. "Health Care Financing and Public Responses: Use of Private Insurance in Western Australia During 1980–2001." *Australian Health Review* 30, no. 1: 73–82.

Moorin, R., and C. D. Holman. 2006a. "Does Federal Health Care Policy Influence Switching between the Public and Private Sectors in Individuals?" *Health Policy* 79, no. 2/3: 284–95. http://dx.doi.org/10.1016/j.healthpol.2006.01.011.

———. 2006b. "Do Marginal Changes in PHI Membership Accurately Predict Marginal Changes in PHI Use in Western Australia?" *Health Policy* 76, no. 3: 288–98. http://dx.doi.org/10.1016/j.healthpol.2005.06.012.

———. 2006c. "The Influence of Federal Health Care Policy Reforms on the Use of Private Health Insurance in Disadvantaged Groups." *Australian Health Review* 30, no. 2: 241–51. http://dx.doi.org/10.1071/AH060241.

———. 2007. "Modelling Changes in the Determinants of PHI Utilisation in Western Australia across Five Health Care Policy Eras between 1981 and 2001." *Health Policy* 81, no. 2/3: 183–94. http://dx.doi.org/10.1016/j.healthpol.2006.05.020.

NHHRC (National Health and Hospitals Reform Commission). 2009. *A Healthier Future for All Australians: Final Report of the National Health and Hospitals Reform Commission.* Canberra: NHHRC.

O'Connell, T. J., D. I. Ben-Tovim, B. C. McCaughan, M. G. Szwarcbord, and K. M. McGrath. 2008. "Health Services under Siege: The Case for Clinical Process Redesign." *Medical Journal of Australia* 188, no. 6 (Suppl.): S9–13.

Palangkaraya, A., and J. Yong. 2005. "Effects of Recent Carrot-and-Stick Policy Initiatives on Private Health Insurance Coverage in Australia." *Economic Record* 81, no. 254: 262–72. http://dx.doi.org/10.1111/j.1475-4932.2005.00260.x.

———. 2007. "How Effective is 'Lifetime Health Cover' in Raising Private Health Insurance Coverage in Australia? An Assessment Using Regression Discontinuity." *Applied Economics* 39, no. 11: 1361–74. http://dx.doi.org/10.1080/00036840500486532.

Paterson, J. P. 2002. "Australian Health Care Agreements, 2003–2008: A New Dawn?" *Medical Journal of Australia* 177: 313–15.

Pearse, J. 1994. *The Outcomes of the 1993 Medicare Agreements.* Proceedings of the 16th Australian Conference of Health Economists, Canberra. Sydney: University of New South Wales.

Petherick, E. S., E. V. Villanueva, J. Dumville, E. J. Bryan, and S. Dharmage. 2007. "An Evaluation of Methods Used in Health Technology Assessments Produced for the Medical Services Advisory Committee." *Medical Journal of Australia* 187, no. 5: 289–92.

Pharmaceutical Benefits Pricing Authority. 2010. *Annual Report.* Canberra: Pharmaceutical Benefits Pricing Authority.

Phillips, P. A., and C. F. Hughes. 2008. "Clinical Process Redesign: Can the Leopard Change Its Spots?" *Medical Journal of Australia* 188, no. 6: 7–8.

Productivity Commission. 2010. *Public and Private Hospitals: Multivariate Analysis—Supplement to Research Report.* Melbourne: Productivity Commission.

Propper, C., M. Sutton, C. Whitnall, and F. Windmeijer. 2008. "Did 'Targets and Terror' Reduce Waiting Times in England for Hospital Care?" *BE Journal of Economic Analysis and Policy* 8, no. 2: 5. http://dx.doi.org/10.2202/1935-1682.1863.

Reid, M. A. 2002. "Reform of the Australian Health Care Agreements: Progress or Political Ploy?" *Medical Journal of Australia* 177: 310–15.

Richardson, J. R. J., S. J. Peacock, and D. Mortimer. 2006. "Does an Increase in the Doctor Supply Reduce Medical Fees? An Econometric Analysis of Medical Fees across Australia." *Applied Economics* 38, no. 3: 253–66. http://dx.doi.org/10.1080/00036840500218513.

Scotton, R. B., and C. R. Macdonald. 1993. *The Making of Medibank.* Sydney: University of New South Wales.

Searles, A., S. Jefferys, E. Doran, and D. A. Henry. 2007. "Reference Pricing, Generic Drugs and Proposed Changes to the Pharmaceutical Benefits Scheme." *Medical Journal of Australia* 187, no. 4: 236–39.

Smith, L., N. Amsing, D. Pilbrow, S. Bird, H. Sinnott, H. Teichtahl, and C. Orkin. 2003. "Providing Better Care for Patients with Chronic Disease." *Australian Journal of Primary Health* 9, no. 3: 119–26. http://dx.doi.org/10.1071/PY03035.

Smith, P. C., A. Anell, R. Busse, L. Crivelli, J. Healy, A. K. Lindahl, G. Westert, and T. Kene. 2012. "Leadership and Governance in Seven Developed Health Systems." *Health Policy* 106, no. 1: 37–49. http://dx.doi.org/10.1016/j.healthpol.2011.12.009.

Spigelman, J. 1967. "Program Budgeting for New South Wales." *Australian Journal of Public Administration* 26, no. 4: 348–67. http://dx.doi.org/10.1111/j.1467-8500.1967 .tb00163.x.

Sundararajan, V., K. Brown, T. Henderson, and D. Hindle. 2004. "Effects of Increased Private Health Insurance on Hospital Utilisation in Victoria." *Australian Health Review* 28, no. 3: 320–29. http://dx.doi.org/10.1071/AH040320.

Sweeny, K. 2009. "The Impact of Copayments and Safety Nets on PBS Expenditure." *Australian Health Review* 33, no. 2: 215–30. http://dx.doi.org/10.1071/AH090215.

Swerissen, H. 2004. "Australian Primary Care Policy in 2004: Two Tiers or One for Medicare?" *Australia and New Zealand Health Policy* 1: 2.

Taylor, M. J., D. Horey, C. Livingstone, and H. Swerissen. 2010. "Decline with a Capital D: Long-Term Changes in General Practice Consultation Patterns across Australia." *Medical Journal of Australia* 193: 80–83.

Tingle, L. 2012. *Great Expectations: Government, Entitlement and an Angry Nation.* Collingwood, VIC: Black.

Tuohy, C. H. 2012. "Reform and the Politics of Hybridization in Mature Health Care States." *Journal of Health Politics, Policy and Law* 37, no. 4: 611–32. http://dx.doi .org/10.1215/03616878-1597448.

Williams, R. 2012. "History of Federal–State Fiscal Relations in Australia: A Review of the Methodologies Used." *Australian Economic Review* 45, no. 2: 145–57. http:// dx.doi.org/10.1111/j.1467-8462.2012.00675.x.

Willis, E., S. Young, and P. Stanton. 2005. "Health Sector and Industrial Reform in Australia." In *Workplace Reform in the Healthcare Industry: The Australian Experience,* edited by P. Stanton, E. Willis, and S. Young, 13–29. Basingstoke, UK: Palgrave Macmillan.

Wooldridge, M. R. L. 1991. "Health Policy in the Fraser Years: 1975–83." MBA thesis, Monash University, Melbourne.

Yong, K., and A. H. Harris. 1999. *Efficiency of Hospitals in Victoria under Casemix Funding: A Stochastic Frontier Approach.* West Heidelberg, VIC: Centre for Health Program Evaluation.

Young, A. F. and A. J. Dobson. 2003. "The Decline in Bulk-Billing and Increase in Out-of-Pocket Costs for General Practice Consultations in Rural Areas of Australia, 1995–2001." *Medical Journal of Australia* 178: 122–26.

seventeen
England
ALAN MAYNARD

Scepticaemia: an uncommon generalised disorder of low infectivity.
Medical school education is likely to confer life-long immunity.
— Skrabanek and McCormick (1992)

Introduction

When analyzing medicine and health-care policy, a strong dose of "scepticaemia" is essential. Since Cochrane's book (1972), the development of the Cochrane Collaboration (www.cochrane.org), and the invention of "evidence-based medicine" (EBM) in the 1990s, the medical community has progressed through an agenda to reduce uncertainty in medical practice (Maynard and Chalmers 1997). However, knowledge of what works for which patients at least cost remains incomplete Maynard (1997). This is particularly so for patients with comorbidities, as evaluation and guidelines remain focused on single diseases. Despite these significant developments and the production of EBM practice guidelines, international evidence of unwarranted variations in clinical practice remains (for an overview of some US evidence, see Wennberg 2010).

Improvements in medical knowledge thus compare favourably with knowledge about the cost-effectiveness of policy interventions. Where is the evidence about the effectiveness and cost-effectiveness of large areas of public and private endeavour such as the judiciary, social work, health care, policing, and education? Campbell (1969) advocated investment in all these policy areas, but funding for the Campbell Collaboration (www.campbellcollaboration.org) remains poor. His hope was to remove the "veil of ignorance" that dominates policymaking. His articulation of quasi-experimental methods when randomized controlled trials were difficult to use has led to a burgeoning literature only in the past decade (Campbell and Russo 1999).

However, health policy development throughout the world continues to be dominated by fashions, opinions, and blind, unevidenced faith rather than hard evidence. For instance, the Americans argue intensely about the cost-effectiveness of competing policy "fashions." During Democrat presidencies the reform effort is focused on supply-side interventions such as health maintenance organizations, now transmogrified into Obamacare-accountable care organizations. During Republican administrations, reform efforts focus on demand-side policies such as deductibles, copayments, and budget caps. Evaluation of these policies tends to be incomplete and, where produced, ineffective in changing the ideological perspectives that determine policy.

English policymakers believe that "re-disorganizing" structures for the delivery of health care will lead to improved processes of care and better patient outcomes. Edwards (2010) details the plethora of NHS organizational reforms since 1974, most of which were based on little or no evidence but implemented with enthusiasm and hope. All policymakers, in public and private health-care systems, waste vast resources with such "faith-based" policymaking. Their failure to evaluate policy initiatives ensures that they continue to formulate policy behind Campbell's veil of ignorance. They fail to accept that such an approach is inefficient—and unethical, as it consumes scarce resources and deprives potential patients of care from which they could benefit.

An essential lesson to be learned from international health-care reform is the need to evaluate every reform and seek evidence of effect and cost-effectiveness. Failure to evaluate reform means that policy is based on faith and unfounded optimism.

The English National Health Service: Some recent history

In the six years between 2004 and 2010, per capita spending of the United Kingdom's National Health Service (NHS) grew from $2,540 to $3,433, with the share of GDP funding health care rising from 6% to 8.2%. After this unparalleled funding growth, the British succeeded in bending the cost curve *upwards*, a phenomenon known as the "Blair bonanza." Then the NHS was promised flat real-term funding for the next four years—the "Cameron crunch" (Appleby, Crawford, and Emmerson 2011). Pay was frozen for all health-care workers for three years from 2010, with a 1% increase in 2013–14.

With demand increasing because of aging of the population and often poorly evaluated developments in technology adding to funding pressures, the coalition government adopted a "report" from the consulting firm McKinsey (2009) that had been commissioned by the previous administration. This report, which consists of a series of PowerPoint slides, is very reminiscent of another document produced in a period of fiscal austerity and published in 1976 (Department of Health and Social Security 1976; Maynard 2013b). The focus of both these documents is variations in clinical and administrative activity and the imperative to reduce dispersion and increase the median of these activity distributions to free up resources.

In the English NHS context, managers are required to save and recycle £20 billion from a current budget of £105 billion over four years to meet increased patient demand. This mandate is called the "Nicholson challenge," after the chief executive of the NHS. The intention was that in addition to the pay freeze, several productivity initiatives would be deployed to produce cost savings, with no deleterious effects on process quality and patient outcomes. Savings were made, but the effects on process quality and outcomes remain unclear.

Another "re-disorganization" of NHS structure

Instead of focusing primarily on this "productivity challenge," the coalition government implemented a radical restructuring of the English NHS. The government came to power in 2010, initially promising "no top down reorganisation" of the NHS. However, the secretary of state in charge of the NHS had been the Opposition spokesman for six years, and he articulated clear plans to reform the organizational structure of the system. Implementation of these reforms was highly contentious because of their focus on an increased role for the private sector in both commissioning and purchasing health care and in its provision. The legislation took nearly two years to implement, with much political turmoil and discord among health-care professionals (Timmins 2012).

The organizational structure, implemented in April 2013, involves significant cuts in managerial capacity and the creation of a qango (quasi-autonomous nongovernmental organization), the NHS Commissioning Board, which will be required to work to an explicit contract from the secretary of state to meet funding and quality targets. The purchaser/provider split is retained, with most NHS hospitals being semi-autonomous "foundation trusts" and primary-care physicians (general practitioners) self-employed private-sector entrepreneurs. The radical element of the reform is the creation of 211 "clinical commissioning groups" (CCGs) to replace primary-care trusts. The CCGs are managed by teams that include primary-care physicians (GPs). It is hoped that these "poachers" can be turned into efficient "gamekeepers," as envisaged 25 years ago (Maynard, Marinker, and Pereira-Gray 1986), and in ways similar to the GP fund-holding reforms of the 1990s (Dusheiko et al. 2006).

In terms of clinical practice, the 2012 legislation changes little. There remains an obligation of the state to provide a comprehensive health-care system that is free at the point of delivery. The further emphasis on private provision of care is a continuation of a policy introduced by the Thatcher administration (1979–91) and continued since then by both the Conservative and Labour governments. As yet this policy has had only a marginal effect on the public/private mix.

These structural reforms imposed significant administrative costs, esti-mated to be in excess of £3 billion. Their nature was nicely summarized by the 1979 NHS Royal Commission (quoted in Department of Health and Social Security 1979), which concluded that the 1974 NHS reform had produced "an immense amount of administrative work in preparation for the new machinery; disruption of ordinary work, both before and after reor-ganisation caused by the need to prepare for and implement the changes; the breakdown of well-established formal and informal networks; the loss of experienced staff through early retirement and resignation; the stresses and strains of having to compete for new jobs."

It appears that little has been learned from history, as English policy-makers insist on focusing their attention on radical structural changes that have unspecified and unevidenced effects on the processes of care, costs, and patient outcomes. The propensity of reformers to ignore the impor-tance of physicians and their teams in efficient resource allocation has survived decades of change. Implementation of the current NHS reforms has diverted managerial capacity away from the practices of these decision-makers, who are crucial in bending the cost curve.

Attempts to increase NHS productivity

What is productivity?

Evidencing increased productivity requires the production of data that show for a given budget that outcomes are improved, or for a given level of patient outcomes that costs are reduced. Attempts to improve produc-tivity tend to focus on processes of care rather than patient outcomes. The belief is that if, as in the US Premier hospital incentive scheme, "well evidenced" process and activity targets can be set and improved upon, patients will be better off. Sadly the evidence from the Premier pay-for-performance (P4P) experiment demonstrated that, while a sample of hospitals improved adherence to clinical practice process guidelines, no mortality benefits resulted (Jha et al. 2012). However, an adaption of the Premier program in the North West region of the English NHS produced improved mortality outcomes in a cost-effective manner (Meacock, Kristensen, and Sutton 2014; Sutton et al. 2012). These effects appear to be related to the English changes to the program, which used larger incentives, such as 4% bonuses on tariffs, compared to 2% bonuses in the United States.

However, mortality is a limited measure of success and failure. Patient-reported outcome measures (PROMs) are expensive to collect but have been developed significantly in England. Since 2009, NHS hospitals have been required to collect data on the physical and psychological functioning of patients before and after four elective procedures: hernia repair, varicose vein surgery, and hip and knee replacements. Two quality-of-life questionnaires are being used in these assessments: a generic measure, Equation 5D (www.euroqol.org), and a specific measure, the Oxford Hip Score. By June 2012, more than 460,000 preoperative questionnaires had been completed—about 70% of total activity—and more than 300,000 post-operative questionnaires had been returned, a response rate of 70%.

Funnel plot analysis of risk-adjusted data identifies providers whose performance is significantly different from the national average. This analysis is conducted for each procedure and each instrument. It facilitates identification of not only "success" and outliers but also differences in treatment thresholds. Currently, success rates for hernia repairs are modest, at around 50%, and for hips and knees in excess of 85%. Providing such data to patients may reduce surgery rates.

PROMs are currently being developed in several other areas, including elective coronary revascularization (CABG) and angioplasty, six chronic disease areas, pelvic cancer, cancer survivorship, musculoskeletal conditions, and secondary-care depression. There remain concerns and debates about the sensitivity of the quality-of-life instruments being used, especially Euro quol 5D.

The immediate challenge is getting this data used by clinicians to drive up performance. The program is expensive, but if used by practitioners to interrogate and improve team performance, PROMs could become an integral part not just of increased productivity and reduced clinical practice variations but also of professional revalidation and performance-related (payment by results) incentive schemes.

Even without the development of PROMs, the NHS has large amounts of often unused administrative data that are not integrated into clinical and nonclinical management. A program of increasing productivity and "bending the cost curve" requires systematic use of evidence of the cost, activity, and outcome characteristics of competing policy options and clinical performance. It is essential to engage the medical profession in the use of linked datasets to ensure that unwarranted clinical practice variations are reduced through transparency and reputation defence.

English NHS programs to increase productivity

Background

The reluctance of managers and clinicians to respond to evidence, particularly in relation to variations in productivity, is replicated in many public and private service and manufacturing industries (Syverson 2011). The UK history of clinical practice variations is well chronicled. Glover (1938) noted a threefold variation in tonsillectomy rates and the lack of evidence for such procedures. The Department of Health and Social Security (1976) pointed out variations in length of stay and the uneven take-up of day-case surgery. Bloor, Venters, and Sampier (1977) explored variations in tonsillectomy and adenoidectomy activity in two regions of Scotland and showed that rates varied because of different "conventional wisdoms" in the two surgical teams.

McPherson and colleagues (1982) applied the Dartmouth College methodology to three countries. They demonstrated that despite differing public and private health-care systems, similar variations were evident. A recent overview of studies of medical practice variations in OECD countries lists 836 papers across surgical specialties. Of these, 51% of the studies were from the United States, 15% from the United Kingdom, and 13% from Canada (Stukel and Corallo 2012). There continues to be vigorous debate about whether all or some of these variations are warranted or not. For instance, Cooper (2009 a, 2009b) asserted that the US variations are a product of differing local health-care needs, which are captured imperfectly by the Dartmouth analytical approach. Sheiner (2013) argued that the Dartmouth results are a product of their selection of the unit of analysis. If the econometric analysis is based on controlling health attributes at the state rather than the individual level, as done in the Dartmouth analysis, much of the variation is removed.

There is continuing debate about the magnitude of these variations. Wennberg and his colleagues continue to assert that the adoption of safe conservative practice would save US Medicare 40% of its budget (Wennberg 2010). Cutler and Sheiner (1999) and Rettenmaier and Wang (2012) are more conservative, estimating that eradicating unwarranted variations could save 10–15% of the US Medicare budget. The US Institute of Medicine reviewed the evidence about clinical variations and concluded that they were ubiquitous at all levels of both the public and private health-care systems (Institute of Medicine 2013). They found that in the private sector, expenditure variations were a product of price discrimination by providers. In the public sector, the variations were a product of variations in clinical practice, and most of the variation was in post-acute care (Newhouse and Garber 2013).

While there is conclusive international evidence of unwarranted clinical practice variations, their reduction remains difficult and slow. With parsimonious funding growth forecast for all health-care systems, can behavioural change be achieved? More particularly, how have the English NHS productivity programs developed this agenda?

Altering the behaviour of primary-care physicians

The contracts of employment for UK general practitioners (GPs) and hospital consultants (specialists) have both been reformed in the past decade, and these reforms increased practitioner income by over 20%. What did British taxpayers get in return?

In 2003 a quality outcomes framework (QOF) was implemented for GPs. The QOF set a series of clinical and organizational targets whose achievement earned group GP practices points, which translated into increased income. The clinical targets were modest (e.g., regular checking of blood pressure of patients identified with hypertension) and in some cases not well evidenced in terms of being related to improved patient outcomes (Fleetcroft and Cookson 2006). The initial activity targets set in the QOF were quickly achieved.

A series of papers using difference in difference (DiD) methods has shown that the QOF was successful in changing clinical behaviour, with the greatest change being among the initial low performers (e.g., Doran et al. 2006). These improvements were achieved with no observable effect on non-incentivized services, although the QOF was introduced in a period of rapid expenditure increases, a situation that no longer prevails (Doran et al. 2011). The evolution of QOF targets is now informed by the National Institute for Clinical Excellence (NICE) advising on improvements in the evidence base. The estimated annual cost of this incentive scheme was £1.2 billion.

An evaluation of a set of QOF indicators showed that the QOF payments were cost-effective (Walker et al. 2010). A nice issue in the debate about the QOF is that most of the targets were what might have been expected from a well-run primary-care organization. So would it have been more cost-effective to penalize those who failed to meet those standards? I will return later to this issue of the choice between bonuses and penalties when seeking to incentivize change.

In any DiD evaluation the collection of accurate baseline data is essential. This is needed to the facilitate comparison with post-intervention data and to ensure that targets are set above current levels of activity. However, this was not always done with the QOF. For instance, it was shown that the hypertension-control targets were already being achieved pre-QOF (Seramuga et al. 2011); that is, the GPs were paid a bonus for what they had already been doing!

Another problem with the QOF is "gaming," or cheating. The scheme was introduced with "light touch" management. Where third-party verification is routine (e.g., hospital blood tests), gaming is minimized. However, when computing success in achieving some targets, self-reporting and the role of exceptions come into play; for example, if you asked patients three or four times to attend for a blood or cholesterol test and they did not show, they were discounted. Such rules create scope for deviance in reporting, some of which has been identified (Gravelle, Sutton, and Ma 2010).

The QOF experience has, however, demonstrated clearly that the incentive schemes did alter practitioners' behaviour and may have been cost-effective.

Altering the behaviour of hospital specialists

Until 2004, NHS consultants (hospital specialists), could opt for a full-time contract with the NHS or a part-time contract that enabled them to work part-time in the private sector. Those who opted for the private sector were often accused of neglecting their NHS work to maximize their private-sector income. However, a study of the comparative activity rates of the two groups showed, counterintuitively, that the maximum part-timers did more NHS work than the full-time consultants (Bloor, Maynard, and Freemantle 2004).

The new consultant contract reflected an unfounded generalized suspicion that NHS consultants were skimping on the job. It required them to opt for new contractual terms in exchange for a pay increase of 27% over three years. The contract required consultants to work ten sessions each of four hours, with the option of contracting for up to two additional sessions. Private work could be done in addition to a part-time or full-time NHS contract. The new contract also encouraged modestly better development of individual work plans for each consultant and a system of annual appraisals.

The contract was accompanied by an agreement that consultant activity would increase by 1.5% per annum. However, this element of the deal was underplayed; one study shows that consultant activity levels have been static at best and have declined in some specialties (Bloor, Freemantle, and Maynard 2012). Thus the new consultant contract was an expensive investment that yielded little or no significant activity benefits and unknown effects on patient outcomes (National Audit Office, 2013).

Altering hospital incentives

Until 2004, hospitals were funded by block grants, but since then a system called "payment by results" (PbR) has been introduced. This is similar to DRG systems in the United States and elsewhere—that is, it is activity based. Currently it funds approximately 60% of NHS hospitals' budgets, with the rest being funded by block grants for services.

The PbR system has been continuously manipulated in an effort to enhance productivity; for example, there is downward adjustment of tariffs of 4% annually. Some service changes have been incentivized by enhanced tariffs such as higher payments for day-case gallbladder removal. The payment system has incentivized investment in improved collection of activity and patient-level costs; local and national cost data remain crude, with large unexplained and unmanaged variations between hospitals for similar procedures.

For purchasers, or what are now called "commissioners of NHS care," PbR is a problem. Annual local contracts between purchasers and providers usually specify theoretical activity levels. However, the system is demand-driven. Thus, if admissions increase because GPs refer more patients, commissioners have to pay even though that may break local budget constraints. An effort to constrain this two-part tariff has been introduced, with full emergency tariffs being paid only up to 2008–09 activity levels, after which the tariffs are reduced to 30%.

Alongside PbR, a system of foundation trust (FT) hospitals has been developed. This is managed by a qango, Monitor (www.monitor-nhsft.gov.uk); its role is to rigorously vet applicants for FT status, to monitor their performance, and to intervene if financial balance and quality are poor (e.g., it can dismiss the board of directors and replace managers). FTs have a greater degree of autonomy, can act as private providers, and are encouraged to be entrepreneurial. Thus far, the success of this policy appears to be modest. Bojke and Goddard (2010) conclude that evidence of cost-effectiveness for this policy is absent.

With no growth in real levels of funding planned for four years, the effects of PbR on FTs and a residual group of more than 100 acute and mental health non-FT hospitals will create significant management challenges. For instance, as PbR tariffs are reduced, the bottom decile, or perhaps the bottom quartile, of FTs may face bankruptcy. This should lead to mergers and closures (though, hopefully, in an evidence-based way!).

Increasing competition by tendering services to the private sector has been a policy theme for a decade, but the evidence is far from conclusive. For instance, during the Labour government the drive to reduce elective waiting times led to the creation of "independent sector treatment centres" (ISTCs) to treat NHS patients. The contracts for these units, which provide largely orthopedic and some general surgery, were fully funded from the outset, but it took some years for referral volume to increase, so the ISTCs were paid even when initially they provided no care. Furthermore, they failed to report activity and outcome data in a systematic manner. What data are available show, unsurprisingly, that they "cream off" uncomplicated patients. Consequently there is a case for their receiving lower PbR tariffs than NHS hospitals that deal with the more complicated patients (Mason, Street, and Verzulli 2010).

In addition to PbR, two other incentive mechanisms have been implemented in NHS hospital systems: "Commissioning for Quality and Innovation" (CQUIN) and "Quality, Innovation, Productivity and Prevention" (QIPP). The former was introduced in 2008 and is "a payment framework that allows commissioners to reward excellence by linking a proportion of providers' income to the achievement of local quality improvement goals" (Department of Health 2010a). Local discretion comes into play in negotiating local CQUIN contracts, which currently put 2% of provider income at risk. Each local contract includes core national targets, which include reducing venous thromboembolism (VTE), improving responsiveness to patient needs, and identifying and appropriately treating dementia patients. A variety of local elements are found in CQUIN contracts—3,300 indicators were used in the 2010–11 contracts—with central review and dissemination of indicators used. The effectiveness and cost-effectiveness of local and national CQUIN indicators have not been evaluated systematically.

The Quality, Innovation, Productivity and Prevention (QIPP) incentive system is focused on saving and recycling £20 billion in NHS funds over four years. QIPP offers a plethora of advice about best practice and seeks to explicitly evidence its advice. The National Institute for Clinical Excellence (NICE) provides evidence-based support for the QIPP program. Evaluation of QIPP is difficult. The annual report of the chief executive of the English NHS (Department of Health 2010a) asserts that the efficiency targets for 2011–12 were met, saving £5.8 billion. This was achieved with a virtually static clinical workforce and slight reductions in activity. While costs were reduced, there are few data to illuminate whether access to care and its quality have been maintained or have deteriorated, that is, whether the NHS is achieving constant returns at a lower unit and total cost. A secondary issue is whether efforts to recycle expenditure savings will exhibit diminishing returns as the "low-hanging fruit" are eliminated.

Overview

Without success in meeting its productivity challenges, the NHS is likely to confront reductions in service unless additional funding is provided by government (Appleby 2012). The current coalition, lobbied by right-wing opponents of continuation of a universal state-funded service, faces a nice dilemma: should it break its public expenditure targets or ration in ways that violate its own legislation? The 2012 *Health and Social Care Act* and the NHS constitution guarantee universal coverage, free at the point of use. The coalition has pledged that it will maintain the real level of NHS funding until 2015. It is doubtful, however, whether this funding will be adequate to meet increasing patient demand and significant concerns about the quality of patient care (Francis Report 2013).

Merely identifying hopefully efficient targets for improving resource allocation is not enough—as the saying goes, you can lead a horse to water but you can't make it drink. Incentives have to be designed and implemented carefully, with a focus on their costs and benefits. The key to improved performance in health care is designing, evaluating, and implementing improved incentives at the level of physicians and hospitals. Percival (1803) and Codman (1916) both emphasized that policies to improve accountability and increase productivity should focus on physician outcomes and comparative performance. Professional reputation may be an efficient engine in the drive for increased efficiency (Maynard 2013a).

How good is the evidence base for pay-for-performance programs? The design of P4P programs internationally is generally poor because of an absence of control groups, little or no consideration of cost-effectiveness, limited or no consideration of the knock-on effects of non-incentivized activity, and gaming (e.g., Maynard 2012; van Herck et al. 2010). The literature also shows a marked preference for bonuses rather than penalties, even though behavioural economics predicts that the latter will be more effective (Kahneman and Tversky 1979). The focus of debate and experimentation with P4P will be on increasing the formerly modest size of bonuses, ensuring that such rewards trickle down to improved clinical service systems of performance data, and comparing financial incentives with non-financial incentives that make comparative performance transparent. Despite continuing efforts by policymakers and researchers, we remain quite ignorant about how to bend the cost curve in ways that are demonstrably cost-effective.

Conclusions

The need for "scepticaemia" about policymakers' innovations to "bend the cost curve" and increase productivity is clearly demonstrated by the large number of reforms worldwide and the poor evidence base they have produced to inform policymaking. There has been little efficient "learning by doing." Instead, decision-makers continually reinvent past failures and repackage them as novelties. England epitomizes this with continuous "re-disorganization" accompanied by little evaluation and learning.

More generally, the international health policy community also reforms with little attention paid to using the evidence base in designing policies, or in evaluating them when implemented! Consequently, for decades clinical practice variations have been documented and there have been arguments about their magnitude and which variations are and are not "warranted." There have been continuous, largely unsuccessful changes in policy to remedy these problems by altering organizational structures, clinical processes, and incentives. Surely to improve future policymaking an improved supply of evidence of cause and effect is essential. Let us progress with scepticaemia, perhaps tinged by a hint of optimism, that is focused on improving knowledge internationally of the cost-effectiveness of incentives in improving clinical practice.

References

Appleby, J. 2012. "A Productivity Challenge Too Far?" *British Medical Journal* 344: e2416.

Appleby, J., R. Crawford, and C. Emmerson. 2011. *How Cold Will It Be? Prospects for NHS Funding: 2011–2017.* London: King's Fund.

Bloor, K., N. Freemantle, and A. Maynard. 2012. "Trends in Consultant Clinical Activity and the Effect of the 2003 Contract Change: Retrospective Analysis of Secondary Date." *Journal of the Royal Society of Medicine* 105, no. 11: 472–79.

Bloor, K., A. Maynard, and N. Freemantle. 2004. "Variation in Activity Rates of Consultant Surgeons and the Influence of Reward Structures in the English NHS." *Journal of Health Services Research and Policy* 9, no. 2: 76–84.

Bloor, M. J., G. A. Venters, and M. L. Sampier. 1977. "Geographical Variations in the Incidence of Operations for Tonsils and Adenoids." *Journal of Laryngology and Otology* 92: 791–801, 883–85.

Bojke, C., and M. Goddard. 2010. *Foundation Trusts: A Retrospective Review.* Research paper no. 58. York, UK: University of York Centre for Health Economics.

Campbell, D. T. 1969. "Reforms as Experiments." *American Journal of Psychology* 24, no. 4: 409–29.

Campbell, D. T., and M. J. Russo. 1999. *Social Experimentation.* Atlanta, GA: Sage.

Cochrane, A. L. 1972. *Effectiveness and Efficiency: Random Reflections on Health Services Research.* London: Nuffield Provincial Hospitals Trust.

Codman, E. A. 1916. *A Study in Hospital Efficiency: As Demonstrated by the Case Report of First Five Years of a Private Hospital.* Boston: Thomas Todd.

Cooper, R. 2009a. "States with More Physicians Have Better Quality Health Care." *Health Affairs* 28, no. 1: w91–102. http://dx.doi.org/10.1377/hlthaff.28.1.w91.

———. 2009b. "States with Better Health Care Spending Have Better Quality Health Care: Lessons from Medicare." *Health Affairs* 28, no. 1: 103–15.

Cutler, D. M., and L. Sheiner. 1999. "The Geography of Medicare." *American Economic Review* 89, no. 2: 228–33, doi: 10.1257/aer.89.2.228.

Department of Health (UK). 2010a. "Achieving World Class Productivity in the NHS 2009/10–2013/14: Detailing the Size of the Opportunity" [McKinsey Report]. DH doc. no. 116520. London: Department of Health.

———. 2010b. *Using the Commissioning for Quality and Health (CQUIN) Payment Framework: A Summary Guide.* London: HMSO.

———. 2012. *Guidance on the New National CQUIN Goals.* London: HMSO.

Department of Health and Social Security (UK). 1976. *Priorities in Health and Social Care.* London: HMSO.

———. 1979. *Patients First: A Consultative Paper on the Structure and Management of the NHS in England and Wales.* London: HMSO.

Doran, T. T., C. Fullwood, H. Gravelle, D. Reeves, E. Kontopantelis, U. Hiroeh, and M. Roland. 2006. "Pay for Performance Programs in Family Practices in the United Kingdom." *New England Journal of Medicine* 355, no. 4: 375–84. http://dx.doi.org/10.1056/NEJMsa055505.

Doran, T., E. Kontopantelis, J. M. Valderas, S. Campbell, M. Roland, C. Salisbury, and D. Reeves. 2011. "Effects of Financial Incentives on Incentivised and Non-incentivised Clinical Activities: Longitudinal Analysis of Data from the UL Quality and Outcomes Framework." *British Medical Journal* 342, no. 1: d3590. http://dx.doi.org/10.1136/bmj.d3590.

Dusheiko, M., H. Gravelle, R. Jacobs, and P. C. Smith. 2006. "The Effect of Financial Incentives on Gatekeeping Doctors: Evidence from a Natural Experiment." *Journal of Health Economics* 25: 449–78. http://dx.doi.org/10.1016/j.jhealeco.2005.08.001.

Edwards, N. 2010. *The Triumph of Hope over Experience: Lessons from the History of Reorganisation.* London: NHS Confederation.

Fleetcroft, R., and R. Cookson. 2006. "Do the Incentive Payments in the New NHS Contract for Primary Care Reflect Likely Population Health Gains?" *Journal of Health Services Research and Policy* 11, no. 1: 27–31. http://dx.doi.org/10.1258/135581906775094316.

Francis Report. 2013. *Report of the Mid-Staffordshire Foundation Trust Public Inquiry* [Francis Report]. Executive summary. House of Commons Papers no. 947. London: HMSO.

Glover, J. A. 1938. "The Incidence of Tonsillectomy in School Children." *Journal of the Royal Society of Medicine* 31: 1219–96.

Gravelle, H., M. Sutton, and A. Ma. 2010. "Doctor Behaviour under a Pay for Performance Contract: Treating, Cheating and Case Finding?" *Economic Journal* 120, no. 542: F129–56. http://dx.doi.org/10.1111/j.1468-0297.2009.02340.x.

Institute of Medicine (US). 2013. *Variations in Health Care Spending: Target Decision Making, Not Geography.* Washington, DC: National Academies Press.

Jha, A. K., K. E. Joynt, E. J. Orav, and A. M. Epstein. 2012. "Long Term Effect of Premier Pay for Performance on Patient Outcomes." *New England Journal of Medicine* 366, no. 17: 1606.

Kahneman, D., and A. Tversky. 1979. "Prospect Theory: An Analysis of Decision under Risk." *Econometrica* 47, no. 2: 263–92. http://dx.doi.org/10.2307/1914185.

Mason, A., A. Street, and R. Verzulli. 2010. "Private Sector Treatment Centres Are Treating Less Complex Patients than the NHS." *Journal of the Royal Society of Medicine* 103, no. 8: 322–31. http://dx.doi.org/10.1258/jrsm.2010.100044.

Maynard, A. 1997. "Evidence Based Medicine: An Incomplete Method for Informing Treatment Choice." *Lancet* 349, no. 9045: 126–28. http://dx.doi.org/10.1016/S0140-6736(96)05153-7.

———. 2012. "The Powers and Pitfalls of Payment for Performance." *Health Economics* 21, no. 1: 3–12, doi: 10.1002/hec.1810.

———. 2013a. "Contracting for Quality in the NHS." Office of Health Economics annual lecture. London: Office of Health Economics.

———. 2013b. "Funding Health Care in Times of Austerity: What Goes Around Comes Around." *Journal of Health Services Research and Policy* 18, no. 1: 1–2. http://dx.doi.org/10.1258/jhsrp.2012.012041.

Maynard, A., and I. Chalmers, eds. 1997. *Non-random Reflections on Health Services Research.* London: BMJ Publishing Group.

Maynard, A., M. Marinker, and D. Pereira-Gray. 1986. "The Doctor, the Patient and Their Contract: Alternative Contracts—Are They Viable?" *British Medical Journal* 292: 1438–40.

McPherson, K., J. E. Wennberg, O. B. Hovind, and P. Clifford. 1982. "Small Area Variations in the Use of Common Surgical Procedures: An International Comparison of New England, England and Norway." *New England Journal of Medicine* 307, no. 21: 1310–14. http://dx.doi.org/10.1056/NEJM198211183072104.

Meacock, R., S. Kristensen, and M. Sutton. 2014. "The Cost Effectiveness of Using Financial Incentives to Improve Provider Quality: A Framework and an Application." *Health Economics* 23, no. 1: 1–13.

Newhouse, J. P., and A. M. Garber. 2013. "Geographic Variation in Health Care Spending in the United States: Insights from an Institute of Medicine Report." *Journal of the American Medical Association* 310, no. 12: 1227–28. http://dx.doi.org/10.1001/jama.2013.278139.

National Audit Office (UK). 2013. *Managing Hospital Consultants.* HC 885. London: HMSO.

Percival, T. 1803. *Medical Ethics: Or, a Code of Institutes and Precepts Adopted to Professional Conduct of Physicians and Surgeons.* Manchester.

Rettenmaier, A., and Z. Wang. 2012. "Regional Variations in Medical Spending and Utilization: A Longitudinal Analysis of US Medicare Population." *Health Economics* 21, no. 2: 67–82.

Seramuga, B., D. Ross-Degnan, A. J. Avery, R. A. Elliott, S. R. Majumdar, F. Zhang, and S. B. Soumerai. 2011. "Effect of Pay for Performance on the Management and Outcomes of Hypertension in the United Kingdom: Interrupted Time Series Study." *British Medical Journal* 342, no. 3: d108. http://dx.doi.org/10.1136/bmj.d108.

Sheiner, L. 2013. *Why the Geographical Variations in Health Care Spending Can't Tell Us Much about the Efficiency or Quality of Our Health Care System.* Finance and Economics discussion series, Divisions of Research and Statistics and Monetary Affairs. Washington, DC: Federal Reserve Board.

Skrabanek, P., and J. McCormick. 1992. *Follies and Fallacies in Medicine*. Glasgow: Tarragon Press.

Stukel, T. A., and A. N. Corallo. 2012. "Medical Practice Variations in OECD Countries: An Overview of Recent Studies." PowerPoint presentation, OECD meeting, April.

Sutton, M., S. Nikolova, R. Boaden, H. Lester, R. McDonald, and M. Roland. 2012. "Reduced Mortality with Hospital Pay for Performance in England." *New England Journal of Medicine* 367, no. 19: 1821–28. http://dx.doi.org/10.1056/NEJMsa1114951.

Syverson, C. 2011. "What Determines Productivity?" *Journal of Economic Literature* 49: 326–65.

Timmins, N. 2012. *Never Again?* London: King's Fund and Institute for Government.

Van Herck, P., D. De Smedt, L. Annemans, R. Remmen, M. B, Rosenthal, and W. Sermeus. 2010. "Systematic Review: Effects, Design Choices and the Context of Pay for Performance Health Care." *BMC Health Services Research* 10, no. 1: 247. http://dx.doi.org/10.1186/1472-6963-10-247.

Walker, S., A. R. Mason, K. Claxton, R. Cookson, E. Fenwick, R. Fleetcroft, and M. Sculpher. 2010. "Value for Money and the Quality Outcomes Framework in Primary Care in the UK NHS." *British Journal of General Practice* 60, no. 574: 213–20. http://dx.doi.org/10.3399/bjgp10X501859.

Wennberg, J. E. 2010. *Tracking Medicine: A Researcher's Quest to Understand Health Care*. New York: Oxford University Press.

eighteen
Nordic Countries

JON MAGNUSSEN

Introduction

Many public health-care systems provide a basket of services to citizens under universal coverage. Copayments are non-existent or very low, with financing based on general taxes and/or mandatory insurance premiums. The term *fiscal sustainability* refers to a system's ability to generate a revenue stream to finance the desired level of public expenditure for the basket of universal services. From a policy point of view it is important to establish both *whether* sustainability will be an issue and also *why* it is expected to be an issue.

Expenditure may grow faster than revenues as a result of increased demand or a reduced willingness or ability to pay for health-care services. Demand may increase as the result of general growth in the population eligible for health care, but also because of changing demographics. Demand is also likely to increase when income increases[1] and may be driven by supply-side innovations such as new drugs, therapies, or technologies. Revenue failure, on the other hand, can be the result of an erosion of the tax base as a result of changing demographics, increased unemployment, economic recession, or unwillingness to increase taxes.

The Council of the European Union has defined its four core values for the health-care sector as universal coverage, solidarity in financing, equity of access, and high-quality care (Thomson et al. 2007). Since 2008 the financial crisis in Europe has put substantial pressure on public finances, strengthening concern about the future sustainability of public health-care systems. However, there are large variations among countries in Europe, both in the organization and delivery of health care and in how countries are affected by the financial crisis. In this chapter we provide a Nordic perspective on the question of sustainability by examining the recent experiences of Norway, Finland, Sweden, Denmark, and Iceland.[2] While health care in

---

1 The literature is not entirely clear on the issue of the size of income elasticity, with estimates ranging from low to high elasticities. See, for example, Baltagi and Moscone 2010.
2 Because of lack of information, not all countries are discussed in all sections.

these countries is based on the same set of values as those proposed by the Council of the European Union, they have some distinctive features that make it relevant to talk about a "Nordic model of health care," one that can be usefully compared to the Canadian model (Magnussen et al. 2009).

The Nordic model of health care[3]

Structural issues

The Nordic countries have a common approach to social welfare, with the central government playing a dominant role in the formation of welfare policies, and decentralized implementation and delivery of policy programs by more local governments and other public bodies. Nordic health-care systems are characterized by tax-based financing, universal access, services that are (almost) free at the point of use, and a strong focus on equity. However, we find important differences in the design and implementation of health-care policy (Table 18.1); we have also included some summery statistics in Table 18.2.

The health-care systems in Nordic countries share many similarities with that of Canada; tax funding, universal access, and focus on equity are all similar features. However, there are also important differences. First, hospital physicians are salaried and thus an integral part of hospitals. Second, the political and fiscal authority and power of Canadian provinces are substantially greater than those of Nordic regions or counties. Third, Canada has a much higher share of private financing than the Nordic countries. Each of these differences may influence health-care spending, and thus also the possibility of bending the cost curve.

Trends in health-care spending

Health-care expenditure as share of GDP (Figure 18.1) is commonly used to describe the "financial burden" of the health-care system. Differences would seem to be quite substantial, with Finland spending less and Denmark well above the OECD average. However, some of these differences reflect that long-term care is accurately included for some (Norway, Denmark, Canada), only partly for one (Finland), and not at all for another (Sweden). In addition, health-care spending as share of GDP will obviously fluctuate with economic cycles in the short run, so it is important to focus on longer-term trends. Finally, two countries may spend an equal share of

---

3 This section builds on the introductory chapter in Magnussen et al. 2009.

Table 18.1 Summary of Nordic health-care systems

	Governance Structure	Political Governance	Purchaser Level	Financing of Purchaser Level	Copayments
Norway	4 state-owned regional health authorities 430 municipalities	State level for specialized care Municipal level for primary and long-term care	Regional health authorities: specialized care Municipalities: primary and long-term care	Regions: mix of capitation and activity-based financing Municipalities: local taxes and state grants	Yes, capped at NOK1,980 ($350) Exemptions for young children, pregnant women, and disabled
Denmark	5 regions 89 municipalities	Through regional elections	Regions: specialized and primary care Municipalities: long-term care	Regions: capitation-based model Municipalities: local taxes and state grants	Only for drugs, decreasing with spending. Capped for chronically ill at DKK3,410 ($640)
Sweden	18 counties, 3 regions 290 municipalities	Through elections	Counties (regions): specialized and primary care Municipalities: long-term care	Mainly local taxes Some income-equalizing state grants	Yes, capped at SEK900 ($140) for health services and SEK1,800 ($280) for drugs Exemptions for children
Finland	336 municipalities 20 hospital districts	Through hospital boards appointed from elected municipal boards	Municipalities, through hospital districts	Local taxes Income-equalizing state grants	Yes, capped at €675 ($860)

Table 18.2 Summary statistics, Nordic countries and Canada

	Denmark	Finland	Norway	Sweden	Canada	OECD
GDP per capita (2005 USD)	32,241	31,310	46,908	34,126	35,223	30,151
Share of GDP to health (%)	11.1	8.9	9.4	9.6	11.4	9.5
Proportion of population over 65 (%)	16.8	17.5	15.1	18.5	14.8	

Source: OECD.

Figure 18.1 Total expenditure on health care as share of GDP, 2010

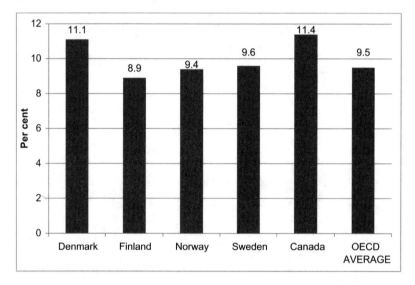

Source: OECD.

GDP on health care, but if GDP differs this may not reflect differences in the availability of health care.

In Figure 18.2 we show public health-care spending per capita in purchase power parity (PPP)–adjusted US dollars. We note that Norway, which has an average spending level when measured as share of GDP, has a substantially higher level of spending per capita. This, of course, reflects a higher level of national income in Norway. Again, such numbers need to be interpreted with substantial care.[4]

---

4 The OECD uses a general deflator, and it is argued (Møinichen-Berstad 2012) that this underestimates the effect of higher wages in Norway.

Figure 18.2 Public spending per capita, 2010 (PPP US dollars)

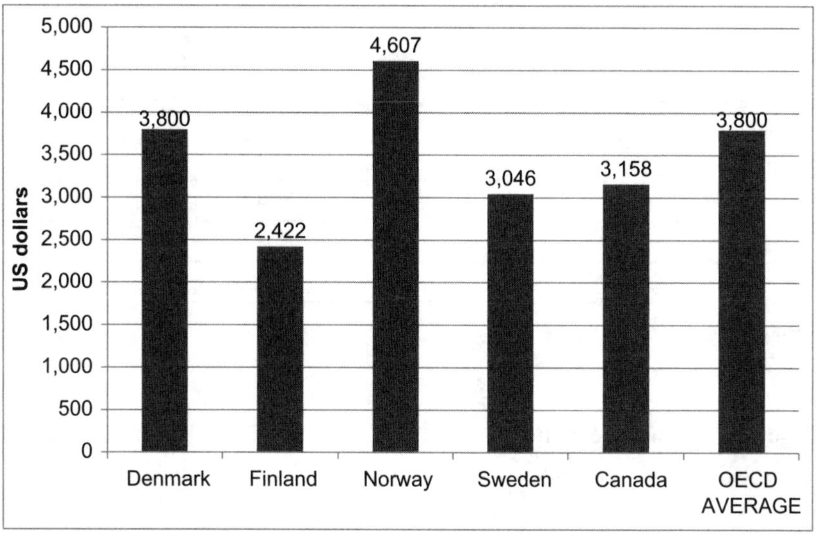

Source: OECD.

The question of fiscal sustainability is generally related to public-sector rather than total expenditures.[5] Di Matteo and Di Matteo (2012) suggest that the ratio of government (public) health expenditure to GDP can be a general macro indicator of fiscal sustainability. In Figure 18.3 we track this indicator from 1990 to 2010 for the Nordic countries.

Norway and Sweden have fairly stable expenditure shares over this 20-year period. Finland went through a severe macroeconomic recession in the early 1990s and is still working gradually to increase its share up to the level before the recession. Denmark has diverged somewhat from its Nordic neighbours since 2000; its spending is now higher than for its neighbouring countries, while Canada's public-sector health spending as share of GDP is close to the levels of Norway and Sweden.

Table 18.3 compares total and public growth in per capita health-care expenditures in real terms in the past decade. Average growth was substantially higher in the first five years, reflecting the impact of the financial crisis in 2008. These numbers also underline that, even though Norway has a higher level of health expenditures, growth there has not been very

---

5 Thomson, Foubister, and Mossialos (2007) make the distinction between *economic* and *fiscal* sustainability. Health-care expenditure as share of GDP thus has more relation to economic sustainability.

Table 18.3 Growth in health-care expenditures in real terms, 2000–2010

	Total		Public	
	2000–05	2005–10	2000–05	2005–10
Denmark	3.6	2.5	3.8	2.7
Finland	5.9	2.1	7.1	1.9
Iceland	4.2	−0.1	4.3	−0.3
Norway	4.3	2.2	4.5	2.7
Sweden	4.8	2.6	3.9	2.6
Canada	4.7	4.2	4.7	4.5

Source: OECD.

Figure 18.3 Public expenditure on health as share of GDP, 1990–2010

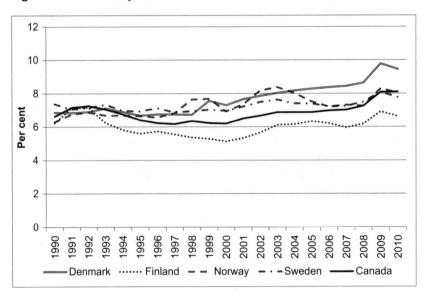

Source: OECD.

different from that in the other countries. While growth in both total and public health-care expenditures has slowed down in the Nordic countries since 2005, this does not appear to have been the case in Canada.

Figure 18.4 shows the share of total health-care spending that is public. Mainly because of a large private occupational health sector, Finland has a lower share than the other Nordic countries. In addition, Finland's public

Figure 18.4 Public share of health-care expenditures, 1990–2010

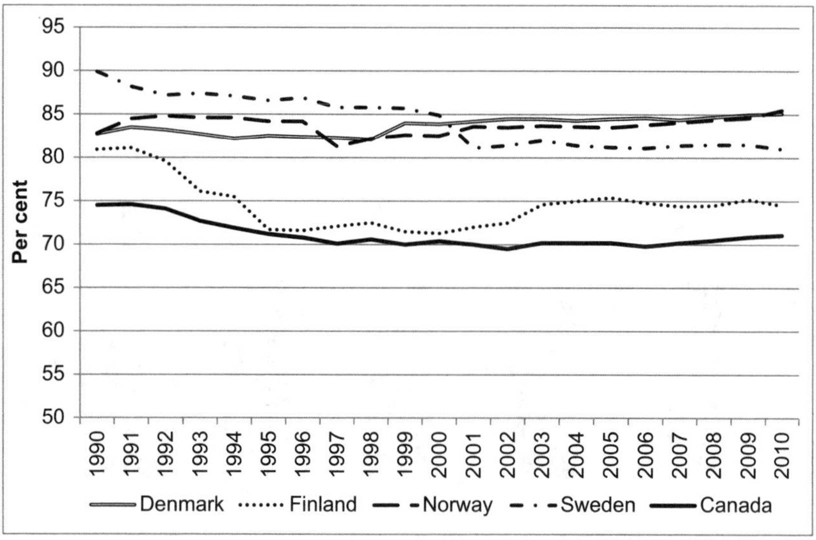

Source: OECD.

spending was reduced dramatically following the macroeconomic recession in the early 1990s. Notably, Sweden experienced a gradual decline in the share of public health-care expenditures in the 1990s but now seems to have reached a stable share. All countries are well above the OECD average of 72.5% in 2010, and also well above the share of public financing in Canada.

Finally, Figure 18.5 shows public health-care expenditures as share of total taxes. There are cyclical fluctuations in tax income, so the share of public health-care expenditures is likely to go up when tax income is reduced. As shown in Figure 18.5, the share of taxes spent on health care increased modestly in Norway, Denmark, and Sweden in this period. Notably, however, in Canada the share increased substantially in the past decade and is now much higher than in the Nordic countries.

The role of private supplementary insurance

If public spending on health care decreased as a result of cost-containing policies, we would expect an increase in the number of people buying supplementary health insurance. Private supplementary insurance has historically played a minor role in all the Nordic countries, but this has changed substantially in the past decade.

Figure 18.5 Public health-care spending as share of total tax revenue, 1990–2010

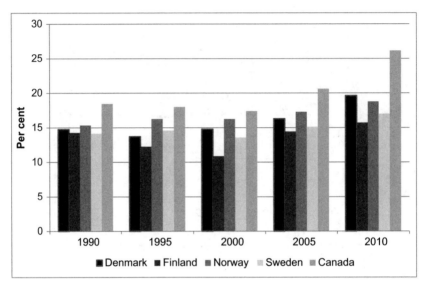

Source: OECD.

Since the turn of the millennium, the share of the population covered by supplementary private insurance has more than quadrupled in Norway, Denmark, and Sweden. In Denmark close to 40% of the workforce is now covered, while the corresponding share in Norway and Sweden is close to 10%. Private insurance is linked predominantly to employment—many employers offer private health insurance as a fringe benefit—and approximately 90% of the policies are group-based policies. The number of individuals signing up for private insurance is nonetheless increasing, albeit at a modest rate. Supplementary insurance does not generally cover copayments but rather guarantees faster access to services or access to services outside of the public health-care benefit package.

The large difference between Denmark, on the one hand, and Norway and Sweden, on the other, may be attributed to private insurance's being tax-exempt in Denmark. A condition for this, however, is that employers offer insurance to all employees. In Sweden, private health insurance is made subject to taxation but at a low level; only 15% of the insurance premium is counted as income. In Norway the whole premium is added as income and also made subject to social security contributions. Notably, Norway had a three-year period (2003–06) during which health insurance was tax-exempt, but a reversal of this policy did not lead to a slowdown in growth of the number of insured.

It is not clear whether the large growth of supplementary insurance is a sign of discontent with the public system, and thus also a measure of the pressure to increase capacity (and costs). Private insurance is relatively inexpensive—the cost of the average policy is approximately 200–300 euros per year in all countries (Berge and Hyggen 2010)—and for employers may be cheaper than offering free health club memberships, cellphones, or similar fringe benefits. From this perspective, the increase in the number of privately insured people may also be interpreted as a result of a competitive labour market, along with effective private-sector marketing.

Bending the cost curve in the Nordic countries

Thomson, Foubister, and Mossialos (2007) suggest three broad paths for securing fiscal sustainability: (1) increasing revenue, (2) weakening obligations (i.e., reducing coverage), and (3) increasing capacity through improved efficiency. Rehnberg and colleagues (2009) draw a distinction between supply-side measures, demand-side measures, and measures to improve the efficiency of the system. This discussion adopts their distinction[6] and provides a brief review of the most relevant health policy measures undertaken to "bend the cost curve" in the Nordic countries. We begin with an examination of the broader fiscal environment in which the five Nordic countries operate.

Fiscal policies[7]

The financial crisis strengthened the focus on the Nordic countries' ability to finance the public sector in the short as well as long term. The combination of high levels of public debt and low levels of future public income has led several countries to reduce their current levels of welfare services as well as other public expenditures. Growth in health-care spending slowed and even fell in response to the financial crisis of 2009 (OECD 2012e); thus a discussion about health-care sustainability must still take into account the general fiscal situation.

Finland has a relatively low level of public deficit and debt but has other, longer-term challenges. These are related to a population that is aging more rapidly compared to the other Nordic countries, as well as a low retirement

---

6 And builds in some parts on their discussion.

7 The Economic Surveys for Denmark, Finland, Norway, and Sweden (OECD 2012a–d) have provided important material for this section.

age. These two factors have produced a combined scenario of lower tax income and higher pension obligations. Thus Finland could well face a situation where it may prove difficult to finance current levels of health care.

Norway has a running surplus, thanks to its substantial petroleum wealth. This wealth is managed thorough the Government Pension Fund (GPF). Fiscal policy dictates that there may be an annual public deficit of non-oil GDP amounting to no more than 4% of the value of the GPF. In reality, Norway is a net saver, and as long as oil reserves are not depleted in the short run and the pension fund generates a healthy return, there is no long-term threat to the fiscal situation in Norway.

Sweden underwent a major recession in 1991–93, to which the central government responded by creating a regime of fiscal discipline that has led to both annual fiscal surpluses and a gradual reduction in public debt. The basic foundation of Sweden's fiscal policy is a combination of a centralized top-down budget process, clear fiscal targets, a ceiling for future government expenditures, and a balanced budget requirement for local governments (Calmfors 2012). While these are not legally enforced, a combination of transparency and consensus seems to be sufficient for local as well as central fiscal control.

Denmark has a relatively good fiscal position, but this is partly due to comparatively high tax rates. Public expenditures (including health care) have increased substantially from levels that were already high. While fiscal control is generally good, the OECD points to "slippage," especially at the sub-national (municipal) level, that needs to be dealt with. Soft budgeting will have an effect both on the public deficit and on the fact that the marginal cost of providing services at the local level will (seemingly) be low, thus creating local pressure for a higher supply of services.

Iceland went through a severe crisis in 2008–09. The debt-to-GDP ratio increased from practically zero in 2007 to 40% in 2009, and the budget deficit went from near balance in 2008 to 10% in 2009. At the time of writing, however, Iceland's economy, as well its fiscal position, had improved and a fiscal surplus was estimated for 2013 (OECD 2011).

Demand-side measures for bending the cost curve

In a system that provides universal coverage for services that are (almost) free at the point of use, there is bound to be pressure on health-care costs.[8] Non-price rationing mechanisms (see below) may alleviate some of this

---

8 The classic argument is that when a service is free, it will be utilized until the marginal benefit to the individual is zero (Pauly 1968).

pressure, but policy measures that can reduce demand are also necessary. Such policies may imply increasing copayments, a gatekeeping system for specialized care, and (in the longer term) shifting focus from treatment to prevention.

Copayments (user charges) can be motivated by a desire to raise revenues or by a wish to reduce spending by limiting demand. Thomson, Foubister, and Mossialos (2010) argue strongly that in the event that user charges are imposed, they need to be value-based, by which they mean directed at making people reduce the use of low-value services. Charging patients for services that we want them to use makes sense only from a fiscal point of view. And in that case the distributional effects of user charges are clearly less desirable than increasing taxes (Thomson et al. 2010).

In line with the Nordic welfare model, copayments have traditionally been kept at a very low level. Furthermore, even when there are copayments, there is an upper limit for individual expenses. Thus, in the Nordic context, copayments are motivated mainly by the desire to curb demand. There are differences between the four countries: Denmark in particular does not have copayments for GP (general practitioner) visits or hospital care; Norway has copayments for GP visits and outpatient (but not inpatient) hospital care; and Finland and Sweden have copayments for both GP visits and hospital care. For long-term care the picture is somewhat different, with all the countries imposing substantially higher copayments for institutionalized care.

Gatekeeping is one of the cornerstones of the Norwegian, Finnish, and Danish systems and is specifically thought of as a mechanism to keep down use of costly specialized services, as well as to provide continuity of care for patients (Pedersen, Andersen, and Søndergaard 2012). In Sweden it is possible to bypass GPs and seek specialist health care directly. However, to encourage patients to first visit a GP, hospital copayments are higher for those who choose to access a specialist directly.

The basic motive behind gatekeeping is that GPs will prevent unnecessary visits to specialists, prevent doctor shopping, and also reduce duplicate testing (Reibling and Wendt 2012). A review by Garrido, Zentner, and Busse (2011) indicates that gatekeeping does lead to fewer and shorter hospital stays, and also to lower health-care costs. The effects do not seem, however, to be strong and straightforward. The crucial point therefore seems to be to provide a set of specific incentives aimed at GPs, together with the general gatekeeping arrangement, to realize its full potential in preventing unnecessary use of hospital services.

Supply-side measures for bending the cost curve

Controlling expenditure growth via the supply side can be done in three ways. First, the delivery system can be reorganized to improve efficiency. Second, the capacity of the system can be limited, in terms of physical capacity and number of personnel but also in terms of introduction of new medical innovations. Third, the scope of public coverage may be reduced.

A specific feature of the Nordic model of welfare has been reliance on a decentralized model of local governance, funding, and delivery. In this model, local authorities have had the opportunity to tax, the responsibility for provision of services, and in many cases also a role as provider (Hagen and Vrangbæk 2009). However, concerns about both geographical inequity and unexploited economics of scale have led the Nordic countries on a path of recentralization. This has been particularly pronounced in Norway and Denmark, where responsibility for specialized health care was transferred from the county level to the state (Norway) or regional (Denmark) level (see Magnussen, Hagen, and Kaarboe 2007; Hagen and Vrangbæk 2009).

Sweden and Finland remain comparatively more decentralized than their two neighbours. In its 2012 economic outlook for Finland, the OECD concluded that "the decentralized structure of the Finnish health care system contributes to inefficiencies" (OECD 2012a). The OECD recommendations are in line with policy in Finland, where the process of merging municipalities into larger, more economically robust entities has been ongoing for some years. No such recentralization has occurred in Sweden, where the role of the state in health policy is traditionally weaker. However, within Swedish counties there are examples of restructuring to exploit perceived economies of scale and thereby improve efficiency.

In addition to recentralization there is also a strong focus on shifting care from specialized to (presumably) less costly primary-care settings. Again Denmark and Norway are leading the way, by introducing a municipal copayment for hospital care and strengthening preventive care. Municipal copayment has been the model in Denmark since 2007; it was introduced as a tool of a much anticipated "coordination reform" in Norway in 2012. In Finland central authorities are currently working to centralize emergency care, a development that is also intended to lead to a better-functioning and more cost-efficient primary-care sector (OECD 2012b). In Sweden, where the organization of primary care varies among the 21 counties, municipalities will pay for patients who are ready to be discharged from hospitals but cannot be admitted to a nursing home.

The combination of expanded choice and legislation (or, in some cases, non-binding guarantees) has been introduced in all Nordic countries as a means to improve efficiency and system integration. Choice (in theory) should increase the flexibility of the system and thus improve efficiency. Using legislation to set the maximum number of days a patient should wait can also be expected to increase demand-side pressure on the system and thereby reduce control over total expenditures.

How different methods of payment affect total health-care expenditure will, among other things, depend on the goals pursued by the hospitals. Nordic hospitals are predominantly publicly owned, with salaried physicians. In this setting it is generally assumed (see, for example, Langenbrunner et al. 2009) that prospective variable-payment systems (e.g., activity-based financing) will provide incentives for increased activity as well as cost consciousness—and therefore efficiency—but might lead to problems with patient selection and treatment quality. Prospective fixed systems (e.g., global budgets) provide incentives for reduced costs and activity but may also generate access problems. This trade-off among quality (selection), cost efficiency, and cost control has resulted in a variety of hospital payment systems across health-care systems, reflecting both differences in the weighting of policy goals and uncertainty about how payment systems actually function.

Norway, and to a lesser extent Denmark, uses activity-based financing not only to pay providers but also to finance purchasers. Thus in Norway since 2014 the regions have received 50% of average DRG cost for somatic-care patients. In Denmark, as noted, the state finances the "planned extra activity" (*merkativitetspuljen*) through activity-based financing, but this accounts for as little as 3% of total income.

Norway, Sweden, and Denmark all pay hospitals through a mixture of activity (DRG)–based financing and a fixed budget. However, only Norway bases the fixed part of the hospital budget on a needs-adjusted capitation. There are two implications of the Norwegian model: First, hospital budgets will reflect the relative need of the population in the hospital's catchment area and thus contribute to equal access. Second, there will be a need for payment mechanisms between hospitals, since there will be a division of tasks between them.

There are also differences related to how budgets are set. Denmark, some counties in Sweden, and some districts in Finland use DRGs to calculate budget levels. Other counties in Sweden and districts in Finland rely more on historical costs. This is somewhat surprising, since retrospective systems are generally believed to be challenging with regards to both cost control and efficiency.

Governance measures for bending the cost curve

Norway is the most centralized of the Nordic countries. This is reflected in a low share of local financing, a common financing system for the regional health authorities (RHAs), and the fact that all RHAs choose similar models for financing hospitals. In Denmark, where we find a similar uniform model for financing the regional level, there are substantial variations between regions in their financing of hospitals. These differences reflect different priorities, different policy challenges, and possibly different policy and value preferences. Similar differences within a country can be found in Sweden and Finland, where devolution is stronger, in the sense that counties and municipalities can also adjust local tax levels.

The differences between Norway and Denmark, as relatively centralized systems, and Sweden and Finland, as politically decentralized systems, are also effectively illustrated in Kalseth et al. (2011). The authors surveyed the public hospital owners[9] in all four countries, analyzing the major challenges in the hospital sector. In Norway the general response is "balance the budget," and keeping costs within budget limits is also presented as the major issue in Denmark. What is striking is the variety of answers from Finland and Sweden, ranging from how to coordinate care across county borders to lack of physicians. Thus the range of challenges reported from Sweden and Finland clearly supports the notion of these two countries as substantially more centralized than Norway and Denmark.

Notably, hospital owners in all four countries report back that deficit spending is a problem. Again countries seem to vary in how these are dealt with. In Norway, deficits have been partly compensated by extra funding from the central government, although budget control seems to have been tightened in the past few years. Denmark has traditionally had fewer problems with deficits but is trying to implement an even tighter regime, demanding that deficits be followed by cuts in subsequent years.

The Danish model has been characterized as balancing on a knife's edge (Bilde, Hansen, and Søgaard 2010). If activity levels exceed planned levels, hospitals may get extra income from the "extra activity pool," but productivity demands will increase the following year. If activity is lower, income is reduced and deficits need to be covered in the subsequent year. Thus the incentive is to reach a targeted activity level. In Finland and Sweden it is again difficult to establish a pattern. Especially interesting

---

9 That is, regions in Denmark, regional health authorities in Norway, counties in Sweden, and hospital districts in Finland.

is the practice in some Finnish hospital districts, where potential deficits are avoided by adjusting DRG reimbursements during the fiscal year. Thus if a deficit is anticipated, the DRG-specific prices are adjusted up, implying that the municipalities in the hospital district bear the cost of the hospital's deficit.

Conclusion

From the discussion above five points have emerged:

1. With the possible exception of Finland, the fiscal situation in the Nordic countries is sound and does not warrant any drastic short-term measures. Notably, however, while the decentralized model seemingly has not led to budget deficits at the local level in Sweden, soft budgeting seems to be a greater concern in Denmark. In a Canadian context it is worth noting that while there are no immediate fiscal concerns at the federal level, provinces may face greater challenges and thus need to curb costs, possibly at a pace more similar to the Nordic countries.

2. Decentralized political governance may contribute to structural inefficiencies, and the policy has therefore been to recentralize political governance and/or merge local authorities into larger, more sustainable units. The exception here is Sweden. There is a lack of hard evidence on to what degree recentralization has actually curbed costs, but anecdotal evidence from Norway and Denmark would suggest that soft budgeting may become less of a problem in a more centralized setting.

3. Payment systems have been refined to include an activity-based component, although the size of this component varies both between and within countries. The effect of this has been improved efficiency (Bjørn et al. 2003), but there may also be resulting higher levels of activity and thus pressure on total health-care spending (Magnussen et al. 2007). Notably, the introduction of the DRG system has also served as a tool for monitoring, and thus has potential for better resource management.

4. Shifting demand (and activity) from specialized to primary health care is a common policy goal. Various measures have been introduced to facilitate this; examples are municipal copayment for hospital care, restructuring of the hospital sector to facilitate more efficient patient pathways, and a stronger focus on prevention. However, there is to date no hard evidence on the effects of this approach.

5. Demand-side measures are few and increased (or reduced) copayment is not being considered. The same applies to reduction in coverage. At the same time, voluntary supplementary private health insurance is growing at a rapid pace. Whether this will lead in turn to the introduction of private complementary insurance, as seen in Canada, and thus reduce the share of publicly financed health care, remains to be seen. At the time of writing, however, the strong focus on equity seems to preclude such a development.

Is there a lesson for Canada here? First, the discussion above would suggest that the fiscal soundness of the Nordic health-care systems is closely linked to the overall fiscal soundness of the Nordic economies. Second, there is an awareness in the traditionally devolved Nordic countries that centralization has its merits, in terms of both fiscal control and a more feasible strategic governance. Thus a feasible strategy seems to be a modest (centralized) supply-side pressure and at the same time a strengthening of the focus on primary care and prevention.

References

Baltagi, B. H., and F. Moscone. 2010. "Health Care Expenditure and Income in the OECD Reconsidered: Evidence from Panel Data." *Economic Modelling* 27, no. 4: 804–11. http://dx.doi.org/10.1016/j.econmod.2009.12.001.

Berge, Ø. M., and C. Hyggen. 2010. *Fremveksten av private helseforsikringer i Norden* [Growth in private health insurance in the Nordic countries]. Fafo notat 2010:11. Oslo: Stiftelsen FAFO.

Bilde, L., A. R. Hansen, and J. Søgaard. 2010. *Økonomi og styring i sygehusvæsenet* [Economy and governance in the hospital sector]. København: Dansk Sundhedsinstitut.

Bjørn, E., T. P. Hagen, T. Iversen, and J. Magnussen. 2003. "The Effect of Activity Based Financing on Hospital Efficiency: A Panel Data Analysis of DEA Efficiency Scores, 1992–2000." *Health Care Management Science* 6, no. 4: 271–83. http://dx.doi.org/10.1023/A:1026212820367.

Calmfors, L. 2012. *Sweden, from Macroeconomic Failure to Macroeconomic Success.* Stockholm: IIES, Stockholm University.

Di Matteo L., and R. Di Matteo. 2012. *The Fiscal Sustainability of Canadian Publicly Funded Healthcare Systems and the Policy Response to the Fiscal Gap.* CHSRF Reports on Financing Models no. 5. Ottawa: Canadian Health Services Research Foundation.

Garrido, M. V., A. Zentner, and R. Busse. 2011. "The Effects of Gatekeeping: A Systematic Review of the Literature." *Scandinavian Journal of Primary Health Care* 29, no. 1: 28–38.

Hagen, T. P., and K. Vrangbæk. 2009. "The Changing Political Governance Structures of Nordic Health Care Systems." In *Nordic Health Care Systems: Recent Reforms and Policy Challenges*, edited by J. Magnussen, K. Vrangbæk, and R. Saltman, 107–25. London: Open University Press.

Kalseth, B., K. S. Anthun, Ø. Hope, S. A. C. Kittelsen, and B. A. Persson. 2011. *Spesialisthelsetjenesten i Norden* [Specialist health care in the Nordic countries]. Report A19615. Trondheim, Norway: SINTEF.

Langenbrunner, J. C., C. Cashin, and S. O'Dougherty, eds. 2009. *Designing and Implementing Health Care Provider Payment Systems: How-To Manuals*. Washington, DC: World Bank and USAID. http://dx.doi.org/10.1596/978-0-8213-7815-1.

Magnussen, J., T. P. Hagen, and O. Kaarboe. 2007. "Centralized or Decentralized? A Case Study of Norwegian Hospital Reform." *Social Science and Medicine* 64, no. 10: 2129–37. http://dx.doi.org/10.1016/j.socscimed.2007.02.018.

Magnussen, J., K. Vrangbæk, and R. Saltman, eds. 2009. *Nordic Health Care Systems: Recent Reforms and Current Policy Challenges*. London: Open University Press.

Møinichen-Berstad, T. L. 2012. "Helseutgiftene i Norge sammenliknet med andre land [Health care expenditures in Norway compared to other countries]." *Samfunnsøkonomen* 2012, no. 3: 12–21.

OECD. 2011. Economic Survey of Iceland 2011. http://www.oecd.org/iceland/economicsurveyoficeland2011.htm.

———. 2012a. Economic Survey of Denmark 2012. http://www.oecd.org/eco/economicsurveyofdenmark2012.htm

———. 2012b. Economic Survey of Finland 2012. http://www.oecd.org/finland/economicsurveyoffinland2012.htm

———. 2012c. Economic Survey of Norway 2012. http://www.oecd.org/norway/economicsurveyofnorway2012.htm

———. 2012d. Economic Outlook: Sweden. http://www.oecd.org/eco/outlook/sweden-economic-forecast-summary.htm.

———. 2012e. "Health: Growth in Health Spending Grinds to a Halt." Newsroom, 28 June. http://www.oecd.org/newsroom/healthgrowthinhealthspendinggrindstoahalt.htm.

Pauly, M. V. 1968. "Comment: The Economics of Moral Hazard." *American Economic Review* 58: 531–37.

Pedersen, K. M., J. S. Andersen, and J. Søndergaard. 2012. "General Practice and Primary Health Care in Denmark." *Journal of the American Board of Family Medicine* 25: S34–38.

Rehnberg, C., J. Magnussen, and K. Luoma. 2009. "Maintaining Fiscal Sustainability in the Nordic Countries." In *Nordic Health Care Systems: Recent Reforms and Current Policy Challenges*, edited by J. Magnussen, K. Vrangbæk, and R. Saltman, 180–97. London: Open University Press.

Reibling, N., and C. Wendt. 2012. "Gatekeeping and Provider Choice in OECD Healthcare Systems." *Current Sociology* 60, no. 4: 489–505. http://dx.doi.org/10.1177/0011392112438333.

Thomson, S., T. Foubister, and E. Mossialos, eds. 2007. *Financing Health Care in the European Union*. Observatory Studies Series no. 17. Brussels: European Observatory on Health Systems and Policies.

———. 2010. "Can User Charges Make Health Care More Efficient?" *British Medical Journal* 341: 487–89.

nineteen

Taiwan and Other Advanced Asian Economies

TSUNG-MEI CHENG

Introduction

Historically, health spending in advanced Asian economies, including Japan, South Korea, Taiwan, Hong Kong, and Singapore, has been lower than health spending in advanced economies in the OECD. In recent years, Japan has become an exception, as health spending has now reached a level at par with the OECD average. Figure 19.1 shows national health spending (NHE) as a percentage of GDP in OECD countries in 2010 (updated to 2011 for Singapore and Taiwan).

In contrast with Europe and North America, where health spending as a percentage of GDP is much higher, the health systems of advanced Asian economies (except Japan), including Taiwan—the focus of this chapter—spend far less. Figure 19.2 shows the percentage of GDP spent on health as a function of GDP per capita in OECD countries.

Figures 19.1 and 19.2 suggest that the question of fiscal sustainability is of less immediate concern in Singapore, South Korea, and Taiwan than in many of the OECD countries with considerably higher health spending relative to per capita GDP, notably the United States and some European countries. The more relevant questions are (a) whether the comparatively lower health spending in advanced Asian economies can be made to yield even greater value—greater cost-effectiveness—in terms of health-care services and population health outcomes, and (b) whether these systems can be made to achieve greater equity in financing without increasing spending to North American and western European levels.

Since it is impossible to discuss the health systems of all these advanced Asian economies in a single chapter—there is no analogue of the "Nordic model of health care" in this instance—this chapter will focus on Taiwan's single-payer health system. Where appropriate, experiences from South Korea and Japan will be touched upon as points of reference; therefore a brief overview of their respective health systems is provided in Table 19.1. It will be shown that Taiwan's health system appears to be able to control health spending relatively effectively, through health systems design and health policy measures.

Figure 19.1 National health expenditure as per cent of GDP in OECD countries, Singapore, and Taiwan, 2011

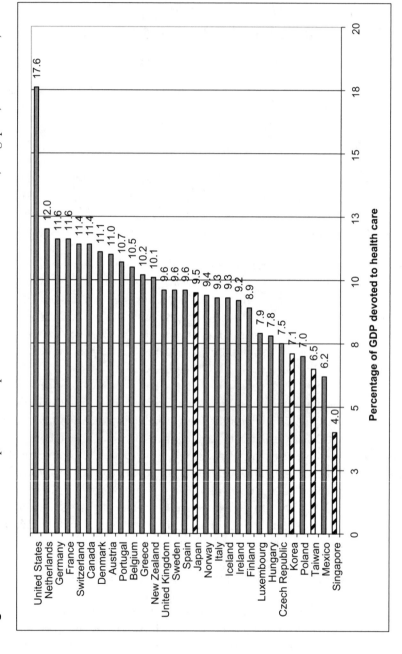

Sources: MOHW 2012; OECD 2012; WHO.

Figure 19.2 Percentage of GDP spent on health care as function of GDP per capita, 2010 (PPP dollars)

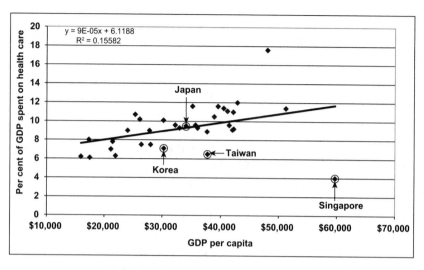

Sources: MOHW 2012; OECD 2012; WHO.

Table 19.1 Overview of selected health systems of Asia

	Japan	Korea	Singapore	Taiwan
Population (millions)	127.5	50.0	5.1	23.3
Population aged 65 or more (%)	22.9	11.4	10.5	10.7
GDP per capita ($)	34,748	31,220	55,790	37,716
Infant mortality	2.3	3	2.0	4.7
Life expectancy at birth				
Female	86	83	84	82
Male	80	77	79	76
Number of health insurers	3,200	1	—	1
NHE as % of GDP	9.6 (2011)	7.4 (2011)	4.0 (2010)	6.6 (2011)
Health spending per capita (PPP $)	2,877	1,980	2,273	2,186
Public health spending as % of NHE	80.0	57.0	36.3	58.0

Sources: OECD 2013a; Singapore 2013 Ministry of Health and Welfare, Taiwan, Republic of China 2011.

This chapter begins with a brief overview of Taiwan's National Health Insurance system (NHI), followed by a description of how health care is financed in Taiwan, the challenges facing health-care financing, and government's response to those challenges. Specific policy instruments, as well as their effectiveness and results, will be discussed. In addition, present and future health reform measures and their expected impact on national health spending and equity of access and affordability will also be examined. The chapter concludes with the observations that Taiwan's single-payer NHI is a case of successful public–private collaboration to serve the health-care needs of Taiwan's population. It also shows how a single-payer health system with universal coverage and broad benefits can both serve social justice and be fiscally sustainable. Some general lessons from Taiwan's experience as a single payer are offered as well.

Taiwan's health-care system at a glance

In the Asian region, Japan was the first to introduce universal health insurance, in 1961, followed by South Korea in 1989. In 1995 Taiwan's government established its single-payer universal National Health Insurance (NHI) program, five years ahead of the scheduled implementation date.

Prior to the NHI there were 13 social insurance schemes in Taiwan, together covering 59% of the population. Overnight, the remaining 41% uninsured—most of whom were vulnerable populations such as women, children, and the elderly—became eligible for full NHI coverage. The factors leading to the NHI's establishment in Taiwan included (a) strong popular demand for more and better health care, (b) an entrenched political party with a parliamentary majority that found itself challenged by a rising opposition party that openly called for universal health insurance, and (c) sustained high economic growth in the preceding decades that made financing for a major social program such as the NHI feasible (Cheng 2003). The confluence of these three conditions created a window of opportunity for Taiwan to create what NHI founding CEO and later health minister Ching-Chuan Yeh called "the most important public policy in fifty years" (Yeh 2002, 31–32).

The NHI is a government-run single-payer system administered by the National Health Insurance Administration (NHIA) under the Ministry of Health and Welfare. The Taiwan government's decision to go the single-payer route in the final planning stage of the NHI in 1990 was based on a recommendation made by Princeton economist Uwe Reinhardt at a high-level planning meeting in Taipei in 1989. He had witnessed the birth of Canada's single-payer health system as a student at the University of Saskatchewan in the 1960s. Reinhardt dubbed it the "single pipe" model, deeming it most suited for Taiwan because (a) it is an ideal platform for egalitarian distribution of health care, to which Taiwan aspired; (b) it endows the government with monopsonistic market power on the payment side whereby it can effectively control overall health-care spending; and (c) it is administratively simple, which makes it relatively inexpensive as well as easily understood by both the public and the providers of health care.

The ability to control health-care spending growth had been a primary goal of Taiwan's health reform. Like the Canadian system, Taiwan's single-payer NHI has the advantage that payments to providers are from a "single pipe" (i.e., a single payer) whose "control valve" can easily manoeuvre the flow of resources (Reinhardt 1991, 17).

Enrolment in the NHI is mandatory. At the end of the first year of implementation, the NHI had enrolled more than 90% of the population. Today more than 99.9% of Taiwan's population of 23.3 million is insured. Approximately 40,000 Taiwan citizens remain "uninsured" not because of lack of ability to pay the premiums; rather, they refuse to join the NHI, opting to freeload or pay out of pocket (Minister of Health and Welfare Chiu Wen-Ta, personal communication). In contrast, as of 2012 an estimated 1.3% of Japan's population was uninsured (Ikegami et al. 2011). In Korea as of 2006, 98.2% of the population was covered under the single-payer Korean National Health Insurance (Kwon 2009, Fig. 1).

Benefits in the NHI are uniform and comprehensive. They include inpatient and outpatient care, laboratory tests, prescription drugs and certain over-the-counter drugs, dental care (excluding orthodontics and prosthodontics), traditional Chinese medicine, daycare for the mentally ill, home nursing care (limited), palliative and end-of-life care, dialysis, and so forth (NHIA 2013, 20). Former health minister Yeh described the NHI's benefits as "all you can eat" (Cheng 2009, 1036).

Patients contribute modest copayments and co-insurance for outpatient and inpatient care and prescription drugs. Copayment for visits to clinics, including traditional Chinese medicine clinics, is currently NT$50 (about US$3 PPP), as are visits to dentists (NHIA 2013, 20); those for large hospitals and medical centres are higher. Copayments and co-insurance account for about 10% of total NHI expenditure (MOHW 2011). Patients also pay a modest registration fee to providers when accessing care, to help pay for administrative expenses associated with the visit. Registration fees also are differentiated by the level of provider organization: lowest for visits to clinics (NT$50) and highest for tertiary medical centres.

To protect patients from undue financial burdens, copayment ceilings apply for both inpatient and outpatient care. In addition, the NHI law (Article 36) stipulates that copayment exemptions apply to specific population groups—residents of remote mountainous areas and offshore islands, veterans and household dependants of diseased veterans, low-income households, children under three, and registered tuberculosis patients under treatment—and to patients with any of 30 catastrophic illnesses (NHIA 2012–13, 21).

Like the health systems of Japan and South Korea, Taiwan's NHI delivery system is largely private: 70.3% of all beds, 84% of all hospitals, and 98% of all clinics are privately operated (Cheng 2012b, 263). The comparable figures for Japan and South Korea are 70% and 85% of all beds and 80% and 90% of all hospitals, respectively (Ii 2012, 210; Kwon 2012, 221). Providers in Taiwan contract with the NHIA to deliver services, for which they are paid by a national uniform fee schedule. As of 2012, 92.62% of Taiwan's providers contracted with the NHIA (NHIA 2012–13, 27).

Unlike the health systems of many OECD countries, including the single-payer systems of Canada and the United Kingdom, there are no waiting lines in Taiwan's NHI. Access to care is easy in Taiwan, and the Taiwanese take full advantage of it. Where Taiwan does have "waiting lines," albeit in the non-traditional sense, is for adoption of new medical technologies, including new drugs. There is usually a delay of two and sometimes five years compared to the United States. Nonetheless, Taiwan introduces 40 to 50 new drugs every year (Cheng 2009, 1037).

Patients in Taiwan enjoy full free choice of providers, including hospitals. The Taiwanese have a penchant for seeking care at tertiary hospitals, especially large academic medical centres. In recent years, to reduce crowding at these facilities, the NHIA introduced a graduated system whereby patients who access tertiary-care facilities without referral pay higher registration fees, copayments, and co-insurance.

Providers receive their remuneration from three sources: (1) the NHIA; (2) patient registration fees, copayments, and co-insurance; and (3) proceeds from the sale of goods and services not covered by the NHI. Prior to December 2012, with the exception of drug-eluting stents, intraocular lenses, and ceramic- and metal-on-metal hip joints, patients were required to use devices and supplies covered by the NHI in order to have their procedures paid for. Providers were not allowed to bill patients extra charges above the NHIA-set fees, as in the Japanese health system, which still does not allow providers to balance-bill patients. Beginning in December 2012, the NHIA began to allow patients to pay out of pocket for more expensive devices and covers the rest of the costs with a diagnostic-related-group (DRG) payment for the particular procedure.

As in Japan and South Korea, fee-for-service payment according to a government-established uniform national fee schedule has been the predominant method of payment to providers in Taiwan. In 2011, however, Taiwan began a major push towards DRG payment for hospitals; as of 2012 there were 154 DRGs. Other methods include pay for performance for diabetes, asthma, breast cancer, hypertension, and tuberculosis, while capitation payment is also being explored.

Public satisfaction with the NHI was in the high 70% range between 2001 and 2008, and has been higher in more recent years. Periods of lower satisfaction—in the 60% range in 2002 and 2006—were associated with a premium rate increase (in 2002) and mere talk of a premium rate increase (in 2006). Since 2008, the year of the global financial crisis, satisfaction has climbed to an average of 85%, despite a second premium rate increase in 2010. This may suggest that during hard economic times the public especially appreciates the NHI as an important social safety net.

NHI financing and spending and the 2008 global financial crisis

Taiwan did not experience the drastic responses to the 2008 global financial crisis of many health systems in OECD countries, which took "the form of indiscriminate cost cuts across the board" or freezing of health and social budgets, stepped-up rationing, and cost shifting to patients (Figueras 2012). OECD data show the dramatic impact of the crisis on the growth rates of health spending in OECD countries. In contrast, health spending in Taiwan continued to grow: at 2.96% in 2008, 5.56% in 2009, and 3.05% in 2010 (MOHW 2010, 86). Taiwan's NHI in this period not only maintained its level of service without benefit cuts or waiting lines, but in fact added benefits and expanded financial assistance for the poor and near-poor. In April 2010 it increased the premium rate from 4.55% to 5.17%, which eliminated the program's cumulative debt and had even built up a small surplus as of early 2012 (Cheng 2012a; NHIA Deputy Director-General Lee Cheng-Hua, personal communication).

Figure 19.3 shows the composition of Taiwan's national health expenditure (NHE) in 2000 and 2010. Its two largest components were the NHI and household out-of-pocket payments. Approximately 50.2% of total NHE flowed into the NHI and paid providers; 43.3% of total health spending was in the private sector, of which household out-of-pocket payments for health care constituted 36.4% (MOHW 2010, 87). In 2002 the NHI

Figure 19.3 Composition of Taiwan's national health expenditure by source of expense, 2000 and 2010

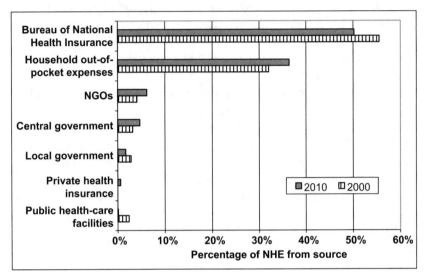

Source: MOHW 2010.

accounted for 55.52% of Taiwan's total national health spending (Cheng 2003, 66).

Financing for the NHI comes from three sources: government (26%), in the form of premium subsidies for various groups of the insured; employers (36%), in the form of premium contributions on behalf of employees; and households (38%), in the form of NHI premium payments (Figure 19.4).

It should be noted that the government as employer accounts for 8.2% of the 36% contribution by employers to the NHI funding pool (Cheng 2012a). Therefore, the de facto total government contribution to NHI funding is 34%; with total government subsidies accounting for 26% of the funding. Taiwan's government planned to increase its contribution to 36% of total NHI funding in 2013 as part of its expanded program to protect disadvantaged populations (Cheng 2012a).

Taiwan's Supreme Court ruled in 1999 that access to care may not be denied those unable to pay the NHI premium and that the government should render appropriate assistance (Supreme Court of the Republic of China 1999). The National Health Insurance Administration (NHIA) makes provisions for those who have difficulty paying premiums, by offering payment by instalments or interest-free loans. The government subsidizes 100% of the NHI premium for low-income households, as well as for other

Figure 19.4 Sources of financing for National Health Insurance, Taiwan

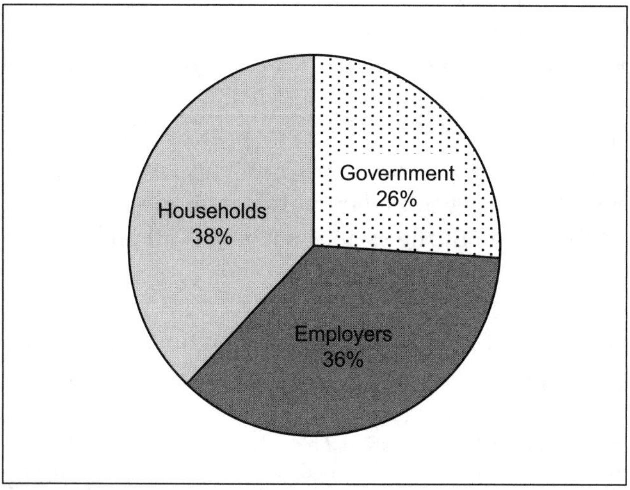

Source: NHIA 2013.

economically disadvantaged individuals, including the physically and mentally impaired, mid- to low-income households with individuals over 70 years old, members of the indigenous population (sometimes referred to as "high mountain tribesmen") under 20 years of age, and unemployed people over 55 years of age (MOHW 2011).

Out-of-pocket (OOP) spending by households for health care in Taiwan increased from 27.82% in 1995 to 32% in 2000, and from 35% in 2008 to 36.43% in 2010, representing a total increase of 8 percentage points over 15 years or a 31% increase in the percentage of OOP—an annual compound growth rate of 1.8% a year (Cheng 2003, 66; Cheng 2012a, 261; MOHW 2010, 90). The trend towards higher OOP over time partly reflects the difficulties that Taiwan's government has experienced in raising NHI premium rates. Interestingly, a 2003 NHIA survey showed that 82% of patients held "positive attitudes toward OOP spending" (NHIA official, personal communication). Taiwan's broad middle class widely views the NHI as inexpensive and beneficial. This implies that there may be room for further increases in OOP spending, provided that provisions are made to ensure that higher OOP does not impair access to care for the poor or the very sick.

In 2012, health spending amounted to 6.6% of Taiwan's GDP, compared to average national health spending in OECD counties of 9.5% (OECD 2012). In US dollar purchasing power parity (PPP) terms, Taiwan's per capita health spending was $2,208 in 2009, compared to $3,035 in Japan, $1,864 in South Korea, $4,316 in Canada, and $7,990 in the United States (MOHW 2010, 194; OECD 2012). Available data on per capita spending in PPP dollars for 2010 show South Korea at $2,035, Canada at $4,445, and the United States at $8,233 (OECD 2012).

Table 19.2 shows growth in Taiwan's national health spending and NHE as a percent of GDP, per capita health spending, and GDP growth for the period 1991–2010. Taiwan's NHE growth rate tells an interesting story about the effects of both the establishment of NHI and the government

Table 19.2 Growth in per capita health spending, national health expenditure, GDP, and NHE as percentage of GDP, Taiwan, 1991–2010

Year	Per Capita Health Spending (NT$)*	Growth in National Health Spending (%)	Growth in GDP (%)	National Health Spending as % of GDP
1991	10,765			4.45
1992	12,512	17.37	11.62	4.68
1993	14,075	13.55	10.40	4.81
1994	15,448	10.74	9.42	4.87
1995	17,971	17.33	8.86	5.25
1996	19,757	10.84	8.64	5.36
1997	21,206	8.29	8.46	5.35
1998	22,874	8.87	7.34	5.43
1999	24,539	8.14	4.83	5.60
2000	25,384	4.26	5.58	5.53
2001	26,130	3.67	−2.52	5.88
2002	27,631	6.32	4.85	5.96
2003	29,154	5.98	2.73	6.15
2004	31,146	7.23	6.25	6.21
2005	32,250	3.93	3.30	6.24
2006	33,591	4.59	4.29	6.26
2007	34,719	3.78	5.45	6.16
2008	35,623	2.96	−2.25	6.49
2009	37,471	5.56	−1.13	6.93
2010	38,510	3.05	9.03	6.55

* 1 New Taiwan (NT) dollar = 0.03 US dollar (2010).
Source: MOHW 2010.

Figure 19.5 National Health Insurance revenue, spending, and deficit/surplus, Taiwan, 1996–2010

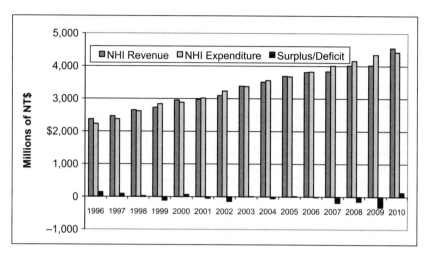

Source: MOHW 2010.

cost-containment strategies implemented since then on containing health-spending growth in Taiwan.

First and foremost, the NHI restrained growth in Taiwan's total NHE from an average of 14.76% per year in the four-year period 1992–95 (13.89% in the three-year period 1992–94, before NHI) to an average of 5.83% per year since NHI's establishment in 1995. In the 10-year period before the implementation of the NHI (1985–94), Taiwan's total national health spending grew 280%. In the 10-year period since the implementation of the NHI (1995–2004), total national health spending grew 71%, a quarter of the growth in the previous 10 years (NHIA 2011a).

For the first three years after implementation (1995–98), the NHI enjoyed a surplus, as revenue exceeded expenditure in that period. From 1996 until 2009, however, except for three years of surpluses (2000, 2003, and 2005), the NHI had annual deficits (Day 2011). Figure 19.5 shows the annual NHI revenue and expenditure figures for the period 1996 to 2010. By the end of 2009, the NHI had accumulated a deficit larger than 10% of its annual operating budget.

The original NHI Act of 1994 allowed the premium rate to be revised every two years as needed, depending on actuarial assessments of NHI finances (Cheng 2003). However, raising premiums turned out to be extraordinarily challenging for successive governments. In the NHI's 19-year history, the government succeeded in raising premium rates only twice, once in 2002 and again in 2010. Each time the disenchanted health minister resigned following the increase. As a consequence, Taiwan's NHI had been running deficits in most years, since its inception in 1995 through to 2010.

Cost-containment measures

In the face of static premiums in the period 1998–2010, the government had to adopt other cost-containment measures. Copayments were increased in July 2001 for certain types of visits, drugs, and inpatient care; prices were cut for 8,961 drugs in 2000, for 10,248 in 2001, and for 1,000 more in 2002 (Cheng 2003, 71). Furthermore, the government introduced its "reasonable outpatient volume" policy in January 2001. Under that policy, the NHIA's payments to doctors decreased according to a sliding scale if set limits on the number of patients seen per doctor were exceeded. The government sought to both reduce outpatient volume and improve quality at hospital outpatient clinics and independent clinics (Cheng 2003, 71). The NHIA also stepped up medical reviews of claims, moved subsidies to medical education to another department, and introduced a limited number of DRGs (Cheng 2003, 52).

By far the most significant and effective cost-containment strategy was the global budget reform that began in 1998 and was completed by 2003. The original design of the NHI had called for the introduction of sectoral global budgets five years after the implementation of the NHI, as one of its founding objectives was cost-containment (Cheng 2003). Borrowing from the experiences of Germany and Canada, the government imposed global budgets—an inflexible cap on spending—on all major sectors in health care, phased in over several years: dental care in 1998, traditional Chinese medicine in 2000, primary care in 2001, and hospitals in mid 2002 (Cheng 2003, 71). Taiwan was experiencing a rapidly rising prevalence of type 2 diabetes among men and women 20 to 40 years of age (especially young men); as a result, in 2003 the government implemented a global budget for dialysis, to provide access to needed care for diabetes and end-stage renal diseases.

The introduction of sectoral global budgets for the dental and traditional Chinese medicine sectors in 1998 and 2000 did not make a significant impact on the overall growth in spending. Those sectors are, relative to the large primary-care and hospital sectors, small ones, together representing 11% of total NHI expenditure. However, the true impact of sectoral global budgets can be seen beginning in 2000, when the sizable primary-care sector was brought under its separate

Figure 19.6 Global budget growth rates by sector, Taiwan National Health Insurance, 2003–2011

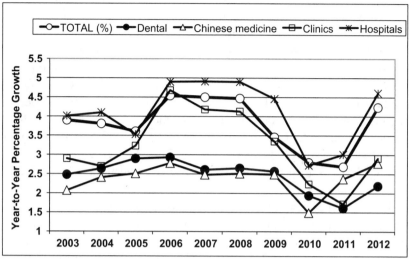

Source: NHIA 2011a.

sectoral global budget. Approximately half of Taiwan's doctors—Western medicine doctors, dentists, and traditional Chinese medicine doctors—practise in independently owned and operated clinics that provide mainly outpatient care. Growth in NHE declined from an average of 8.43% per year, for the three-year period before the imposition of the primary-care global budget, to 4.26% in 2000 and 3.67% in 2001.

In the hospital sector, costs continued to grow through 2004, despite imposition by the government of the hospital global budget in the fall of 2002. The government did not want to shock the hospital sector in the wake of the premium rate increase in the summer of 2002, but eventually the global budget reform did bring hospitals costs down, as Figure 19.6 illustrates.

By contrast, South Korea has not been able to establish a global budget for its single-payer National Health Insurance program because of strong provider resistance. As a result, Korea had the highest rate of increase in health expenditure among OECD countries for the period 2000–09, averaging 9.3% a year (OECD 2013b).

In the early 2000s, when the NHI was experiencing its first financial crisis, the NHIA had introduced limited (52) DRGs in an attempt to contain cost (Cheng 2003). In January 2010 the NHIA expanded its DRG program to a total of 164 DRGs. These accounted for 28.6% of the total Taiwan-DRG program and approximately 17.4% of total hospital expenditure. In 2012 the NHIA had planned to introduce five major diagnostic categories (MDCs), consisting of 225 additional DRGs and accounting for an additional 18.1% of the total Taiwan-DRG program and 11% of total hospital expenditure (Day 2011). However, provider resistance caused postponement of the plan's implementation to 2014, when 254 DRGs were scheduled to be implemented. This delay resulted in delayed implementation of the full Taiwan-DRG program, originally scheduled for 2013. When fully implemented, this comprehensive program—1,017 DRGs—will account for 61% of total hospital expenditure in Taiwan (Day 2011). Some time will need to elapse before it will be possible to evaluate the DRG reform's ultimate impact on costs.

The use of key health technologies is also regulated to save cost. Certain procedures, medical supplies, and drugs that are high-risk, expensive, and prone to overuse and misuse by providers require preauthorization by the Bureau of National Health Insurance (BNHI). Some examples are heart transplants, artificial knee joints, and cancer drugs such as Erbitux. Failure to obtain preauthorization results in nonpayment by the BNHI, with exceptions made in cases of emergencies (Day 2011).

Fiscal sustainability of Taiwan's health system

The fiscal sustainability of any health system depends critically on the equilibrium of its revenues and expenditures. As earlier discussions show, inadequate financing in much of the NHI's history was the Achilles heel of its longer-term financial sustainability. At the heart of the NHI's financial troubles was the narrow premium base (only payroll). For more than a decade the government sought to broaden that base. It succeeded with implementation of the so-called Second-Generation NHI (G2-NHI) in January 2013. Premiums under the G2-NHI consist of a basic contribution, calculated on 4.91% of wages or salary, and a 2% supplemental premium contribution, based on six types of non-payroll income. These latter include bonuses exceeding four months' salary, earnings from second and third jobs, stock dividends, interest, rent, and earnings from businesses such as entertainment and modelling (one top model who earned millions a year paid virtually nothing for health insurance). The new financing scheme is expected to ensure the NHI's financial stability through 2016, at which time a third-generation version is expected to take its place.

Opening up new sources of revenue is but one avenue to longer-term fiscal sustainability in any health system. Cost containment is another important avenue. Cost-containment strategies in Taiwan have relied on both supply-side controls (e.g., global budgets and regulated prices) and demand-side controls (e.g., premium rate increases). Available data to date show that Taiwan has successfully contained health-care costs; in fact, the NHI is enjoying a surplus at present. By comparison, in Japan the main cost-containment strategy has relied mostly on government regulation of fee schedules, and Japan's health-care system is currently "facing a financial crisis" (Ii 2012, 209). In South Korea there have been proposals concerning the introduction of global budgets and payment (DRG) reforms, but as of this writing, neither cost-containment measure has been put in place. In terms of "bending the cost curve," Taiwan appears to have been more successful than its East Asian neighbours.

Taiwan's success has put it in the enviable position of being able to spend more on health care because of its economic strength. Indeed, President Ma Ying-jeou has on numerous occasions called for health-care spending to increase to 7.5% of Taiwan's GDP, as has the author since 2003 (Cheng 2003). Taiwan's general public, often egged on by parliamentary representatives and nongovernmental watchdogs and pundits, expects ever more services from the NHI, including numerous heroic high-tech end-of-life medical interventions and drugs. However, the populace have only reluctantly permitted two premium rate increases and the addition of one small supplemental premium rate in the NHI's 19-year history.

The public insists that the NHIA first eliminate "waste" before asking for premium rate increases. That demand, of course, is not without merit, if one considers the overuse, misuse, underuse, and induced demand for services that are prevalent in most modern health systems. However, eliminating waste in any health system is far easier said than done. All health insurance systems that have relatively low cost-sharing at the time of using health care sooner or later must act out the tragedy of the commons (Hiatt 1975; Cheng 2003, 73).

Conclusion

Single-payer health systems may vary in the way they are financed and the way services are delivered. In terms of financing, single payers may be tax-financed, as in the UK National Health Service (NHS) or Canada's medicare. These systems can also be premium-financed, as in the national health insurance programs of Taiwan and South Korea. Whether a single-payer system is tax- or premium-financed, it is the government alone that administers the payment system. In terms of service delivery, single-payer systems may have predominantly public delivery systems such as the NHS, which runs a vast network of public hospitals, or a private/public mixed system of delivery facilities such as those of Taiwan, South Korea, and Canada, where public and private facilities exist side by side.

Several lessons emerge from Taiwan's two decades of experience. First and foremost, Taiwan's NHI shows that a single-payer health system with universal coverage and broad benefits can both serve social justice and be fiscally sustainable, in part because the single-payer approach is known to be able to control costs, and therefore overall health spending, better than multi-payer systems and private commercial health insurance systems such as those of the United States and Switzerland. At the same time, Taiwan's NHI is also a case of successful public–private collaboration that serves the health-care needs of an entire population, without waiting lines or rationing of care. In addition, Taiwan NHI's IT-supported low administrative cost—1.6% of total NHI expenditure in 2012 (NHIA 2013, 28)—means that more money can be—and is—spent on services (and profits). And perhaps because overall health spending has been maintained at an easily affordable level, equity can be maintained easily; affordable prices for services help make it possible for everyone to receive identical benefits and services, unlike in the United States.

There are also other lessons that emerge from Taiwan's experience as a single-payer health system. First, copayments are acceptable when prices are "affordable" for the general public and provisions are made to protect access to needed care for those with serious illnesses. Second, high satisfaction with the NHI suggests that Taiwan's public does not mind not having a choice of health insurer—what counts is having free choice of providers. Finally, drawing comparative lessons from best practices in other health systems, as Taiwan did when first planning the system and continues to do, is both important and beneficial.

A final word of caution is in order. A single-payer system will not work well unless it is administered by a cadre of well-educated and highly motivated civil servants supported by excellent leadership at the top. Furthermore, there is always the danger that, to balance the government budget, a single-payer system may at times be underfunded, as Taiwan's NHI once was. That will lead to public dissatisfaction and could potentially affect the quality of care. And, if protracted, it could eventually split the system into different tiers, undermining its original policy objectives of providing care on the basis of need rather than ability to pay.

References

Cheng, T.-M. 2003. "Taiwan's New National Health Insurance Program: Genesis and Experience So Far." *Health Affairs* 22, no. 3: 61–76. http://dx.doi.org/10.1377/hlthaff.22.3.61.

———. 2009. "Lessons from Taiwan's Universal National Health Insurance: A Conversation with Taiwan's Health Minister Ching-Chuan Yeh." *Health Affairs* 28, no. 4: 1035–44. http://dx.doi.org/10.1377/hlthaff.28.4.1035.

———. 2012a. "Innovative Financing. Case 5: Taiwan." In *Closing the Cancer Divide: A Blueprint to Expand Access in Low and Middle Income Countries,* edited by F. Knaul, J. Frenk, and L. Shulman, 190–91. Boston: Global Task Force on Expanded Access to Cancer Care and Control in Developing Countries (GTFCCC), Harvard Global Equity Initiative.

———. 2012b. "Taiwan Province of China's Experience with Universal Health Care Coverage." In *The Economics of Public Health Care Reform in Advanced and Emerging Economies,* edited by B. Clements, D. Coady, and S. Gupta, 253–79. Washington, DC: International Monetary Fund.

Chiu, S.-S. [2009/2010]. *Report on the 2007 Cancer Registry.* Taiwan: Health Promotion Administration, Ministry of Health and Welfare.

Chou, S.-Y., M. Grossman, and J.-T. Liu. 2011. "The Impact of National Health Insurance on Birth Outcomes: A Natural Experiment in Taiwan." NBER working paper no. 16811. Cambridge, MA: National Bureau of Economic Research.

Day, G.-Y. 2011. "Implementing Second-Generation National Health Insurance: Going Forward with Financing and Payment Reform." Presentation to Taiwan Health Insurance Association, 20 August. Taipei: NHIA, Ministry of Health and Welfare.

Figueras, J. 2012. "Health Care in Europe after the Financial Crisis of 2008." Paper presented at "Bending the Cost Curve in Health Care in Canada," Saskatoon, 28 September.

Hiatt, H. H. 1975. "Protecting the Medical Commons: Who Is Responsible?" *New England Journal of Medicine* 293: 235–41.

Huang, Y.-F. 2012. "Second-Generation National Health Insurance Supplementary Premium Revenues Estimates Indicate Large Differences." *United Evening News* (Taipei), 31 August. http://mag.udn.com/mag/life/storypage.jsp?f_ART_ID=409990#ixzz2G1L7YG7H.

Ii, M. 2012. "Challenges in Reforming the Japanese Health Care System." In *The Economics of Public Health Care Reform in Advanced and Emerging Economies,* edited by B. Clements, D. Coady, and S. Gupta, 209–20. Washington, DC: International Monetary Fund.

Ikegami, N., B.-K. Yoo, H. Hashimoto, M. Matsumoto, H. Ogata, A. Babazono, R. Watanabe, K. Shibuya, B.-M. Yang, M. R. Reich, and Y. Kobayashi. 2011. "Japanese Universal Health Care Coverage: Evolution, Achievements, and Challenges." *Lancet* 378, no. 9796: 1106–15. doi:10.1016/S0140-6736(11)60828-3.

Kwon, S. 2009. "Thirty Years of National Health Insurance in South Korea: Lessons for Achieving Universal Health Care Coverage." *Health Policy and Planning* 24, no. 1: 63–71. http://dx.doi.org/10.1093/heapol/czn037.

———. 2012. "Coverage Expansion and Cost Containment in the Republic of Korea." In *The Economics of Public Health Care Reform in Advanced and Emerging Economies,* edited by B. Clements, D. Coady, and S. Gupta, 221–32. Washington, DC: International Monetary Fund.

MOHW (Republic of China Ministry of Health and Welfare). 2007. *Health Statistical Trends*. Taipei: Ministry of Health and Welfare.

———. 2010. *Republic of China Health Statistical Trends*. Taipei: Ministry of Health and Welfare.

———. 2011. *National Health Insurance in Taiwan*. Taipei: Ministry of Health and Welfare.

NHIA (National Health Insurance Administration). 2011a. *National Health Insurance in Taiwan: 2011 Annual Report*. Taipei: Ministry of Health and Welfare.

———. 2011b. *Towards Equity, Efficiency, and Quality: Second-Generation National Health Insurance Reform*. Taipei: Ministry of Health and Welfare.

———. 2013. *National Health Insurance in Taiwan: NHI 2012–2013 Annual Report*. Taipei: Ministry of Health and Welfare.

OECD (Organisation for Economic Co-operation and Development). 2012. "Health: Growth in Health Spending Grinding to a Halt." OECD Newsroom, 28 June. Accessed 7 January 2013. http://www.oecd.org/newsroom/healthgrowthinhealth spendinggrindstoahalt.htm.

———. 2013a. "Health Status." StatExtracts [database]. Accessed 4 March 2013. http://stats.oecd.org/index.aspx?DataSetCode=HEALTH_STAT.

———. 2013b. "OECD Health Statistics." http://www.oecd-ilibrary.org/social-issues -migration-health/data/oecd-health-statistics_health-data-en.

Reinhardt, U. 1991. "Providing Access to Health Care and Controlling Costs: The Universal Dilemma." In *New Perspectives in Health Care Economics*, edited by U. E. Reinhardt and F. Pinto, 12–27. London: Medio.

Singapore. Department of Statistics. 2013. "Population Trends 2013." www.singstat.gov.sg.

Supreme Court of the Republic of China. 1999. Ruling no. 472, 29 January.

Taiwan Shin-Sheng Bao. 2010. "Editorial: G2 NHI Good Prescription for Solving the 'Taiwan Crisis'?" *Taiwan Shin-Sheng Daily News*, 12 April.

WHO (World Health Organization). "Singapore." http:/www.who.int./countries/sgp/en/.

Yeh, C.-C. 2002. *The Legend of the National Health Insurance:* Taipei: Tung Foundation.

Index